G. Puddu · A. Giombini · A. Selvanetti (Eds.)
Rehabilitation of Sports Injuries

Springer
Berlin
Heidelberg
New York
Barcelona
Hong Kong
London
Milan
Paris
Singapore
Tokyo

G. Puddu · A. Giombini · A. Selvanetti (Eds.)

Rehabilitation of Sports Injuries

Current Concepts

With 172 Figures in 212 Parts and 45 Tables

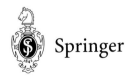 Springer

Giancarlo Puddu, MD, Prof.
Clinica "Valle Giulia"
Via de Notaris 2 b, 00197 Rome, Italy

Arrigo Giombini, MD
Sports Science Institute, Department of Medicine
Service of Rehabilitation and Functional Reconditioning
Via dei Campi Sportivi 46, 00197 Rome, (Italy)

Alberto Selvanetti, MD
Sports Science Institute, Department of Medicine
Service of Rehabilitation and Functional Reconditioning
Via dei Campi Sportivi 46, 00197 Rome, (Italy)

ISBN 3-540-67475-6 Springer-Verlag Berlin Heidelberg New York

Library of Congress Cataloging-in-Publication Data
Rehabilitation of sports injuries : current concepts / [edited by] Giancarlo Puddu, Arrigo
Giombini, Alberto Selvanetti.
p. ; cm.
Includes biographical references and index.
ISBN 3540674756 (alk. paper)
1. Sports injuries. 2. Sports injuries – Patients – Rehabilitation. 3. Sports physical therapy.
I. Puddu, Giancarlo. II. Giombini, Arrigo, 1960– III. Selvanetti, Alberto, 1962–
[DNLM: 1. Athletic Injuries – rehabilitation. QT 261 R3447 2001]
RD97.R438 2001
617.1'027 – dc21   00-061188

Springer-Verlag Berlin Heidelberg New York
a member of BertelsmannSpringer Science+Business Media GmbH

© Springer-Verlag Berlin Heidelberg 2001
Printed in Germany

Cover Design: E. Kirchner, D-69121 Heidelberg
Typesetting: FotoSatz Pfeifer GmbH, D-82166 Gräfelfing
Printed on acid-free paper – SPIN: 10730055   24/3130 – 5 4 3 2 1 0

3-19-03

Preface

Over the last few years, in the field of sports science and medicine, empirical theories about the treatment and rehabilitation of injured athletes have been gradually supported by a rapid growth of research data and scientific literature. This has permitted a better knowledge of the healing process from injury and/or surgery, and a more appropriate understanding of the biomechanical behavior of several biological structures to load and exercise.

We agree with the opinion that development and advancement through a rehabilitation program should be based on the type and severity of the lesion, healing time of the injured structures, individual pain tolerance level, possible adopted surgical procedure, and sport-specific biomechanical demands.

Currently, the most recent theories on rehabilitation of the injured athlete emphasize the concepts of a multidisciplinary approach, a functional recovery instead of symptomatic improvement, and an early mobilization with the implementation of an individualized program treating the entire body kinetic chains.

Among different methods of rehabilitation, the physician should choose those revealing their clinical appropriateness, founded on a validated scientific data and/or proven clinical efficacy.

Our goal has been to provide a comprehensive coverage of principles and practical applications of the rehabilitation methods of the most common sports injuries, and we have tried to combine the variety of expertise and backgrounds of a multidisciplinary group of contributing authors.

The editors would like to thank each of the contributors and express their appreciation and gratitude to the publisher for giving them the opportunity to develop and realize their ambitious project.

Giancarlo Puddu, MD
Arrigo Giombini, MD
Alberto Selvanetti, MD

Contents

Contributors

Paolo Aglietti, MD, Prof.
First Orthopaedic Clinic, University of Florence
Largo P. Palagi 1, 50139 Florence, Italy

GianCarlo Aisa, MD
Orthopaedic Clinic Terni, Ospedale S. Maria, University of Perugia
Piazzale T. di Joannuccio, 05100 Terni, Italy

James R. Andrews, MD, Prof.
American Sports Medicine Institute, 1313 13th Street South, Birmingham, AL 35205,
USA

Carmelo Bosco, PhD, DU, D Hon C
School of Specialization in Physical Medicine and Rehabilitation
University of Tor Vergata, c/o Fondazione Don Gnocchi ONLUS
V. Maresciallo Caviglia 30, 00194 Rome, Italy

Auro Caraffa, MD
Orthopaedic Clinic of Terni, Ospedale S. Maria, University of Perugia
Piazzale T. di Joannuccio, 05100 Terni, Italy

Ignazio Caruso, MD, Prof.
School of Specialization in Physical Medicine and Rehabilitation
University of Tor Vergata, c/o Fondazione Don Gnocchi ONLUS
V. Maresciallo Caviglia 30, 00194 Rome, Italy

Antonio Castagnaro, MD
Servizio Chirurgia Della Mano, Ospedale Belcolle, Strada Sanmarinese,
01100 Viterbo, Italy

Giuliano Cerulli, MD, Prof.
Director of Orthopaedic and Traumatology Department, Silvestrini Hospital
University of Perugia, Piazzale T. di Joannuccio, 05100 Terni, Italy

Guglielmo Cerullo, MD
Clinica "Valle Giulia", Via G. Dé Notaris 2B, 00197 Rome, Italy

Kai-Ming Chan, MD, Prof.
The Chinese University of Hong Kong, Department of Orthopaedics and Trauma-
tology, Room 724029 5/F, Clinical Science Building, Prince of Wales Hospital
Shatin, New Territories, Hong Kong

Dario Dalla Vedova, PT
Sports Science Institute, Department of Physiology, Via dei Campi Sportivi 46,
00197 Rome, Italy

Nick A. Evans, BSc, FRCS (Orthop)
Orthopaedic and Sports Medicine Clinic of Nova Scotia, 5595 Fenwick Street,
Suite 311, Halifax, Nova Scotia B3H 4M2, Canada

Piero Faccini, MD
Sports Science Institute, Department of Physiology, Via dei Campi Sportivi 46,
00197 Rome, Italy

Vittorio Franco, MD
Clinica "Valle Giulia", Via G. De Notaris 2b, 00197 Rome, Italy

Freddie H. Fu, MD
Musculoskeletal Research Center, Department of Orthopaedic Surgery
University of Pittsburgh, Pittsburgh, PA 15213, USA

William E. Garrett, Jr, MD, PhD
Department of Orthopaedics, University of North Carolina, 236 Burnett-Womack
Building, CB No. 7055, Chapel Hill, NC 27599, USA

Enrico Giannì, MD
Clinica "Valle Giulia", Via G. Dé Notaris 2B, 00197 Rome, Italy

Arrigo Giombini, MD
Sports Science Institute, Department of Medicine, Service of Rehabilitation
and Functional Reconditioning, Via dei Campi Sportivi 46, 00197 Rome, Italy

Francesco Giron, MD
First Orthopaedic Clinic, University of Florence, Largo P. Palagi 1, 50139 Florence,
Italy

Carl Gustafson, PT
Division of Sports Medicine, Boston Children's Hospital, 319 Longwood Avenue
Boston, MA 02115, USA

Pierre A. d'Hemecourt, MD
Division of Sports Medicine, Boston Children's Hospital, 319 Longwood Avenue
Boston, MA 02115, USA

Donald T. Kirkendall, PhD
Department of Orthopaedics, University of North Carolina, 236 Burnett-Womack
Building, CB No. 7055, Chapel Hill, NC 27599, USA

Lars Konradsen, MD
Department of Orthopedic Surgery, Gentofte Hospital, University of Copenhagen
Denmark

Mario Lamontagne, PhD
School of Human Kinetics and Department of Mechanical Engineering
University of Ottawa, 125 University Street (MNT341), Ottawa, Ontario KIN 6N5,
Canada

Jean-Pierre Liotard, MD
Clinique Sainte Anne Lumière, 85 Cours Albert Thomas, 69003 Lyon, France

Nicola Maffulli, MD, MS, PhD, FRCS (Orth)
Department of Orthopaedic Surgery, University of Aberdeen Medical School
Polwarth Building, Foresterhill, Aberdeen AB25 2ZD, UK

Lee J. Mi, MD
Musculoskeletal Research Center, Department of Orthopaedic Surgery
University of Pittsburgh, Pittsburgh, PA 15213, USA

Lyle J. Micheli, MD, Prof.
Division of Sports Medicine, Boston Children's Hospital
319 Longwood Avenue, Boston, MA 02115, USA

Fabrizio Ponteggia, MD
Lecturer in Physical Medicine and Rehabilitation, CTO, University of Florence
Largo P. Palagi 1, 50139 Florence, Italy

William E. Prentice, PhD
Department of Physical Education, Exercise and Sport Sciences, University
of North Carolina, Chapel Hill, NC 27599, USA

Giancarlo Puddu, MD, Prof.
Clinica "Valle Giulia", Via G. de Notaris 2B, 00197 Rome, Italy

Bal Rajagopalan, MD
Orthopaedic and Sports Medicine Clinic Of Nova Scotia, 5595 Fenwick Street,
Suite 311, Halifax, Nova Scotia B3H 4M2, Canada

Per F.A.H. Renström, MD, PhD
Department of Orthopedics, Sports Medicine and Arthroscopy
Karolinska Hospital, SE-17176 Stockholm, Sweden

Andrea Scala, MD
Department of Orthopaedic, S. Camillo Hospital, Via Portuense 332, 00152 Rome,
Italy

Alberto Selvanetti, MD
Sports Science Institute, Department of Medicine, Service of Rehabilitation
and Functional Reconditioning, Via dei Campi Sportivi 46, 00197 Rome, Italy

William D. Stanish, MD, FRCS (C)
Orthopaedic and Sports Medicine Clinic Of Nova Scotia, 5595 Fenwick Street,
Suite 311, Halifax, Nova Scotia B3H 4M2, Canada

Gilles Walch, MD, Prof.
Clinique Sainte Anne Lumière, 85 Cours Albert Thomas, 69003 Lyon, France

Kevin E. Wilk, PT
American Sports Medicine Institute, 1313 13th Street South, Birmingham, AL 35205,
USA

Eric K. Wong, BS
Musculoskeletal Research Center, Department of Orthopaedic Surgery
University of Pittsburgh, Pittsburgh, PA 15213, USA

Savio L-Y. Woo, MD, PhD, DSc (Hon)
Ferguson Professor and Director, Musculoskeletal Research Center, Department of
Orthopaedic Surgery, University of Pittsburgh, PO Box 71199, Pittsburgh, PA 15213,
USA

Masayoshi Yagi, MD
Musculoskeletal Research Center, Department of Orthopaedic Surgery
University of Pittsburgh, Pittsburgh, PA 15213, USA

Sabrina Zanolli, PT
Sports Science Institute, Department of Physiology, Via dei Campi Sportivi 46,
00197 Rome, Italy

CHAPTER 1

Ligaments of the Knee in Sports Injuries and Rehabilitation

Savio L-Y. Woo, Eric K. Wong, J. Mi Lee, Masayoshi Yagi, Freddie H. Fu
Supported in part by NIH grants AR39683 and AR41820

Introduction

Increased athletic participation in high impact and high risk sports has increased the occurrence of soft tissue injuries in the knee. It has been estimated that the annual incidence of knee ligament injuries in the United States is 70,000 anterior cruciate ligament (ACL), 40,000 medial collateral ligament (MCL), and 20,000 combined ACL/MCL injuries [1, 2]. Seventy percent of all ACL injuries are sports-related [3]. In fact, an ACL injury occurs during every 1500 h of football, basketball, and soccer that are played [4]. A study from 1972 to 1987 concluded that an ACL tear occurs on approximately 1 out of 20,000 skier days [5]. Overall, 72% of all ACL injuries occur in males because they participate in sports more than females [6]. However, females have a proportionally much higher rate of ACL injury than males. Almost three times as many female basketball players and over two times as many female soccer players as their male counterparts injure their ACL [7]. Overall, the serious knee injury rate in all female athletes has increased to twice the level of that in males [8]. As the management of such ligamentous injuries occurs with greater frequency, elucidation of ligament function has become more emergent.

Whereas ligaments are static stabilizers of the knee (guiding the joint through its motions), muscles are dynamic structures that generate the necessary forces for movement. Nevertheless, the two must work harmoniously. An analogy to describe this is demonstrated in Fig. 1. The muscles act like a hammer that exerts large dynamic forces; the ligaments are represented as the hand that holds the nail (other soft tissues in and around the joint). If the hand (ligament) is not there to stabilize the nail, a strike by the hammer (muscle) may destroy the nail. Thus, without ligament function, the

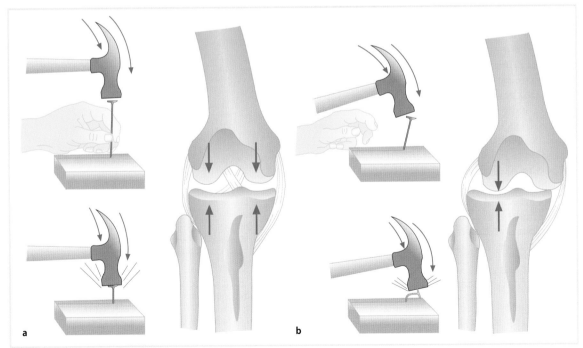

Fig. 1. An analogy of muscles, ligaments, and the knee joint as represented by the hammer and nail. **a,** Intact joint; **b,** displaced joint when ligaments are injured

knee joint is in danger of progressive damage, even if proper activation of the muscles occurs. Thus, severe ligament injuries can produce chronic instability of the knee and may result in long-term or even premature degenerative changes [1, 4, 9].

The sequelae of injury to the knee ligaments have directed the exploration into their function and biomechanical properties. In turn, the clinician is able to identify and optimize variables that restore joint stability when managing ligamentous injuries. This chapter will review the function of the ligaments of the knee with particular emphasis on the ACL and MCL. The basic mechanical properties and viscoelastic behaviors of normal knee ligaments will be covered as well as the structural properties of their respective bone-ligament-bone complexes. This is followed by a review of the current knowledge on ligament healing, with a focus on the MCL, and a discussion of the clinical and experimental results of ACL reconstruction including the variables that affect surgical outcomes and rehabilitation protocols. A discussion of the future direction in research and management of ligamentous injuries will conclude the chapter.

Biomechanical Properties of Ligaments

Anatomy and Structure

Ligaments are white, shiny, band-like structures of highly specialized, dense tissues that connect bones to each other. They are relatively hypocellular, with few fibroblastic cells interspersed within the tissue matrix. Knee ligaments such as the ACL and MCL are composed of abundant collagen fibers that are nearly parallel with the long axis of the ligament. Under polarized light microscopy, these fibrils have a sinusoidal wave pattern or crimp which is thought to have significance in the nonlinear functional properties [10, 11].

The attachments of the ligaments to bones occur as direct or indirect insertions. In the former, there is a gradual transition through four distinct zones: ligament, uncalcified fibrocartilage, calcified fibrocartilage, and bone [12]. For indirect insertions, the superficial portion of the ligament connects with the periosteum while the deeper layers connect to bone via the Sharpey's fibers. A prime example of a ligament that exhibits both types of insertions is the MCL of the knee. Its attachment to the femoral side is a direct insertion while that to the tibial side is an indirect insertion [13].

Biochemistry of Ligaments

Water comprises 60%–70% of the total weight in ligaments [12]. Of the dry weight, 70%–80% is collagen. Ninety percent of this is type I and the remaining 10% is made up of type III and other minor types of collagen [14–16]. Other, noncollagenous constituents include

proteoglycans, elastin, fibronectin, and glycoproteins. Although proteoglycans form less than 1% of the dry weight, their hydrophilic nature plays an integral part in the viscoelastic properties of ligaments [10, 17]. Additionally, elastin molecules can resist tension by reverting from globular to coiled form under stress.

Tensile Properties of Ligaments

As a tensile load is applied to a bone-ligament-bone complex, the relationship between load and elongation is initially nonlinear (Fig. 2a). The nonlinear region is referred to as the toe region and characterized by large elongations with only small increases in load. This is attributable to the straightening of crimped collagen fibers within the ligament [11]. As the applied load continues to increase, the fibers become taut and the slope increases until a linear region is reached. The slope of the linear portion of the curve, defined between two limits of elongation, is the stiffness of the complex. With further loading, the load-elongation curve demonstrates a slight decrease in slope as individual fibers start to fail. Failure of the ligament occurs when the ultimate tensile load is reached. The area under the entire load-elongation curve constitutes the energy absorbed to failure. The stiffness, ultimate tensile load, and energy absorbed to failure are the structural properties of the bone-ligament-bone complex.

During the same tensile test, the mechanical properties of the ligament substance are represented by its stress-strain curve. The stress in a ligament is defined as load per cross-sectional area (N/mm^2), while strain is defined as the change in length (ΔL) divided by the initial length (L_o) of a ligament ($\Delta L/L_o$). The cross-sec-

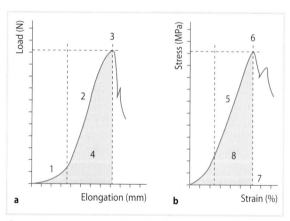

Fig. 2. a Structural properties of the bone-ligament-bone complex during uniaxial tensile test. *1* Nonlinear region referred to as the toe region, *2* stiffness, *3* ultimate tensile load, *4* energy absorbed to failure. **b** Mechanical properties of ligament substance during uniaxial tensile test. The stress-strain curve delineates parameters of the ligament substance such as *5* modulus, *6* tensile strength, *7* ultimate strain, and *8* the strain energy density.

tional area can be measured using a laser micrometer system, which uses a laser beam and light sensor to determine the width of the specimen through 180° of rotation [18, 19]. The strain can be determined using a video technique which tracks markers on the surface of the ligament as they separate during the tensile test [11, 20, 21]. The advantage of both of these methods is that no contact is made with the specimen during measurement sets. Similar to the load-elongation curve, the stress-strain curve of the ligament substance is also nonlinear (Fig. 2b). The stress-strain curve delineates parameters of the ligament substance such as modulus (slope of the linear portion between two defined limits of strain), tensile strength (stress at which tissue failure occurs), ultimate strain (strain at which tissue failure occurs), and the strain energy density (the area under this curve).

Additional considerations during biomechanical testing of ligaments are discussed below.

Specimen Age and Orientation

Skeletal maturity can have profound effects on the structural and mechanical properties of ligaments [22]. For example, the rabbit femur-MCL-tibia complexes (FMTCs) in age groups of 1.5, 4–5, 6–7, 12–15, 36, and 48 months were tested. The structural properties were found to increase until 12–15 months, reach a plateau between 15–36 months, and subsequently decline until 48 months [23–25]. The largest differences were apparent between the 7- to 12-month-old groups. During this period, skeletal maturity occurred with the closing of the epiphyses. Prior to this interval, all specimens failed at the tibial insertion site, but after skeletal maturation, all failures occurred as midsubstance tears. Thus, age of the animal has a significant effect on the strength of the FMTC [22]. In the human femur-ACL-tibia complex (FATC), the structural properties declined rapidly with specimen age [26, 27]. The older specimens (60–97 years) showed 26%, 70%, and 85% drops in stiffness, ultimate load, and energy absorbed to failure, respectively, when compared to younger specimens (22–35 years).

Because of the complex geometry of the FATC, the direction of applied force and the initial orientation of the ligament during tensile testing have large effects on the behavior of the ACL. To determine the structural properties of an FATC, the specimen should be oriented such that tensile loads can be aligned with the most collagen bundles. For example, the structural properties for specimens tested in the anatomical orientation (tensile load aligned with the long axis of the ACL) were approximately 20% higher than specimens tested in tibial orientation (tensile load applied along the long axis of the tibia) [27]. Thus, specimen age and ligament orientation are important when reporting the properties of knee ligaments.

Minor Effect of Strain Rates

Contrary to the dogma that strain rate affects the mechanical properties of ligaments, it has been demonstrated that strain rate actually plays a relatively minor role [28, 29]. Strain rates of over four decades (0.011%/s to 222%/s) were used to test the mature rabbit MCL. The stress-strain curves for all rates were similar [29]. In another study on the rabbit ACL, the same was true of mechanical properties, which did not significantly change over a wide range of strain rates [28]. Thus, one may conclude that strain rate does not affect the mechanical properties of ligaments during tensile testing.

Nonhomogeneity

Some ligaments are comprised of discrete bundles and are nonhomogenous. The human ACL is divided into the anteromedial (AM) and posterolateral (PL) bundles. Some advocate that there is also an intermediate (IM) bundle between the AM and PL bundles [30, 31]. The posterior cruciate ligament (PCL) consists of the anterolateral (AL) and posteromedial (PM) bundles [32, 33]. Previous studies have shown that the bundles are loaded differentially at varying knee positions, particularly when changing flexion angles [31–34]. Due to the complex geometry of cruciate ligaments, the mechanical properties of each ligament bundle have been evaluated separately. In the human ACL, it was found that the AM and IM bundles had higher values for modulus, tensile strength, and strain energy than the PL bundle [30]. However, in rabbit ACL, the mechanical properties of the medial and lateral bundles were found to be similar [35]. In human PCL, the AL bundle was found to have stiffness and ultimate tensile load values more than double those of the PM bundle [36]. Thus, the individual structural and mechanical properties of the ligament bundles must be appreciated when knee function is determined or ligament reconstruction is performed.

Viscoelastic Properties of Ligaments and Replacement Grafts

Ligaments are viscoelastic tissues that exhibit time- and history-dependent viscoelastic behavior. During a cycle of loading and unloading between two limits of elongation, the loading and unloading curves of a ligament follow different paths. The area enclosed by these two curves is called the area of hysteresis, which represents the energy loss. Other viscoelastic properties of ligaments include stress-relaxation behavior, i.e., decrease in stress when subjected to constant elongation, and creep behavior, i.e., a time-dependent elongation when subjected to a constant load. Tendons, which are commonly used as replacement grafts in ACL reconstructions, also exhibit these viscoelastic properties.

Consideration of the viscoelastic behavior of a tendon is crucial when it is utilized for ACL reconstruction. Clinically, the phenomenon of stress-relaxation predicts that the initial tension applied to a replacement graft in an ACL reconstruction can decrease 30%–60% over the course of surgery. However, it has been shown that cyclic stretching of primate patellar tendon grafts prior to graft tensioning reduced the amount of stress-relaxation [37]. Hence, preconditioning of a graft will attenuate the loss of tension that may occur after graft fixation.

Although stress-relaxation is reduced via preconditioning, the replacement graft continues to demonstrate cyclic stress-relaxation. For example, a large number of cyclic loads, such as during running, reduces stress in the graft with each elongation cycle. Fortunately, this behavior is recoverable. Also, cyclic stress relaxation contributes to prevention of graft failure. The viscoelastic behavior also illustrates the importance of warm-up exercises prior to physical activity in order to decrease maximal stresses in the ligamentous tissue.

Effects of Immobilization and Exercise

Traditional management of orthopedic ailments included rigid immobilization of joints. Prolonged immobilization can lead to joint stiffness and damage of healthy ligaments as a result of synovial adhesions [38]. In a rabbit model, the structural properties of an FMTC decreased drastically after 9 weeks of knee immobilization [39]. The ultimate load of the FMTC was 33% and the energy absorbed at failure was only 16% in the contralateral, nonimmobilized control. The elastic modulus and ultimate tensile strength of the MCL were also reduced. Histologic evaluation revealed marked disruption of the deeper fibers which attach to the MCL on the tibia by osteoclastic bone resorption in the subperiosteum. This disruption correlated with an increasing occurrence of immobilized FMTCs that failed by tibial avulsion. Similar decreases occurred in the FATC of rabbits, where resorption was observed at both the femoral and tibial insertions [40]. After remobilization of the knee, the structural properties of the FMTC were significantly lower than those of the control and slow to recover to the original state [39]. This observation was also seen in the structural properties of primate and rat FATC [41, 42]. The data also demonstrate that the ligament substance recovers more quickly from immobilization than the ligament insertions. Overall, a rehabilitation protocol comprised of months of remobilization is necessary for full recovery. Conversely, exercise has been known to strengthen the ligament, yet this in-

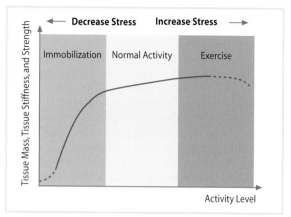

Fig. 3. A hypothetical curve to describe the nonlinear homeostatic characteristics of ligaments (Woo, J Biomech, 1997)

crease is small [43] (Fig. 3). Fortunately, normal daily activity provides enough stimulus to maintain ligament homeostasis.

Ligament Healing

Healing of Isolated MCL Injury

In recent years, both laboratory and clinical studies have demonstrated that isolated MCL injuries are capable of healing spontaneously and can result in excellent knee function [44]. Studies on dogs demonstrated that primary repair of a transected MCL with immobilization resulted in higher valgus rotations of the knee when compared to knees managed without primary repair or immobilization [45–47]. The structural properties of the FMTC from the latter group were also closer to the control values throughout the 1-year study period. Nevertheless, the mechanical properties of all the experimental MCLs were considerably different from those of the control. The modulus improved minimally with time, while the tensile strength reached only 60% of the control level at 1 year [47]. These findings fortify the argument for nonoperative management of grade III (complete) MCL injuries with controlled early mobilization and bracing.

A model more representative of MCL injury than simple transection was created to evaluate the effects of primary repair versus nonoperative treatment in the rabbit MCL [24, 45, 48]. In this model, the MCL was undermined and a rod was used to rupture the MCL by creating a "mop-end" tear of the ligament substance while simultaneously injuring the insertion sites. Primary repair of the torn MCL initially decreased the varus-valgus rotation of the knee, but after 6 weeks there was no difference between the repaired and nonrepaired groups. After 52 weeks, the varus-valgus rotation of both groups was similar to that of the control.

Additionally, there was no significant difference in stiffness of the FMTC between both groups and the control. However, the mechanical properties of the repaired and nonrepaired groups remained significantly lower, only approaching 50% of the control (Fig. 4). Thus, the injured MCL substance did not completely return to the normal state after either repair or nonrepair [24, 48]. The healed MCL was sufficient for knee function due to the larger cross-sectional area of the healed ligament.

The initial contact of the injured ends of the MCL also affects the subsequent properties of the healed ligament. A rabbit knee model was used to compare the healing of "contact" and "gap" injuries of the MCL [49]. By 40 weeks after injury, the ultimate tensile load for the "contact" group was indistinguishable from that of the control ligament. However, the "gap" group recovered only 65% of the strength and was significantly weaker than the control group. Thus, it appears that the healing of contact injury in the MCL is superior to that of gap injury.

To elucidate the healing of gap injuries in the MCL, a long-term study was conducted to examine the effects

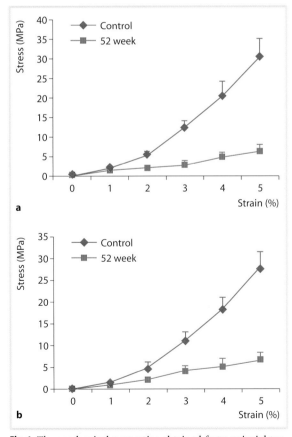

Fig. 4. The mechanical properties obtained from uniaxial tensile test of **a** repaired and **b** nonrepaired rabbit medial collateral ligament for control and 52 weeks postinjury (Ohland, Trans ORS and ASME, 1991)

of gap size [50]. Wider gap injuries healed with significantly lower structural properties over a long time interval (104 weeks) than smaller gap injuries. It was suggested that larger gaps between the ligament ends may cause a detectable weakness in the healed ligament due to differences in tissue remodeling.

Combined MCL and ACL Injury

In knee injuries that involve both the MCL and ACL, reconstruction of the ACL is usually performed, but surgical repair of the MCL is still debated. A combined injury model in rabbits was used to evaluate the repair of mop-end tears of the MCL in combination with an ACL reconstruction. After 6 and 12 weeks, both repair and nonrepair of the MCL injury yielded mechanical properties that were far below those of the control MCL [51]. At the 12-week period, the mechanical properties of the repair group were only slightly better than in the group managed with nonrepair. However, the modulus of the nonrepaired group was only 10% of the control MCL at both time periods. This is consistent with the less successful clinical outcomes of combined injuries of the MCL and ACL compared to isolated MCL injury [52, 53].

At longer-term healing of combined injury of the MCL and ACL (52 weeks), there was no significant difference between repair and nonrepaired MCL groups for any biomechanical properties measured. Similarly, the biomechanical properties of the healed MCL were not different in the two groups [54]. These data support clinical findings that the MCL can heal successfully with conservative treatment, even in combined injury of the MCL and ACL when the ACL is reconstructed.

Methods to Improve the Healing of Knee Ligaments

Growth factors have been introduced to the injured MCL because they are thought to augment or accelerate the healing process. A variety of growth factors have been screened through in vitro cell culture studies. Epidermal growth factors (EGF) and platelet-derived growth factors (PDGF-BB) were found to stimulate fibroblast proliferation while transforming growth factor beta-one (TGF-β_1) was found to promote collagen synthesis [55–58].

These growth factors were then used in an in vivo rabbit study. Their effect on healing of a ruptured MCL as well as dosage effects were examined. At 6 weeks, the structural properties of the FMTC that received only a high dose of PDGF-BB (20 µg) had ultimate load and energy absorbed to failure values that were 1.6 and 2.4 times greater respectively than in the group without any growth factor ($p < 0.05$) [59]. A low dose of PDGF-BB (400 ng) resulted in no significant increase, implying that PDGF-BB has an effect on MCL healing that is dosage-dependent. The addition of TGF-β_1 did not enhance the structural properties of the FMTC. Other studies confirmed that PDGF-BB and basic fibroblast growth factor (bFGF) may promote ligament healing, but TGF-β_2 had no effect [60–63].

It should be noted that the data in all these studies are preliminary. Long-term effects need to be investigated before growth factors can be utilized safely and effectively in humans. Furthermore, the rapid decay of growth factors has warranted the development of methods for repeat delivery of growth factors. Ultimately, the mechanism by which growth factors foster healing must be elucidated further. Collagen scaffolding, gene transfer technology (both viral and nonviral), mesenchymal stem cell therapy, mechanical stimulation, and manipulation of cells are other methods on the horizon to be investigated in hopes of enhancing the mechanical properties of healing MCL [64–67].

Anterior Cruciate Ligament Reconstruction

While the MCL has the capacity to heal without intervention, midsubstance tears of the ACL generally will not heal. Primary surgical repair has also been proven to fail. In order to restore knee stability after such an injury, reconstruction of the ACL has become the accepted option. Nevertheless, the choice of ACL replacement graft and the optimization of the surgical technique are still widely debated.

Functional Properties of the ACL

To obtain a better understanding of the function of the ACL, the in situ force in the ACL and its contribution to knee kinematics have been investigated. The term "in situ force" is used to describe the force in the ligament in its normal location and native environment in the knee. Approaches used to measure force and strain in the ACL include the attachment of mechanical devices such as buckle [68] and implantable transducers [69, 70]. Alternatively, noncontact methods include external force transducers [71], roentgenograms [72], and a kinematic linkage/materials testing machine system [20, 73].

In our research center, a robotic/universal force-moment sensor (UFS) testing system has been developed to measure knee kinematics accurately in multiple degrees of freedom and to determine directly the in situ force in a ligament without making physical contact with the ligament [74–76]. The robot can reproduce a previously recorded path of knee motion, such as those of intact and ACL-deficient knees. Thus, the difference in forces and moments in response to an externally applied load before and after ACL transection is the in situ force of the ACL, based on the principle of superposition. After ACL reconstruction, the in situ

forces in the ACL replacement grafts can be measured using the same specimen by repeating the identical path of the motion of the intact knee. As a result, the interspecimen variability is eliminated and the statistical power of the experiments significantly increased.

Using the robotic/UFS testing system, the in situ force in the human ACL in response to a 134-N anterior tibial load was highest at 15° of knee flexion (130±30 N) but decreased as it approached 90° of flexion (90±37 N) (Fig. 5a). Further, the distribution of in situ force between the AM and PL bundles was also measured. For the AM bundle, it remained relatively constant after peaking at 60° of flexion (66±35 N), while that for the PL bundle was highest at full extension (89±29 N). A "crossover" point (where the AM and PL bundles both had a similar magnitude of force) appeared at 30° of knee flexion [31, 34]. In addition, the function of these ACL bundles in response to a simulated pivot shift load (combined 5 Nm internal tibial torque and a 10-Nm valgus torque) was also examined. It was found that the in situ force in the AM bundle was 25% greater than that of the PL bundle at 30° of flexion, but both bundles played an equal role at 15° of flexion (approximately 21 N) (Fig. 5b). These data suggest the importance of both bundles of the ACL, which should taken into consideration during an ACL reconstruction.

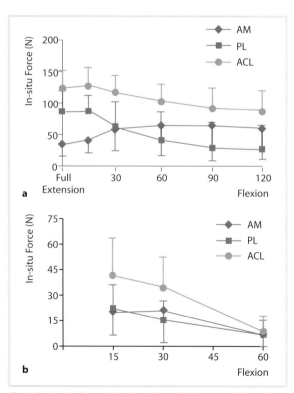

Fig. 5a,b. In situ force in the bundles of the human ACL vs. flexion angle **a** during 134 N anterior tibial load and **b** during a simulated pivot shift. ($n=6$, mean±SD)

Factors Affecting ACL Reconstructions

The literature suggests a 5% – 25% failure rate after 4 – 9 years for ACL reconstructions using autologous bone-patellar tendon-bone (BPTB) [4, 77]. Also, a higher incidence of osteoarthritis may be apparent in ACL-reconstructed knees [9]. In various animal studies, the structural properties of autologous BPTB grafts were less than 45% of those for intact ACL after 1 or 2 years [78 – 80]. Data in the canine model showed that the stiffness and ultimate load were much lower than in controls and comparable to findings from earlier studies using rabbit knees [81, 82]. These findings demonstrate that the ACL graft may never reproduce the stiffness and strength of the intact ACL.

Many ACL reconstruction techniques have been designed to replicate the function of the knee, and numerous associated variables have been identified. Due to space limitations, only graft fixation and graft healing will be discussed here.

Graft Fixation

With the advent of interference screws, the BPTB graft has gained popularity because the bone plugs on the graft can heal quickly to the bone in the tunnel. The biodegradable interference screw has also gained popularity, as its initial fixation strength is similar to that of the metal interference screw [83]. For a semitendinosus/gracilis tendon (ST/G) graft, a combined titanium button and polyester loop technique is commonly used for femoral fixation, while the tibial fixation is usually achieved through use of a soft-tissue washer and post, interference screw, or staples. Recently, the titanium button/polyester loop device was demonstrated to produce large motion of the graft within the femoral tunnel [84, 85]. Thus, early postoperative rehabilitation should take into account this motion and the consequences of delayed healing and failure.

There is no consensus as to which device provides the best clinical outcome. When choosing a fixation device, one should consider the biomechanical behavior of the overall graft and fixation complex. Viscoelasticity of the tissue, stiffness of the device, and bone interface are important factors when prescribing an accelerated rehabilitation protocol.

Graft Healing

Semitendinosus/gracilis tendon graft healing within the bone tunnel has been the subject of intense study [86, 87]. Based on a canine extra-articular model, the mechanical strength of the graft interface increased after 6 – 8 weeks of healing. Bone morphogenic protein-2 (BMP-2) was localized to mesenchymal cells at the tendon-bone interface at 3 days and its exogenous application may poten-

tially be used to enhance healing at the interface. In our research center, bone-to-bone healing and tendon-to-bone healing were studied at the femoral and tibial tunnels, respectively, using a goat model [88]. Histological examination showed that at 6 weeks there was complete incorporation of the bone block but not the tendon. The failure mode during tensile loading consistently was pull-out of the tendon from the tibial tunnel. Based on these results, rehabilitation protocols should consider the delayed graft incorporation of the ST/G graft. Nevertheless, further scientific and clinical studies are needed.

Rehabilitation After ACL Reconstruction

The commencement of rehabilitation after ACL reconstruction has been a subject of heated debate in recent years [69, 89, 90]. While some advocate an aggressive approach including full knee extension, immediate walking with full weight-bearing, and a return to light sports by 8 weeks, others prefer more conservative rehabilitation such as bracing for 1 month before ambulation [90]. In vivo studies revealed that the strains of a BPTB graft were significantly greater for active extension of the knee with weight-bearing than without [69]. This suggests that rehabilitation programs including immediate postoperative weight-bearing have the potential to endanger ACL grafts. Furthermore, no significant differences in the maximum ACL graft strain values were found between closed-chain (weight-bearing) kinetic exercise and open-chain (nonweight-bearing) kinetic exercise [91]. However, laboratory investigation revealed the importance of hamstring contraction on the kinematics of the knee and in situ force in the ACL [92]. The addition of antagonistic hamstring load to the quadriceps load significantly reduced both anterior tibial translation and internal tibial rotation and consequently reduced the in situ force of the ACL by 30% – 40% (Fig. 6). These data

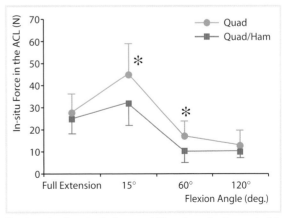

Fig. 6. In situ force in the human ACL vs. knee flexion angle following application of either a quadriceps load or a combination quadriceps/hamstring load ($n = 10$, mean ± SD) ($p < 0.05$)

suggest that rehabilitation should be performed at higher flexion angles of the knee in order to reduce the in situ force in the ACL graft. Nevertheless, further research is needed so that rehabilitation protocols can be based on scientific findings.

Summary and Future Directions

In this chapter, ligament properties including viscoelastic behavior have been reviewed. For the MCL, immobilization has proven to be detrimental to the properties of the ligament. A torn MCL has the potential to heal with conservative treatment, yet the functional ligament possesses mechanical properties inferior to those of the intact MCL. Current efforts to accelerate and augment this healing process have explored methods such as gene therapy to deliver growth factors. There are also many possibilities to address these injuries with consideration of fibroblasts and the interaction between the cell and matrix.

While ACL reconstructions are successful for many patients, significant research is required for the remaining 10%–20% of unsatisfactory surgical outcomes. The BPTB grafts have the advantage of rapid incorporation, but the properties do not reach those of the intact ACL. There is less morbidity with ST/G grafts, but greater tunnel motion dictates a slower rehabilitation protocol. Variables such as the ideal graft fixation technique, tunnel position, and the number of reconstruction graft bundles still raise debate. Gene therapy may be a powerful tool to enhance the process of graft incorporation.

In the future, a more anatomic ACL reconstruction such as double bundle reconstruction should be examined to determine if knee kinematics and in situ forces of normal ACL can be approximated during complex loading conditions. Also, more physiologic loading conditions that simulate rehabilitation protocols and/or activities of daily living need to be incorporated into experimental protocols. To address these goals, our research center has installed a higher-capacity robot (FANUC S-900 W) with a higher payload so that simulation of full body weight compression and high impact loads (exercise simulation) are possible. It is possible to analyze the effect of rehabilitation protocols not only on ligaments but also on cartilage, menisci, and bone.

Computer simulation and visualization of joint motion is another avenue to be pursued. Once validated, these models can simulate more realistic and complex loading conditions to study the mechanism of ligamentous injuries. Use of this technology would yield more precise and accurate methods of characterizing the functions of cruciate ligaments and their reconstructions. Ultimately, this approach can be used for preoperative planning for each patient in the hopes that more successful long-term outcomes will result.

Acknowledgements. We are grateful for the financial support from U.S. National Institutes of Health grants AR39683 and AR41820 and the assistance of Rich Debski, Serena Chan-Saw, Steve Abramowitch, and Kirstin Woo in writing this chapter.

References

1. Hirshman H, Daniel D, Miyasaka K (1990) The fate of unoperated knee ligament injuries. In: Daniel D, Akeson W, O'Connor J (eds) Knee ligaments: Structure, function, injury and repair. Raven Press, New York, pp 481–503
2. Miyasaka KC, Daniel DM, Stone ML et al (1991) The incidence of knee ligament injuries in the general population. Am J Knee Surg 4:3–8
3. Johnson RJ (1988) Prevention of cruciate ligament injuries. In: Feagin JA (ed) The Crucial Ligaments. Churchill Livingstone, New York, pp 349–356
4. Daniel DM (1994) Anterior cruciate ligament injuries. In: DeLee J (ed) Orthopaedic Sports Medicine. W.B. Saunders, Philadelphia
5. Johnson RJ, Pope MH (1991) Epidemiology and prevention of skiing injuries. Ann Chir Gynaecol 80:110–115
6. Ireland ML (1999) Anterior cruciate ligament injury in female athletes: Epidemiology. J Athl Train 34:150–154
7. Arendt E, Dick R (1995) Knee injury patterns among men and women in collegiate basketball and soccer: NCAA data and review of literature. Am J Sports Med 23:694–701
8. Huston LJ, Wojtys EM (1996) Neuromuscular performance characteristics in elite female athletes. Am J Sports Med 24:427–436
9. Gillquist J (1990) Knee stability: Its effect on articular cartilage. In: Ewing DD (ed) Articular Cartilage and Knee Joint Function: Basic Science and Arthroscopy. Raven Press, New York
10. Frank C, Amiel D, Woo SL-Y et al. (1985) Normal ligament properties and ligament healing. Clin Orthop 196:15–25
11. Woo SL-Y, Gomez MA, Seguchi Y et al. (1983) Measurement of mechanical properties of ligament substance from a bone-ligament-bone preparation. J Orthop Res 1:22–29
12. Woo SL-Y, Maynard J, Butler D et al. (1988) Ligament, tendon, and joint capsule insertions to bone. In: Woo SL-Y, Buckwalter JA (eds) Injury and Repair of Musculoskeletal Soft Tissues. American Academy of Orthopaedic Surgeons, Chicago, pp 133–166
13. Woo SL-Y, An KN, Arnoczky SP et al. (1994) Anatomy, biology, and biomechanics of tendon, ligament, and meniscus. In: Simon SR (ed) Orthopaedic Basic Science. American Academy of Orthopaedic Surgeons, Park Ridge, pp 45–87
14. Niyibizi C, Sagarriga Visconte C, Kavalkovich K et al. (1995) Collagens in adult bovine medial collateral ligament: Immunofluorescence localization by confocal microscopy reveals that type XIV collagen predominates at the ligament-bone junction. Matrix Biol 14:743–751
15. Niyibizi C, Sagarriga Visconti C, Gibson G et al. (1996) Identification and immunolocalization of type X collagen at the ligament-bone interface. Biochem Biophys Res Commun 222:584–589
16. Sagarriga Visconti C, Kavalkovich K, Wu JJ et al. (1996) Biochemical analysis of collagens at the ligament-bone interface reveals presence of cartilage-specific collagens. Arch Biochem Biophys 328:135–142
17. Woo SL-Y, Gomez MA, Akeson WH (1981) The time and history-dependent viscoelastic properties of the canine medial collateral ligament. J Biomech Eng 103:293–298

18. Lee TQ, Woo SL-Y (1988) A new method for determining cross-sectional shape and area of soft tissues. J Biomech Eng 110:110–114

19. Woo SL-Y, Danto MI, Ohland KJ et al. (1990) The use of a laser micrometer system to determine the cross-sectional shape and area of ligaments: A comparative study with two existing methods. J Biomech Eng 112:426–431

20. Hollis MJ, Takai S, Adams DJ et al. (1991) The effects of knee motion and external loading on the length of the anterior cruciate ligament: A kinematic study. J Biomech Eng 113:208–214

21. Woo SL-Y, Akeson WH, Jemmott GF et al. (1976) Measurement of nonhomogeneous directional mechanical properties of articular cartilage in tension. J Biomech 9:785–791

22. Woo SL-Y, Orlando CA, Gomez MA et al. (1986) Tensile properties of the medial collateral ligament as a function of age. J Orthop Res 4:133–141

23. Inoue M, Woo SL-Y, Amiel D et al. (1990) Effects of surgical treatment and immobilization on the healing of the medial collateral ligament: A long-term multidisciplinary study. Connect Tissue Res 25:13–26

24. Ohland KJ, Weiss JA, Anderson DR et al. (1991) Long-term healing of the medial collateral ligament (MCL) and its insertion sites. Trans Orthop Res Soc 16:158

25. Woo SL-Y, Ohland KJ, Weiss JA (1990) Aging and sex-related changes in the biomechanical properties of the rabbit medial collateral ligament. Mech Ageing Dev 56:129–142

26. Noyes FR, Grood ES (1976) The strength of the anterior cruciate ligaments in humans and rhesus monkeys. Age-related and species-related changes. J Bone Joint Surg Am 58A:1074–1082

27. Woo SL-Y, Hollis JM, Adams DJ et al. (1991) Tensile properties of the human femur-anterior cruciate ligament-tibia complex: The effect of specimen age and orientation. Am J Sports Med 19:217–225

28. Danto MI, Woo SL-Y (1993) The mechanical properties of skeletally mature rabbit anterior cruciate ligament and patellar tendon over a range of strain rates. J Orthop Res 11:58–67

29. Woo SL-Y, Peterson RH, Ohland KJ et al. (1990) The effects of strain rate on the properties of the medial collateral ligament in skeletally immature and mature rabbits: A biomechanical and histological study. J Orthop Res 8:712–721

30. Butler DL, Guan Y, Kay MD et al. (1992) Location-dependent variations in the material properties of the anterior cruciate ligament. J Biomech 25:511–518

31. Girgis FG, Marshall JL, Al Monajem ARS (1975) The cruciate ligaments of the knee joint: Anatomical and experimental analysis. Clin Orthop 106:216–231

32. Fuss FK (1989) Anatomy of the cruciate ligaments and their function in extension and flexion of the human knee joint. Am J Anat 184:165–176

33. Harner CD, Livesay GA, Kashiwaguchi S et al. (1995) Comparative study of the size and shape of human anterior and posterior cruciate ligaments. J Orthop Res 13:429–434

34. Sakane M, Fox RJ, Woo SL-Y et al. (1997) In situ forces in the anterior cruciate ligament and its bundles in response to anterior tibial loads. J Orthop Res 15:285–293

35. Woo SL-Y, Newton PO, MacKenna DA et al. (1992) A comparative evaluation of the mechanical properties of the rabbit medial collateral and anterior cruciate ligaments. J Biomech 25:377–386

36. Harner CD, Xerogeanes JW, Livesay GA et al. (1995) The human posterior cruciate ligament complex: An interdisciplinary study. Am J Sports Med 23:736–745

37. Graf BK, Vanderby RJ, Ulm MJ et al. (1994) Effect of preconditioning on the viscoelastic response of primate patellar tendon. Arthroscopy 10:90–96

38. Woo SL-Y, Matthews JV, Akeson WH et al. (1975) Connective tissue response to immobility. Correlative study of biomechanical and biochemical measurements of normal and immobilized rabbit knees. Arth Rheum 18:257–264

39. Woo SL-Y, Gomez MA, Sites TJ et al. (1987) The biomechanical and morphological changes in the medial collateral ligament of the rabbit after immobilization and remobilization. J Bone Joint Surg Am 69A:1200–1211

40. Newton PO, Woo SL-Y, Mackenna DA et al. (1995) Immobilization of the knee joint alters the mechanical and ultrastructural properties of the rabbit anterior cruciate ligament. J Orthop Res 13:191–200

41. Larsen NP, Forwood MR, Parker AW (1987) Immobilization and retraining of cruciate ligaments in the rat. Acta Orthop Scand 58:260–264

42. Noyes FR (1977) Functional properties of knee ligaments and alterations induced by immobilization: A correlative biomechanical and histological study in primates. Clin Orthop 123:210–242

43. Woo SL-Y, Kuei SC, Gomez MA et al. (1979) The effect of immobilization and exercise on the strength characteristics of bone-medial collateral ligament-bone complex. ASME Biomechanics Symposium, Niagara Fally, NY, pp 67–70

44. Baker CL, Liu SH (1994) Collateral ligament injuries of the knee: Operative and nonoperative approaches. In: Fu FH, Harner CD, Vince KG (eds) Knee Surgery. Williams and Wilkins, Baltimore, pp 787–808

45. Weiss JA, Woo SL-Y, Ohland KJ et al. (1991) Evaluation of a new injury model to study medial collateral ligament healing: Primary repair versus nonoperative treatment. J Orthop Res 9:516–528

46. Woo SL-Y, Gomez MA, Inoue M et al. (1987) New experimental procedures to evaluate the biomechanical properties of healing canine medial collateral ligaments. J Orthop Res 5:425–432

47. Woo SL-Y, Inoue M, McGurk-Burleson E et al. (1987) Treatment of the medial collateral ligament injury II: Structure and function of canine knees in response to differing treatment regimens. Am J Sports Med 15:22–29

48. Ohland KJM, Woo SL-Y, Weiss JM et al. (1991) Healing of combined injuries of the rabbit medial collateral ligament and its insertions: A long-term study on the effects of conservative vs. surgical treatment. Adv Bioeng 20:447–448

49. Chimich D, Frank C, Shrive N et al. (1991) The effects of initial end contact on medial collateral ligament healing: A morphological and biomechanical study in a rabbit model. J Orthop Res 9:37–47

50. Loitz-Ramage BJ, Frank CB, Shrive NG (1997) Injury size affects long-term strength of the rabbit medial collateral ligament. Clin Orthop 337:272–280

51. Ohno K, Pomaybo AS, Schmidt CC et al. (1995) Healing of the medial collateral ligament after a combined medial collateral and anterior cruciate ligament injury and reconstruction of the anterior cruciate ligament: Comparison of repair and nonrepair of medial collateral ligament tears in rabbits. J Orthop Res 13:442–449

52. Fetto JF, Marshall JL (1978) Medial collateral ligament injuries of the knee. Clin Orthop 132:206–218

53. Warren RF, Marshall JL (1978) Injuries of the anterior cruciate and medial collateral ligaments of the knee. A long-term follow-up of 86 cases – part II. Clin Orthop 136:198–211

54. Yamaji T, Levine RE, Woo SL-Y et al. (1996) Medial collateral ligament healing one year after a concurrent medial collateral ligament and anterior cruciate ligament injury: An interdisciplinary study in rabbits. J Orthop Res 14:223–227

55. Deie M, Marui T, Allen CR et al. (1997) The effects of age on rabbit MCL fibroblast matrix synthesis in response to TGF-$\beta 1$ or EGF. Mech Ageing Dev 97:121–130

56. Marui T, Niyibizi C, Georgescu HI et al. (1997) The effect of growth factors on matrix synthesis by ligament fibroblasts. J Orthop Res 15:18–23

57. Scherping SC Jr, Schmidt CC, Georgescu HI et al. (1997) Effect of growth factors on the proliferation of ligament fibroblasts from skeletally mature rabbits. Conn Tissue Res 36: 1–8

58. Schmidt CC, Georgescu HI, Kwoh CK et al. (1995) Effect of growth factors on the proliferation of fibroblasts from the medial collateral and anterior cruciate ligaments. J Orthop Res 13:184–190

59. Hildebrand KA, Woo SL, Smith DW et al. (1998) The effects of platelet-derived growth factor-BB on healing of the rabbit medial collateral ligament. An in vivo study. Am J Sports Med 26:549–554

60. Batten ML, Hansen JC, Dahners LE (1996) Influence of dosage and timing of application of platelet-derived growth factor on early healing of the rat medial collateral ligament. J Orthop Res 14:736–741

61. Letson AK, Dahners LE (1994) The effect of combinations of growth factors on ligament healing. Clin Orthop 308:207–212

62. Spindler KP, Dawson JM, Stahlman GC et al. (1996) Collagen synthesis and biomechanical response to TGF-β_2 in the healing rabbit MCL. Trans Orthop Res Soc 21:793

63. Weiss JA, Beck CL, Levine RE et al. (1995) Effects of platelet-derived growth factor on early medial collateral ligament healing. Trans Orthop Res Soc 20:159

64. Gerich TG, Fu FH, Robbins PD et al. (1996) Prospects for gene therapy in sports medicine. Knee Surg Sports Traumatol Arthrosc 4:180–187

65. Hildebrand KA, Deie M, Allen CR et al. (1999) Early expression of marker genes in the rabbit medial collateral and anterior cruciate ligaments: The use of different viral vectors and the effects of injury. J Orthop Res 17:37–42

66. Lazarus HM, Haynesworth SE, Gerson SL et al. (1995) Ex vivo expansion and subsequent infusion of human bone marrow-derived stromal progenitor cells (mesenchymal progenitor cells): Implications for therapeutic use. Bone Marrow Transplant 16:557–564

67. Young RG, Butler DL, Weber W et al. (1998) Use of mesenchymal stem cells in a collagen matrix for achilles tendon repair. J Orthop Res 16:406–413

68. Lewis JL, Lew WD, Hill JA et al. (1989) Knee joint motion and ligamental forces before and after ACL reconstruction. J Biomech Eng 111:97–106

69. Beynnon BD, Fleming BC, Johnson RJ et al. (1995) Anterior cruciate ligament strain behavior during rehabilitation exercises in vivo. Am J Sports Med 23:24–34

70. Holden JP, Grood ES, Korvick DL et al. (1994) In vivo forces in the anterior cruciate ligament: Direct measurements during walking and trotting in a quadruped. J Biomech 27:517–526

71. Markolf KL, Gorek JF, Kabo JM et al. (1990) Direct measurement of resultant forces in the anterior cruciate ligament. J Bone Joint Surg Am 72A:557–567

72. Vahey JW, Draganich LF (1991) Tensions in the anterior and posterior cruciate ligaments of the knee during passive loading: Predicting the ligament loads from in-situ measurements. J Orthop Res 9:529–538

73. Takai S, Livesay GA, Woo SL-Y et al. (1993) Determination of the in-situ loads on the human anterior cruciate ligament. J Orthop Res 11:686–695

74. Fujie H, Mabuchi K, Woo SL-Y et al. (1993) The use of robotics technology to study human joint kinematics: A new methodology. J Biomech Eng 115:211–217

75. Fujie H, Livesay GA, Woo SL-Y et al. (1995) The use of a universal force-moment sensor to determine in-situ forces in ligaments: A new methodology. J Biomech Eng 117:1–7

76. Rudy TW, Livesay GA, Woo SL-Y et al. (1996) A combined robotics/universal force sensor approach to determine in-situ forces of knee ligaments. J Biomech 29:1357–1360

77. Shelbourne KD, Gray T (1997) Anterior cruciate ligament reconstruction with autogenous patellar tendon graft followed by accelerated rehabilitation. A two- to nine-year follow-up. Am J Sports Med 25:786–795

78. Jackson DW, Grood ES, Goldstein JD et al. (1993) A comparison of patellar tendon autograft and allograft used for anterior cruciate ligament reconstruction in the goat model. Am J Sports Med 21:176–185

79. McPherson GK, Mendenhall HV, Gibbons DF et al. (1985) Experimental, mechanical and histologic evaluation of the Kennedy ligament augmentation device. Clin Orthop 196:186–195

80. Yoshiya S, Andrish JT, Manley MT et al. (1986) Augmentation of anterior cruciate ligament reconstruction in dogs with prostheses of different stiffnesses. J Orthop Res 4:475–485

81. Ballock RT, Woo SL-Y, Lyon RM et al. (1989) Use of patellar tendon autograft for anterior cruciate ligament reconstruction in the rabbit – a long term histological and biomechanical study. J Orthop Res 7:474–485

82. Beynnon BD, Johnson RJ, Toyama H et al. (1994) The relationship between anterior-posterior knee laxity and the structural properties of the patellar tendon graft: A study in canines. Am J Sports Med 22:812–820

83. Rupp S, Krauss PW, Fritsch EW (1997) Fixation strength of a biodegradable interference screw and a press-fit technique in anterior cruciate ligament reconstruction with a BPTB graft. Arthroscopy 13:61–65

84. Hoher J, Sakane M, Vogrin TM et al. (1998) Viskoplastische Elongation eines gevierfachten Semitendinosussehnenkonstrukts mit Tape-und Fadenfixierung unter zyklischer Belastung. Arthroskopie 11:52–55

85. Hoher J, Livesay GA, Ma CB et al. (1999) Hamstring graft motion in the femoral bone tunnel when using titanium button/polyester tape fixation. Knee Surg Sports Traumatol Arthrosc 7:215–219

86. Grana WA, Egle DM, Mahnken R et al. (1994) An analysis of autograft fixation after anterior cruciate ligament reconstruction in a rabbit model. Am J Sports Med 22:344–351

87. Rodeo SA, Arnoczky SP, Torzilli PA et al. (1993) Tendonhealing in a bone tunnel. J Bone Joint Surg 75-A:1795–1803

88. Papageorgiou CD, Ma CB, Withrow JD et al. (1999) The multidisciplinary study of the healing of an intra-articular ACL replacement graft. 25th Annual Meeting of the American Orthopaedic Society for Sports Medicine, Traverse City, p 446

89. Fu FH, Woo SL-Y, Irrgang JJ (1992) Current concepts for rehabilitation following anterior cruciate ligament reconstruction. ACL Surg Rehab 15:270–278

90. Shelbourne KD, Nitz P (1990) Accelerated rehabilitation after anterior cruciate ligament surgery. Am J Sports Med 18:292–299

91. Beynnon BD, Johnson RJ, Fleming BC et al. (1997) The strain behavior of the anterior cruciate ligament during squatting and active flexion-extension. A comparison of an open and a closed kinetic chain exercise. Am J Sports Med 25:823–829

92. Li G, Rudy TW, Sakane M et al. (1999) The importance of quadriceps and hamstring muscle loading on knee kinematics and in-situ forces in the ACL. J Biomech 32:395–400

Chapter 2

Methods of Functional Testing During Rehabilitation Exercises

Carmelo Bosco

Testing Muscle Functions

The assessment of muscle strength and power as well as range of motion, stiffness, and flexibility is important in exercise science. Similarly, evaluation of neuromuscular behaviour is extremely relevant in the rehabilitation of sport injuries. Consequently, several tests, methods, and techniques have been used to provide information regarding the relevance of strength and power to various physical pursuits and to monitor progress of rehabilitation from injuries [63]. Physical characteristics are dependent on several factors, including structure and function of the nervous system, structure and biochemical profile of skeletal muscle, mechanics of the joints and levers, and external mechanics. Each of these components has its specific influence on a given performance, but more importantly, they are all interdependent. Proper integrative function is of great relevance to neuromuscular performance. Therefore, the development and refinement of valid and reliable tests of muscular function are one of the pillars upon which rehabilitation from sport injuries is based.

It should be stressed that during conditions of injury and after surgery, satisfactory results can be obtained only through the combined efforts of surgeon, patient, and therapist. A rehabilitative plan is based upon consideration of the effects of disuse and immobility on musculoskeletal tissues and knowledge of the healing requirements following injury and the specific surgical procedure [56]. A balance must be found between simultaneous demands for protection against undue stress to facilitate healing and the need for stress to retard atrophy of musculoskeletal tissue. The physical approach to sport rehabilitation is based upon a logical progression through the succession of immobility, range of motion, progressive weight bearing, and strengthening exercises. The latter category can be subdivided into its own progression from isometric, isotonic (isoinertial load), and functional exercises through isokinetic exercises. The ultimate goal and final phase is a safe return to full activity.

On the other hand, it has been suggested that, in clinical practice, postimmobilisation rehabilitation should be early and effective [42]. To help in this long process from injured conditions to normal physiological behaviour, rehabilitation programs can be effectively helped by the assessment of muscle behaviour. This should be performed periodically during the training period for monitoring the effect of training on neuromuscular functions and specific performances. Furthermore, in case of injuries or surgery, the evaluation utilised to follow up the training program could be used as general clinical data for assisting and planning rehabilitation exercises. To provide this information, it is important that the test modality has relevance to the performance of interest. In this context, both dynamic and isometric muscular activation have been employed for tests and evaluation assessments. However, the testing protocol should be reliable enough that measurements for training- or injury-induced changes in muscle strength cannot be attributed to instrument or testing error.

Isometric Test

Isometric evaluation of muscle behaviour, which measures a muscle's maximum capacity to produce static force, has proceeded with different and often conflicting results [7, 29, 32, 45, 49, 66, 74]. One of the major limitations of such tests is that they are not specific to the performance of most human movements, which require dynamic activation of musculature through a movement range. Additionally, in previous research there have been large variations in the angles used for isometric assessment. For example, isometric leg extension tests have been performed with a large range of knee angles ($90° - 140°$) [35, 62, 65]. However, recent research indicates that, whenever such tests are used as predictors of performance, the joint angle should not be arbitrary. In fact, the relationship between the various isometric tests themselves and with performance varies substantially as a function of the angle [52]. These authors have recommended that these tests should be performed at the angle at which peak force is achieved in the performance of interest. In contrast, it has been suggested [63] that isometric testing be performed at joint angles which correspond to the peak of the strength curve for the particular muscle group to reduce the variability associated with small errors in the determination of joint angle.

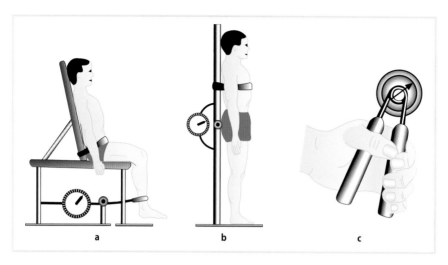

Fig. 1a–c. Examples of different methods utilised for assessment of maximal isometric strength

Although isometric measurements can be performed using not only one joint angle (Fig. 1a), but multiple ones (Fig. 1b,c), isometric force appears poorly related to dynamic performance [7, 49, 50]. In a longitudinal study performed with the Finnish national male volleyball team, it was noted that a decrease in heavy resistance training and the utilisation of jumping drills induced enhancement of jumping performance, which was accompanied by a reduction in isometric force [7]. Also, no relationship between jumping performance and isometric force has been reported in several publications [74, 81]. The rise of tension development (RTD) (which most probably represents the point in the force-time curve where the amount of active motor units and/or their firing frequency is maximal) calculated during concentric movement was superior to isometric RFD in its relationship to dynamic performance [60, 74].

It was suggested that there might be differences between isometric and dynamic activation in the neural activation of muscles. Furthermore, the isometric rate of force development test was ineffective in monitoring training-induced changes in performance of the triceps brachii and pectoralis major of 24 male subjects [50]. Such results support the suggestions that specific recruitment patterns be developed for dynamic contractions and that these patterns differ according to motor unit recruitment during isometric activity [3]. Consequently, alterations in training programs for athletes should be based on changes in actual performance, as opposed to muscular function tests. These findings appear due to the large neuronal and mechanical differences between dynamic and isometric muscular actions. In light of the above observations, it is recommended that isometric assessment of dynamic performance should be avoided and dynamic forms of muscle assessment should be employed. However, since isometric evaluations are popular, tests to en-

hance their reliability and validity are recommended [76], such as:

1. Study participants to undergo a separate familiarisation session prior to the collection of data
2. Several repeat trials to be performed, particularly if accurate RTD data is required
3. Clear and appropriate instructions to be given
4. Negligible pretension to be allowed prior to testing
5. The tests be performed in a position specific to the performance of interest
6. The angle which involves the highest force output in the performance of interest be used in the isometric test. Alternatively, a number of joint angles could be assessed

Isokinetics

Since the inception of the isokinetic concept [37], this form of exercise has been considered a valuable tool for assessment and evaluation of muscular function and pathology. Isokinetic devices allow individuals to exert as much force and angular movement they can generate. Some of the advantages that have been advocated in isokinetic exercise and assessment are:

1. They allow the isolation of muscle groups
2. Single joint assessment allows better isolation of specific diagnostic problems than multijoint tests, making it desirable for the identification of specific problems
3. They provide accommodating resistance to maximal exercise throughout the range of motion
4. Quantifiable data can be collected for analysis
5. They allow for the examination of muscle output at certain submaximal velocities (25% of V_{max}) throughout the movement range and are there-

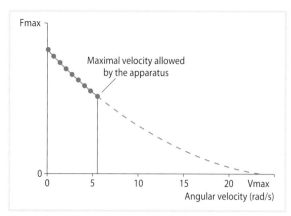

Fig. 2. Schematic representation of the torque/velocity relationship using isokinetic devices. The maximal speed allowed by these apparatus represents not more than 25% of that developed in ballistic motion

fore often considered more specific to human physical performance than isometric assessment

6. Allow development of the torque/velocity (T/V) relationship (Fig. 2)

7. Allow high reproducibility ($r = 0.82 - 0.96$) of test protocols [59, 77] if gravity correction and patient setup are properly considered [78]

On the other hand, several limitations are connected with this particular muscular activity:

1. Isokinetic motion shows nonspecificity with typical human movement characterised by the acceleration and deceleration of a constant mass [17].

2. Isokinetic tests have not always provided data which accurately differentiate performance between athletes of varying skill levels [29, 38]

3. The maximum velocity allowed by isokinetic apparatus reaches only 25% of the maximal velocity (Fig. 2) which can be developed by leg extensor muscles during ballistic motion [15] and only 10% of the maximum velocity obtained by the shoulder during throwing motion [55]

4. Exercise occurs primarily from nonweight-bearing open kinetic chain (OKC) positions, even if nowadays many isokinetic dynamometers can be used as a closed kinetic chain (CKC) [48]

5. Recent results [30] support the belief that isokinetic strength does not correlate strongly with functional tasks

6. The inability of the isokinetic dynamometer to detect increases in quadriceps performance has been also presented [2, 80]. Those findings should be seriously considered, since isokinetic values are frequently used as criteria for a return to functional activities

Although isokinetic tests have been extensively employed, recent observations strongly question the real effectiveness of such evaluation. In this connection, new approaches for assessment of muscle functions in planning sport activity and rehabilitation exercises have been applied using isoinertial evaluation.

Isoinertial Testing

From the physiological and functional points of view, the best tests of muscular behaviour are those using isoinertial loads. Among these, dynamometers, which utilise rotator inertial masses, have been built only for research purposes and therefore were not commercially available [40, 73]. Only recently, the assessment of muscle function in dynamic conditions has been performed against a constant mass rather than a constant velocity using commercial dynamometers. Several apparatus have been utilised for this purpose, from a force platform [11] to a special sledge built ad hoc to study the stretch-shortening cycle (SSC) [41]. An electronic processing unit which can be used with any muscular machine using gravitational forces as external resistance (e.g. leg presses, dips, pull-down, barbells, etc.) has been recently developed [8, 9, 19, 20]. This apparatus (Muscle Lab, Langensund, Norway) allows detecting and amplifying internal muscular biological processes. This usually unavailable information is thus made available in a way that is meaningful, rapid, precise, and consistent. Wherever raising or lowering a load involves a muscular activity, the apparatus can measure with an encoder and record the displacement in function of time. In addition, all derived parameters can be synchronised with four EMG channels. It should be reminded that with the Muscle Lab it is possible to monitor not only the raising or lowering of an isoinertial mass but also any ballistic motion like jumping or throwing. With this new apparatus, it is possible to measure, record, and analyse single and multiple joint movements. These in turn may be performed in all types of muscular activation: (a) concentric, (b) eccentric, or (c) a combination of both in SSC performance, which represents most human physical efforts in the gravitational field.

Physiological activities of mammals on the Newtonian level manifest primarily as movement, spatial displacement, or postural maintenance in the gravity field [53]. Thus it can be said that the earth's field of gravity has played a part in the evolutionary development of neuromuscular and motor systems in mammals [67, 82]. In light of the above observations, the utilisation of isoinertial evaluation represents the most natural assessment which can be performed during both pathologic and physiologic conditions. In this respect, it has been pointed out that the most unbiased monitoring of training occurs when the same regime (same equip-

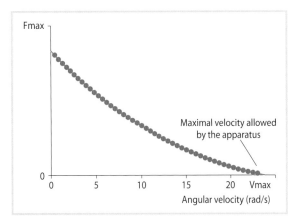

Fig. 3. Schematic representation of the force/velocity relationship using isoinertial apparatus. The apparatus allows recording of the maximal velocity which can be developed in ballistic motion

ment and same movement pattern) is used for both training and testing [64]. It should be remembered that the Muscle-Lab makes it possible to monitor muscular activation in the whole range of force-velocity relationships, since it allows the evaluation of muscular behaviour which can be performed with extremely light or heavy external resistance (Fig. 3).

Some advocate the following to be the advantages of isoinertial exercise and assessment [19, 51]:

1. The ability to isolate muscle groups
2. Better isolation than multijoint tests in that they allow single joint assessment, desirable for identification of specific problems
3. The ability to perform multijoint assessment
4. Measurement of SSC exercises
5. OKC and CKC can both be assessed
6. Collect quantifiable data for analytic evaluation
7. Allow the examination of muscle output in all velocities (1% – 95% of V_{max}) throughout the movement range. These conditions are more specific to human physical performance than isokinetic or isometric assessments
8. Allow determination of force/velocity (F/V) relationships (Fig. 3).
9. Present high reproducibility ($r = 0.85 – 0.97$) of test protocols [9, 19, 51]

It is likely that assessment of dynamic characteristics using isoinertial loads present few limitations, since the most natural muscular activity is utilised. However, if the subjects are not well familiarised with the test to be performed, some difficulties can be found. In addition, some claim [57] that one difficulty in this system is that the amount of resistance is limited to the weakest point in the range of motion. This point is determined by biomechanical characteristics of the joint. Actually

this is not a relevant question, since we are dealing with a kinetic chain, and in Newtonian physics the strength of a chain is determined by the weakest link. For each muscle or muscle group, there is an optimal condition during a range of motion which allows the development of maximum torque. This condition is strongly influenced by muscle length and the leverage from the joint the muscle is activating.

Isometric, Isokinetic, and/or Isoinertial Measurements

Muscle function can be measured by a variety of methods characterised as the isoinertial, isokinetic, semi-isokinetic, and isometric testing modalities. Further, the type of muscle activity (concentric, eccentric, or isometric) and velocity may vary in testing. In addition, more confusion arises if we compare the various testing methods presented by the literature [44]. The problem is related to the question of whether assessments of muscle behaviour should be general or specific.

Since it has been shown that strength and explosive-power training had a specific effect on the biological structures activated [18, 33, 34], a pertinent answer to the above question has been suggested by Sale and MacDougal [64], who pointed out that the most important criterion in selecting a test is specificity. The weak relationship between dynamic and isometric tests [7, 49, 50] indicates that muscular measurements are not general qualities but specific to the test modality. The lack of correlation between changes in dynamic performance and isometric test that was observed by many authors [7, 65, 72, 81] suggests that different mechanisms may underlie the changed performance of these two measures of strength. This would seem to indicate that training-induced speed-strength adaptations are also specific. Consequently, isometric tests or testing at a certain speed may not be valid for monitoring neuromuscular adaptations meant to be induced through dynamic training [3, 7]. On the other hand, there are strong indications to suggest that the pattern of motor unit recruitment at moderate knee angular velocity is velocity-dependent, regardless of the muscle activity involved (isokinetic vs. ballistic motion) [17]. Finally, it should be noted that the effect of prestretching cannot be measured properly with isokinetic apparatus, while this muscle behaviour is the most natural pattern of human locomotion and can be easily monitored with an isoinertial apparatus.

Neural Considerations

Even if it has been suggested that there may be preferential recruitment of certain motor units at certain positions or angles as a muscle moves through a range of motion [22, 70], the neural recruitment pattern observed during isokinetic muscle activation seems to differ from those observed during isoinertial contraction (Fig. 4).

High motor unit activation characterised the beginning of the effort of half-squat exercises; however, as subjects moved through the motion range, a parallel decrease in neural activation was noted. The exact mechanism which caused this reduction is not clear. In this connection, it has been suggested that the high tension required at the beginning of a motion to overcome inertial force may trigger some inhibition from the Golgi tendon organs (GTO) [1, 14]. In contrast, in isokinetic contraction the leg extensor muscle maintained the same magnitude of myoelectrical activity along the whole range of motion, as expected [25, 37]. This finding is no surprise, since one advantage of isokinetic exercises has been indicated to be the possibility of maintaining maximum nervous activity through the whole range of motion [37]. In half-squat activity, even when a drastic decrease in EMG occurred at the end of motion, the level was higher than in the isokinetic exercise, even if the same external resistance was used.

The different structural aspects of the two exercises could also modify the neural recruitment pattern, and hence the force output of the musculature may be affected accordingly. The dynamic squat is often performed with the toes pointing slightly outwards, while the isokinetic leg extensor test is performed with the toes pointing straight ahead. A difference in position affecting the line of pull that has been shown in other muscle groups alters neural recruitment patterns [71, 75].

Mechanical Considerations

Several mechanical factors characterise the behaviour of muscle functions during exercises performed with isoinertial resistance and in isokinetic conditions. Thus, the assessment of skeletal muscle working capacity is specific for the motion executed and depends on the test used.

Prestretch

One factor which strongly differentiates isoinertial and isokinetic assessments is the possibility of utilising the SSC pattern in the first activity, while in the latter exercises effective prestretching is almost impossible. The performance of eccentric muscular action followed immediately by a concentric action is a common feature of movement executed in the gravitational field. The use of SSC augments the concentric phase of movement, resulting in increased work and power [14, 24] and enhanced movement efficiency [15, 23] compared to similar movements performed without prior stretching. The reported augmentation of concentric action is typically ascribed to the reuse of elastic energy [23, 24] in combination with neural facilitation induced by stretch reflex [16]. The effect of prestretch also depends on the length of the coupling time, which reflects the transient period between the eccentric and the concentric phases [13]. If this transient period is too long (>100 ms) the stored elastic energy can be lost as heat [28]. Similarly the facilitation induced by stretch reflex can be lost with long coupling times [11]. Thus, the length of the transient period between the eccentric and concentric phases is of fundamental importance for the efficacy of SSC. However, even though modern

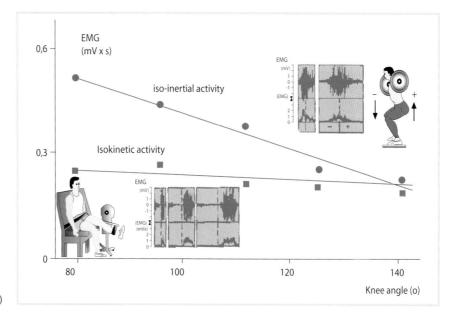

Fig. 4. Electromyographic (EMG) activity of the leg extensor muscles recorded from the same subjects during an isokinetic test (*square symbols*) and during an isoinertial test (half squat performed with an extra load) (*round symbol*) of similar external resistance. In the isokinetic evaluation, EMG activity remained at the same level through the range of movement. In contrast, during isoinertial assessment, the EMG activity demonstrated a dramatic burst at beginning of the movement followed by a parallel decrease of neural input as the motion continued to the end. (Modified from [35, 46])

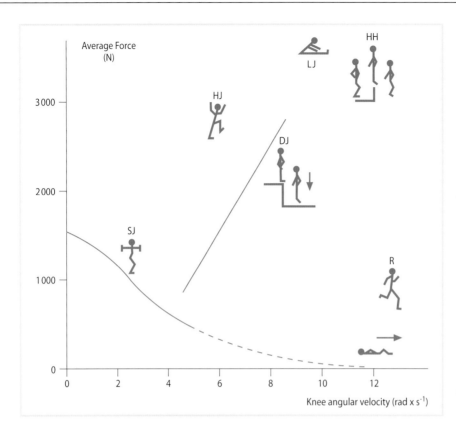

Fig. 5. Force/velocity relationships presented for two different conditions: vertical jump performed during simple concentric work (*SJ*) and after prestretching (*DJ*). In SJ, the force is developed mainly by the contractile component of the muscles, while in DJ the effect of prestretching is a remarkable increase in force through neural potentiation and the reuse of elastic energy. The forces developed during several sport disciplines are also presented in function of the average knee angular velocity: *HJ*, high jump; *LJ*, long jump; *HH*, jumping over the hurdle; *R*, running. (Modified from [10, 11])

isokinetic dynamometers allow SSC exercises, it is rather difficult to note an increase in EMG after prestretching [69]. In fact, it is almost impossible to build any electromechanical apparatus which allows reversal of motion from eccentric to concentric in less than 50–100 ms. In contrast, as it occurs in running [39] or jumping [12], the coupling time in normal motion can be in the order of 10 ms. In light of the above considerations, the validity of an isokinetic apparatus to monitor muscle behaviours which in real-life situations are almost exclusively performed with SSC must be questioned. The forces developed under SSC conditions are demonstrated always to be dramatically greater than those which rely only on the shortening contraction. The force/velocity curves shifted to the right whenever the concentric contractions followed prestretch activity as in running or jumping (Fig. 5). Thus, during normal daily activity or ballistic performances, the effect of prestretching enhances force output in the function of shortening velocity [10].

Force/Velocity Relationship

The use of an isoinertial apparatus [19] and isokinetic dynamometers [58] allows one to reconstruct F/V and torque/velocity (T/V) relationships. Both represent more sophisticated diagnostic assessment of muscle function than isometric testing. The mechanical be-

haviour of skeletal muscle is better described and analysed using F/V values than T/V ones. The F/V relationship can be described through recording several exercises performed with different loads, allowing from 3 to more than 100 measurements. Consequently, dramatic variations in velocity (from 0.5 rad/s up to 13 rad/s) can be reached in response to external loads, for example during leg extensor muscle tests [11, 19]. Unfortunately, the isokinetic dynamometers allow only few (not more

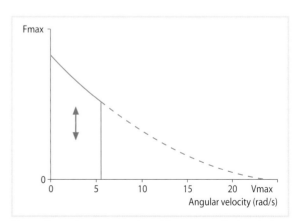

Fig. 6. Schematic representation of the torque/velocity relationship using an isokinetic device. *Arrow* represents changes registered by the isokinetic dynamometer. With such a device, only torque magnitude can be recorded

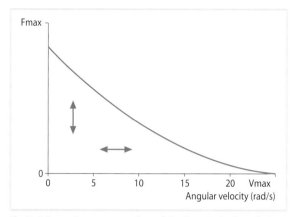

Fig. 7. Schematic representation of the force/velocity relationship obtained with an isoinertial load device. *Arrow* represents the physiological variable which can be detected and recorded with the dynamometer. Note that both speed and force can be varied in the effort performed

than 8 or 9) measurements [58], limiting the velocity range to 0.5 rad/s – 5 rad/s. Furthermore, with isoinertial measurements, the voluntary effort is modulated by changing both velocity and force (Fig. 7). Since velocity in the isokinetic test is already preset by the operator, it is only possible to detect changes in torque production (Fig. 6). In conclusion, with an isoinertial dynamometer it is possible to analyse and discriminate muscle tension developed against low or high external resistance, while only high resistance can be measured with the isokinetic test.

Assessment of Muscle Strength and Pain Tolerance

Muscle Function and Pain Threshold

Athletes with any type of injury should be able to return to activity quickly and safely with appropriate surgery, treatment, and rehabilitation. The rehabilitation programme should emphasise decreasing inflammation, restoring motion, increasing strength, and a safe return to competition. This can begin preoperatively and progress postoperatively through a programmed treatment and intervention protocol supported by functional evaluation and clinical diagnosis of muscular behaviour. Since the last phase of an athlete's rehabilitation programme usually involves isokinetic training, most of the muscular evaluation assessments have been performed with isokinetic apparatus. Unfortunately, such an evaluation system presents a strong and dramatic limitation. In fact, in both preoperative and postoperative conditions, evaluation of the maximum torque capacity requires the development of at least 60% of the maximum strength from the patient/athlete, even at the highest speed allowed by the isokinetic

apparatus. This high level of muscle tension does not represent the full neuromuscular performance but is strongly influenced by pain thresholds. Thus, during an evaluation assessment, high force is required and a tension-limiting mechanism may occur. Consequently, it is likely that the strength output results from many factors including pain sensibility, reduction of neural drive, and the effects of disuse and immobility on musculoskeletal tissues. It has been suggested that, during eccentric load conditions, joint kinaesthetic receptors of a Golgi type [68], free nerve endings in the muscle, and cutaneous and joint receptors may also participate in the reduction of neural drive [79]. This tension-regulating mechanism would contribute to the limitation of muscle tension and preservation of muscle integrity, not only during eccentric work but also during injury and the postoperative phase. It means that the true maximum effort and maximum force output depend on the individual pain threshold, and the measured torque does not reflect true muscle function but also the ability of the patient to stand the pain.

Assessment of Muscle Function Using Light Loads

In light of the above observations, the isoinertial assessment test which allows the measurement of muscle function against very light loads, seems to be the most appropriate evaluation system. In fact, in both pre- and postoperative conditions, it could be possible the measure the muscular behaviour using only light loads (e.g. 1% – 5% of maximum strength). Therefore, the development of low force at high speed may avoid the negative influence induced by pain and eliminate intervention of the tension-regulating mechanism. The isoinertial dynamometer can be used for evaluation of both CKC and OKC to asses a patient's strength and readiness to progress to higher functional levels. Even CKC evaluation tests have been promoted as more functional, appropriate, and safe than OKC tests.

With the isoinertial load dynamometer, it is also possible to measure skeletal muscle group functions postoperatively during OKC. In this respect, Muscle Lab was used to assess and calculate the power developed during leg extension exercises using only 5 kg as external resistance. The measurements from female basketball and female volleyball players collected 2 and 50 weeks after ACL surgery, respectively, are shown in Figs. 8 and 9. The isoinertial apparatus allowed detection of a dramatic loss of power (220%) for the basketball player (182 W vs. 82 W, nonoperated vs. operated leg). In the volleyball player, a strong rapid recovery was noted in the postsurgery period, and the power developed was 195 W vs. 166 W for nonoperated and operated legs, respectively. The EMG, recorded simultaneously with leg extension power measurements in the vastus lateralis and medialis of both legs, showed that

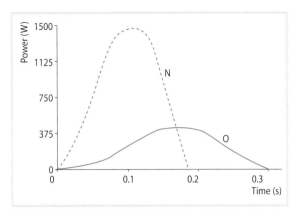

Fig. 8. Power developed during leg extension exercises performed by a female basketball player with a total load of 10 kg (including weight estimated for the thigh), presented in function of time. The operated leg (O) demonstrated lower power requiring longer development time than the other leg (N)

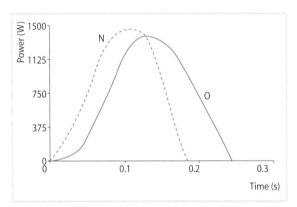

Fig. 9. Power developed during leg extension performed by a female volleyball player with a total load of 10 kg (including weight estimated for the thigh), presented in function of time. The operated leg (O) demonstrated lower power than the other leg (N)

low power output of the operated leg was related to low EMG activity (only 27% of the nonoperated leg). These results indicate the occurrence of strong neural drive inhibition [26]. In contrast, the operated leg of the volleyball athlete demonstrated neuromuscular efficiency. In fact, its EMG activity was 200% higher than in the nonoperated leg, while the power output showed only a modest reduction (17%) compared to the nonoperated one. In light of these results, a more specific rehabilitation programme could be facilitated. Although those measurements were performed with OKC, it could be possible as well to use CKC. Exercises performed on leg press or any similar machine which utilises gravitational loads as external resistance or no loads such as squats or squat jumps can be monitored with the Muscle Lab. The latter test exercises have been recently emphasised in the international literature to be more functional in assessment of muscle behaviour in the rehabilitation setting [5, 30, 54].

The Effect of Vibration on EMG Activity of Skeletal Muscle

In recent decades, the assessment of neuromuscular behaviour has experienced great improvement through the evolution of diagnostic technique. This was made possible by the creation of new instruments and equipment used mainly in the field of rehabilitation and sport medicine. However, the assessment of neuromuscular function is far from sufficient for covering the large spectrum of biological changes which occur with injuries and after surgery. In fact, a high percentage of patients show weakness of the leg extensor muscles after long follow-up periods, most likely due to the severing of proprioceptors during surgery [27]. Thus, even though such problems are well known, due to the proprioceptors' inability to function properly there is no specific and adequate evaluation technique to allow quantification and assessment of the impairment. In this respect, a pilot investigation was conducted to analyse the possibility of detecting and quantifying proprioceptor function on the operated knee joint. For this purpose, a new diagnostic technique consisting of monitoring muscular EMG activity during vibration was applied for identifying altered neural strategies of motoneuron pool recruitment. Previous EMG findings recorded in the biceps brachii of boxers [20] showed a significant enhancement ($p < 0.001$) of neural activity during the vibration treatment period over normal conditions.

Similar results were noted in EMG activity of the leg extensor muscles (left and right vastus lateralis and left and right vastus medialis) of a healthy athlete during vibration treatment (Fig. 10). Facilitation of the spinal reflex was elicited through vibration to the quadriceps muscle [21]. The possibility that vibration may elicit excitatory inflow through muscle spindles and alpha motoneuron connections in the overall motoneuron inflow was suggested previously [47]. It has been demon-

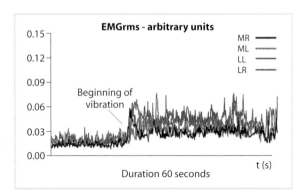

Fig. 10. Electromyographic (EMG) activity recorded from leg extensor muscles (right and left vastus lateralis and vastus medialis of both left and right legs) before and during entire vibration treatment. A remarkable enhancement of the EMG was recorded

strated that vibration drives alpha motoneurons via a Ia loop, producing force without reducing motor drive [61]. In addition, it has been shown that vibration induced activation of muscle spindle receptors, not only in the muscle to which vibration was applied but also to neighbouring muscles [43]. Mechanical vibration (10 Hz – 200 Hz) applied to muscle belly or tendon can elicit reflex contraction [31]. This response has been named "tonic vibration reflex" (TVR). It has been also argued that, in the presence of TVR, vibration-induced suppression of motor output in maximal voluntary contractions probably does not depend on voluntary commands [6]. It was suggested that a contributing mechanism might be vibration-induced presynaptic inhibition and/or transmitter depletion in the group Ia excitatory pathways, which constitute the afferent link of the gamma loop [6]. In light of the above findings, a pilot study was planned to introduce a new assessment strategy for identifying muscle behaviour and possibly dysfunction.

EMG Analysis and Vibration for Assessment of Proprioceptor Function

To evaluate the proprioceptors' capacity to function properly, several subjects who had been previously operated in one leg (at least 1 year before) were exposed to vertical sinusoidal whole body vibration (WBV) for 60 s. During the vibration treatment, EMG activity of the leg extensor muscles (left and right vastus lateralis and left and right vastus medialis) was monitored simultaneously in normal and operated legs. The subjects stood on a vibration platform (Nemes, Bosco System) in a half-squat position (knee angle 90°) while the frequency of vibration was settled at around 40 Hz for a total of 60 s (Figs. 11, 12). When the EMGs were com-

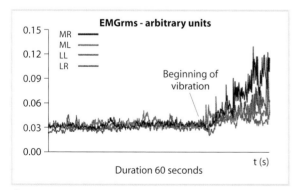

Fig. 11. EMG activity recorded from leg extensor muscles of a male athlete (right and left vastus lateralis and medialis of both left and right legs) before and during vibration treatment. During the vibration period, higher EMG activity was noted in both legs than in normal conditions. However, a remarkable enhancement of the EMG was noted in the postoperated leg (right vastus lateralis and left vastus medialis) compared to the healthy one

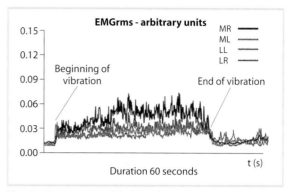

Fig. 12. Electromyographic (EMG) activity recorded from leg extensor muscles of a female athlete (vastus lateralis and medialis of both left and right legs) before and during vibration treatment. During administration of vibration, higher EMG activity was noted in both legs. However, a remarkable enhancement of the EMG was noted in the postoperated leg (right vastus lateralis and left vastus medialis) compared to the healthy one

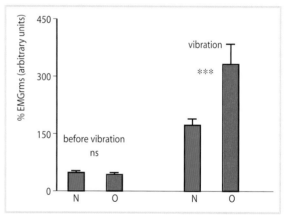

Fig. 13. Mean ± SD of the electromyogram root-mean square given as percentage of baseline values recorded from vastus lateralis and medialis in both nonoperated (N) and operated (O) legs of eighteen subjects before and during vibration treatment. No significant statistical difference was observed between N and O before vibration treatment (ns) while, during vibration, the O legs demonstrated a statistical significant difference from N legs ($p < 0.002$, Student's t-test for paired observations)

pared, remarkably higher activity could be observed in the postoperated leg during vibration treatment. Statistical analysis confirmed this (Fig. 13). Therefore, since it is likely that a severing of proprioceptors may occur during surgery, it is tempting to suggest that the high EMG activity of the operated leg might be caused by inadequate proprioceptor function. It is likely that one function of the proprioceptors is to filter and modulate neural drive from central command. Therefore, if the proprioceptors were severed during surgery [27], this capacity could be lost, resulting in hyperactivity during vibration treatment. However, although it is no easy task to find a proper explanation, these findings could help in detecting the function of proprioceptors. It should be noted that 100% of the subjects studied ($n = 18$) demonstrated higher EMG activity in the muscles of operated legs than in the contralateral, healthy legs in response to vibration. These findings suggested that, if a rehabilitation programme can claim to be successful, describing the physiological assessment of muscle functions only by mechanical evaluation of force or torque output is not enough. There is still a lack of adequate, specific evaluation techniques for assessing impairment due to the proprioceptors' inability to function properly.

New Diagnostic Method for Prediction of Hamstring Injuries

Hamstring strains are among the most common injuries (and reinjuries) in athletes. Hamstring muscle tear takes place during eccentric exercise when the muscle develops tension while lengthening. The isokinetic strength test has usually been employed to determine the relation of hamstring and quadriceps muscle strength and imbalance to hamstring injury [57]. It is generally thought that, to prevent hamstring injuries, the H:Q ratio assessed with an isokinetic device should not be less than 60%. Unfortunately, this is a poor evaluation for predicting possible hamstring injuries. In fact, strength assessment with a constant speed device at low speed (3–4 rad/s) cannot be compared with the force developed during eccentric work at extremely high speed [14]. In this connection, it has been noted that isokinetic strength testing does not predict hamstring injury in athletes [4]. Consequently, a new functional test was developed which allows assessment of leg extensor muscle function during ballistic motions such as the vertical jump. During a vertical jump performed from half-squat position, hamstring and quadriceps cocontraction has been documented and explained via a cocontraction hypothesis. This hypothesis provides for a stabilising force at the knee by producing a posteriorly directed force on the tibia to counteract the anterior tibial force imparted by the quadriceps.

To determine muscle recruitment patterns of knee extensor and flexor muscles, EMGs were made of the right and left hamstrings (hr, hl) and left rectus femoris (rfl). Fig. 14 presents an example of a female sprinter revealing that both rfl and hl were strongly engaged during vertical pushoff, while the hr demonstrated only moderate activity at the end of the pushoff. The high activity noted in the hl was associated with a previous hamstring injury. On the other hand, the hr showed a low level of activity, reflecting the low demand placed on it to counter anteriorly the shear force acting at the proximal tibia. This altered neural strategy reflects changes in neural input to the motoneuron pools rec-

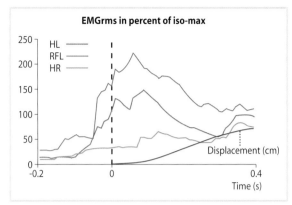

Fig. 14. EMG root-mean square recorded in the left (*HL*) and right hamstrings (*HR*) and left rectus femoris (*RFL*) of a female sprinter during vertical jump performance. Also shown is the displacement in cm during the beginning of the jump. The high activation of the hl was related to the claim of problems felt by the athlete in that muscle

ruited in generating specific motor tasks. Trying to detect possible dysfunction, the EMG activity of Q was compared with that of H. Preliminary results revealed that when the EMG Q:H ratio is greater than 1, no problems could be noted in the hamstring. On the other hand, if the ratio was lower than 1, some symptom of hamstring injury was claimed by the athletes. Similar procedures have been suggested recently to assess muscle dysfunction [26]

References

1. Angel RW (1974) Electromyography during voluntary movement: The two burst pattern. Electroenc Neurophysiol 36:493–498
2. Augustsson J, Esko A, Thomee R et al (1998) Weight training of the thigh muscles using closed vs. open kinetic chain exercises: A comparison of performance enhancement. J Orthop Sports Phys Ther 27(1):3–8
3. Baker D, Wilson G, Carlyon B (1994) Generality versus specificity: A comparison of dynamic and isometric measures of strength and speed-strength. Eur J Appl Physiol 68:350–355
4. Bennell K, Wajswelner H, Lew P et al (1998) Isokinetic strength does not predict hamstring injury in Australian rules footballers. Br J Sports Med 32(4): 309–331
5. Blackburn JR, Morrissey MC (1998) The relationship between open and closed chain strength of the lower limb and jumping performance. J Orthop Sports Phys Ther 27(6):430–435
6. Bongiovanni LG, Hagbarth KE, Stjenberg L (1990) Prolonged muscle vibration reducing motor output in maximal voluntary contractions in man. J Physiol (Lond) 423:15–23
7. Bosco C (1981) New tests for measurement of anaerobic capacity in jumping and leg extensor muscle.Volleyball, I.F.V.B. Official Magazine 1:22–30
8. Bosco C (1991a) Nuove metodologie per la valutazione e la programmazione dell'allenamento. SDS Rivista di Cultura Sportiva 22:13–22
9. Bosco C (1991b) Nuovi metodi di pianificazione dei carichi di lavoro. In: Riabilitazione del traumatizzato e preparazio-

ne fisica dello sportivo. Edn Erre Come Riabilitazione, Rome 109:109–123

10. Bosco C (1992) Strength assessment with the Bosco's test. Società Stampa Sportiva, Rome

11. Bosco C, Komi PV (1979) Potentiation of the mechanical behaviour of the human skeletal muscle through pre-stretching. Acta Physiol Scand 106(4):467–472

12. Bosco C, Luhtanen P, Komi PV (1976) Kinetics and kinematics of the take-off long jump. In: Komi PV (ed) Biomechanics 5B. University Park Press, Baltimore, pp 174–180

13. Bosco C, Komi PV, Ito A (1981) Pre-stretch potentiation of human skeletal muscle during ballistic movement. Acta Physiol Scand 111(2):135–140

14. Bosco C, Viitasalo JT, Komi PV et al (1982a) Combined effect of elastic energy and myoelectrical potentiation during stretch-shortening cycle exercise. Acta Physiol Scand 114 (4):557–565

15. Bosco C, Ito A, Komi PV et al (1982b) Neuromuscular function and mechanical efficiency of human leg extensor muscles during jumping exercises. Acta Physiol Scand 114(4): 543–550

16. Bosco C, Tarkka I, Komi PV et al (1982c) Effect of elastic energy and myoelectrical potentiation of triceps surae during stretch-shortening cycle exercise. Int J Sport Med 3:137–140

17. Bosco C, Mognoni P, Luhtanen P (1983) Relationship between isokinetic perfromance and ballistic movement. Eur J Appl Physiol 51:357–364

18. Bosco C, Komi PV, Bosco E, Nicol C, Pulvirenti G, Caruso I (1994) Influence of training on mechanical and biochemical profile's muscles. Coaching Sport Sci J 1(1):8–13

19. Bosco C, Belli A, Astrua M et al (1995) A dynamometer for evaluation of dynamic muscle work. Eur J Appl Physiol 70:379–386

20. Bosco C, Cardinale M, Tsarpela O (1999) Influence of vibration on mechanical power and electromyogram activity in human arm flexor muscles. Eur J Appl Physiol 79(4):306–311

21. Burke JR, Schutten MC, Koceja DM et al (1996) Age-dependent effects of muscle vibration and the Jendrassik maneuver on the patellar tendon reflex response. Arch Phys Med Rehabil 77(6):600–604

22. Caldwell G, Jamison J Lee S (1993) Amplitude and frequency measures of surface electromyography during dual task elbow torque production. Eur J Appl Physiol 66:349–356

23. Cavagna GA, Saibene FP, Margaria R (1964) Mechanical work in running. J Appl Physiol 19(2):249–256

24. Cavagna GA, Dusman B, Margaria R (1968) Positive work done by a previously stretched muscle. J Appl Physiol 24(1):21–32

25. Counsilman J (1971) New approach to strength building. Scholastic Coach 41:50–52

26. Edgerton VR, Wolf SL, Levendowski DJ et al (1996) Theoretical basis patterning EMG amplitudes to assess muscle dysfunction. Med Sci Sports Exerc 28(6):744–751

27. Engel A, Petschnig R, Baron R et al (1990) The effect of meniscectomy on the strength of the femoral quadriceps muscle after more than 3 years. Wien Klin Wochenschr 102(22):663–666

28. Fenn WO, Marsh BS (1934) Muscular force at different speeds of shortening. J Physiol Lond 85:277–297

29. Fry AC, Kraemer WJ, Weseman CA et al (1991) Effects of an off-season strength and conditioning program on starters and non-starters in women's collegiate volleyball. J Appl Sport Sci Res 5:174–181

30. Greenberger HB, Paterno MV (1995) Relationship of knee extensor strength and hopping test performance in the assessment of lower extremity function. J Orthop Sports Phys Ther 22(5):202–206

31. Hagbarth KE, Eklund G (1965) Motor effects of vibratori stimuli. In: Granit R (ed) Muscular afferents and motor control. Proceedings of the First Symposium. Almqvist and Wiksell, Stockholm, pp 177–186

32. Hakkinen K, Alen M, Komi PV (1984) Neuromuscular, anaerobic, and aerobic performance characteristics of elite power athletes. Eur J Appl Physiol 53:97–105

33. Hakkinen K, Alen M, Komi PV (1985a) Changes in isometric force- and relaxation-time, electromyographic and muscle fiber characteristics of human skeletal muscle during strength training and detraining. Acta Physiol Scand 125:573–583

34. Hakkinen K, Alen M, Komi PV (1985b) Effect of explosive type strength training on isometric force- and relaxation-time, electromyographic and muscle fiber characteristics of leg extensor muscles. Acta Physiol Scand 125:587–600

35. Hakkinen K, Komi P, Kauhanen H (1987) Scientific evaluation of specific loading of the knee extensors with variable resistance, isokinetic and barbell exercises. In: Marconet P, Komi P (eds) Medicine and sport science. Kargel, Basel, pp 224–237

36. Hakkinen K, Pakarinen A, Alen A et al (1987) Relationship between training volume, physical performance capacity, and serum hormone concentrations during prolonged training in elite weight lifters. Int J Sports Med 8:61–65

37. Hislop HJ, Perrine JJ (1967) Isokinetic concept of exercise. Phys Ther 47:114–117

38. Hurley JM, Hagberg JM, Holloszy BF (1988) Muscle weakness among elite power lifters. Med SciSports Exerc 20:S81

39. Ito A, Komi PV, Sjodin B (1983) Mechanical efficiency of positive work in running at different speed. Med Sci Sports Exerc 15(4):299–308

40. Kaneko M (1971) Dynamic of human muscle with special reference to explosive power output. Kyrin Book Co., Tokio

41. Kaneko M, Komi PV, Aura O (1984) Mechanical efficiency of concentric and eccentric exercises performed with medium to fast contractions rate. Scand J Sport Sci 6:15–22

42. Kannus P, Jozsa L, Kvist M et al (1998) Effects of immobilisation and subsequent low-high-intensity exercise on morphology of rat calf muscles. Scand J Med Sci Sports 8(3):160–171

43. Kasai T, Kawanishi, Yahagi S (1992) The effects of wrist muscle vibration on human voluntary elbow flexion-extension movements. Exp Brain Res 90:217–220

44. Knuttgen E, Kraemer W (1987) Terminology and measurement in exercise performance. J Appl Sports Sci Res 1:1–10

45. Komi P, Karlsson J, Tesh P et al (1982) Effects of heavy resistance and explosive type strength training methods on mechanical, functional, and metabolic aspects of performance. In Komi PV (ed) Exercise and sport biology. Human Kinetics, Champaign, pp 90–102

46. Kuntz H, Unold A (1986) Zielgerichtetes Krafttraining, Magglingen TLG, ETS. Trainer Information 247

47. Lebedev MA, Peliakov AV (1991). Analysis of the interference electromyogram of human soleus muscle after exposure to vibration. [Russian.] Neirofiziologia 23(1): 57–65

48. Levine D, Klein A, Morrissey M (1991) Reliability of isokinetic concentric closed kinematic chain testing of the hip and knee extensors. Isokinetic and Exercise Science 1:146–152

49. Mero A, Luhtanen P, Viitasalo J et al (1981) Relationships between the maximal running velocity, muscle fiber characteristics, force production and force relaxation in sprinters. Scand J Sport Sci 3:16–22

50. Murphy AJ, Wilson GJ (1996) Poor correlation between isometric tests and dynamic performance: Relationship to muscle activation. Eur J Appl Physiol 63:352–357

51. Murphy AJ, Wilson GJ, Pryor JF (1994) Use of iso-inertial

force mass relationship in the prediction of dynamic human performance. Eur J Appl Physiol 69:250–257

52. Murphy AJ, Wilson GJ, Pryor JF et al (1995) Isometric assessment of muscular function: The effect of joint angle. J Appl Biom 11:205–215

53. Organov VS, Skuratova SA, Potapov AN et al (1981) Physiological mechanism of adaptation of skeletal muscles of mammals to the weightless state. Adv Physiol Sci 24 :17–24

54. Ostenberg A, Roos W, Ekdahl C et al (1998) Isokinetic knee extensor strength and functional performance in healthy female soccer players. Scand J Med Sci Sports 5(1):257–264

55. Pappas AM, Zawaki RM, Sullivan TJ (1985) Biomechanics of baseball pitching: A preliminary report. Am J Sport Med 13:216–222

56. Paulos LE, Wnorowski DC, Beck CL (1991) Rehabilitation following knee surgery. Sport Med 11:257–275

57. Perrin DH (1993) Isokinetic exercise and assessment. Human Kinetics, Champaign

58. Perrine JJ, Edgerton R (1978) Muscle force-velocity and power-velocity relationships under isokinetic loading. Med Sci Sports Exerc 10:159–166

59. Pincivero DM, Lephart SM, Karunakara RA (1997) Reliability and precision of isokinetic strength and muscular endurance for quadriceps and hamstrings. Int J Sport Med 18:113–117

60. Pryor JF, Wilson GJ, Murphy AJ (1994) The effectiveness of eccentric, concentric and isometric rate of force development tests. J Hum Mov Stud 27:153–172

61. Rothmuller C, Cafarelli E (1995). Effects of vibration on antagonist muscle coactivation during progressive fatigue in humans. J Physiol 485:857–864

62. Ryushi T, Hakkinen K, Kauhanen H et al (1988) Muscle fibre characteristics, muscle cross-section area and force production in strength in athletes, physically active males and females. Scand J Sports Sci 10:7–15

63. Sale DG (1991) Testing strength and power. In: MacDougall J, Wenger H, Green H (eds) Physiological testing of the high performance athlete, 2nd edn. Human Kinetics, Champaign, pp 21–106

64. Sale DG, MacDougall D (1981) Specificity in strength training: A review for coach and athlete. Can J Appl Sport Sci 6:87–92

65. Sale DG, Martine JE, Moroz DE (1992) Hypertrophy without increased isometric strength after weight training. Eur J Appl Phsyiol 64:51–55

66. Secher NH (1975) Isometric rowing strength of experienced and inexperienced oarsmen. Med Sports Exerc 7:280–283

67. Smith AT (1975) Foundations of gravitational biology. In: Foundation of space biology and medicine. Nauka II, Moscow, pp 141–175

68. Solomonow M, Baratta R, Zhou BH et al (1988) Electromyogram co-activation patterns of the elbow antagonist muscles during slow isokinetic movement. Exp Neurol 100:470–477

69. Svantesson U, Sunnerhagen SK (1997) Stretch-shortening cycle in patients with upper motor lesions due to stroke. Eur J Appl Physiol 75:312–318

70. Ter Haar Romeny B, Denier van der Gon J, Gilen C (1982) Changes in recruitment order of motor units in the human biceps brachii. Exp Neurol 78:360–368

71. Ter Haar Romeny B, Denier van der Gon J, Gilen C (1984) Relation between location of motor units in the human biceps brachii and its critical firing levels for different tasks. Exp Neurol 85:631–650

72. Thorstensson A, Hulten B, Karlsson J (1976). Effects of strength training on enzyme activities and fibre characteristics in human skelatal muscle. Acta Physiol Scand 96:392–398

73. Tihanyi J, Apor P, Feket G (1982) Force-velocity-power characteristics and fiber composition in human knee extensor muscles. Eur J Appl Physiol 48:331–343

74. Viitasalo JT, Hakkinen K, Komi PV (1981) Isometric and dynamic force production and muscle fibre composition in man. J Hum Mov Stud 7:199–209

75. Wagman I, Pierce D, Burges R (1965) Proprioceptive influence in volitional control of individual motor units. Nature 207:957–958

76. Wilson GJ, Murphy AJ (1996) The use of isometric test of muscular function in athletic assessment. Sport Med 22(1):19–37

77. Wilson GJ, Walshe AD, Fisher MR (1997) The development of an isokinetic squat device: Reliability and relationship to functional performance. Eur J Appl Physiol 75:455–461

78. Winter DA, Wells RP, Orr GW (1981) Error in the use of isokinetic dynamometers. Eur J Appl Physiol 46:397–408

79. Westing SH, Seger JY, Thorstensson A (1990) Effect of electrical stimulation on concentric and eccentric torque-velocity relationships during knee extension in man. Acta Physiol Scand 140:17–22

80. Worrel TW, Borchert B, Erner K, Fritz J, Leerar P (1993) Effect of lateral step-up exercise protocol on quadriceps and lower extremity performance. J Orthop Sports Phys Ther 18(6):646–653

81. Young WB, Bilby GE (1993) The effect of voluntary effort to influence speed of contraction on strength, muscular power and hypertrophy development. J Strength Cod Res 7:172–178

82. Zenkevich LA (1944) Assay on evolution of the motor system of animals. J Obshch Biol 5:129

CHAPTER 3

Proprioceptive Training in the Prevention of Sports Injuries

Giuliano Cerulli, Fabrizio Ponteggia, Auro Caraffa, GianCarlo Aisa

The Proprioceptive System

We must first define some words and concepts to know better what the proprioceptive system is [25]. The concept of proprioception is commonly described as the conscious and subconscious ability to know the position of one's body segment in space. Kinesthesia is the ability to feel movement and its direction. Integrated with tactile, visual, and vestibular information, proprioception and kinesthesia [2, 3, 21] comprise the proprioceptive system. Its function is necessary for body posture and joint movement. Commonly, the word "proprioception" is used to mean the entire proprioceptive system.

Mechanoreceptors and free nerve endings have been demonstrated in many joints (ankle, knee, hip, spine, shoulder, elbow, wrist, finger) [29]. To our knowledge, Abbott [1] was the first to describe sensory innervation in the ligaments of the knee joint. Freeman and Wike classified the receptors, naming types I (Ruffini's endings), II (Pacini's corpuscle), III (Golgi's tendon organs), and IV (free nerve endings) [22].

There is a physiological distinction between phasic and tonic receptors [5]. The rapidly adapting receptors ("phasic", Pacini) begin to generate impulses immediately at the onset of stimulus and quickly end their function even though the stimulus remains present: the role of these receptors is to be sensitive to a change of state (initiation or termination of a movement). The slowly adapting receptors ("tonic", Ruffini, Golgi) send their impulses until the stimulus is present (position of a body segment during a movement). Like other body functions, the proprioceptive system deteriorates with age [19, 28, 48, 56].

Measurement Methods

There is no device for measuring the effectiveness of the proprioceptive system in its entirety. Proprioception can be measured using a modified isokinetic machine: from a starting position, a passive joint movement is performed ending at a certain joint angle and then returning to starting position; the subject must accurately reproduce the previous joint angle in which the passive movement was stopped, with or without visual aid. This test is called reproduction of passive positioning (RPP).

Kinesthesia can be quantified using a modified isokinetic machine by measuring the threshold to detect passive motion (TTDPM): a joint is moved with a modified isokinetic device at very low angular velocity; the subject must feel the movement and its direction as soon as possible without visual aid. Another test to evaluate part of the proprioceptive system is reflex muscle contraction latency recorded with electromyography; this is useful in determining the activity level and arisement time of muscle reaction after a sudden joint movement and is in our opinion the most useful

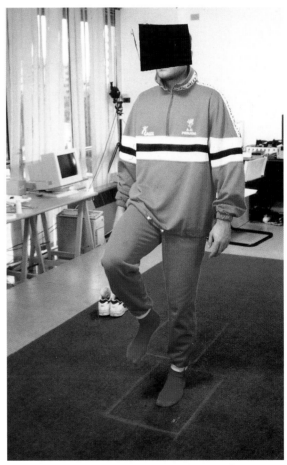

Fig. 1. Proprioceptive evaluation using a force platform

test to analyze in vivo the correlation between the proprioceptive system and sport-specific movements.

Force platforms (stabilometry) (Figs 1, 2) are used mostly to test patient posture (including visual, neurological, and vestibular afferents) [20, 24, 43, 63], while

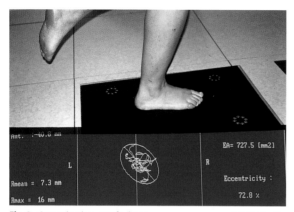

Fig. 2. Quantitative result (trace, sway area, eccentricity) of a proprioceptive test performed on a force platform

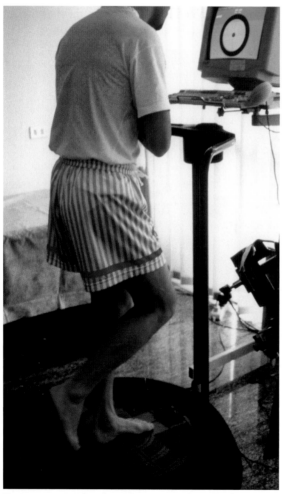

Fig. 3. An example of a computerized unstable board: the KAT2000 kinesthetic ability trainer

the unstable board (Fig. 3) (such as the KAT2000 kinesthetic ability trainer) is useful not only for evaluation but also for training. It is important to remember that the training method and the measurement device must be different because if the athlete always uses the same tool, a "training effect" could appear in quantitative evaluation – a methodological error. Due to the different rationales of the devices mentioned, it is impossible to compare their function [27]. We can state that, except for reflex muscle contraction latency, the other tests are for the laboratory and not the field. Only in biomechanical laboratories is it possible to perform several synchronized examinations to study an athlete's movement. Every type of measurement requires attention to give valid results (for example distraction of the patient during examination provokes worse results) [58].

The Knee and the Proprioceptive System

Many authors demonstrated the existence of mechanoreceptors and free nerve endings in several parts of the knee joint. In 1984, Schultz [52] described receptors like Golgi's tendon organs in the anterior cruciate ligament (ACL) suggesting a role in a proprioceptive reflex arc for protecting the joint from extreme movement. Two years later, an Italian study [15] discovered Ruffini's and Pacini's corpuscles, placed mostly in the middle and proximal thirds of the ACL. The neural anatomy of the ACL and its sensory role were better described a few years later [32, 53]. Mechanoreceptors are described also in the posterior cruciate, lateral collateral, and medial collateral ligaments (PCL, LCL, and MCL, respectively) [17, 51].

The presence of type I and II mechanoreceptors and nerve tissue within the meniscus and in perimeniscal connective tissue has been reported by several authors [4, 33, 45, 46]. Free nerve endings were also found in the distal iliotibial tract: this finding is important to warn surgeons of that area [39]. A clinical study on the influence of medial meniscus lesions on knee proprioception was performed by Jerosch in 1996 [30]: an RPP test showed less proprioception in patients with meniscus lesions than in a healthy control group. Values returned to normal level after partial meniscectomy.

We do not know why meniscectomy improves proprioception. It could result from the pain reduction, as hypothesized by the study's authors. Neurophysiological intraoperatory experience shows that, by stimulating the meniscus with an arthroscopic probe, it is possible to record EMG signals due to muscle response from the vastus medialis and the biceps femoris [16]. According to these results, we always recommend a conservative surgical approach to resect only small parts of the meniscus and not alter its proprioceptive and biomechanical functions.

Stimulation of the ACL with evoked potentials in animal [42] and human studies [49] caused a recordable electric response of the thigh muscles (quadriceps and hamstrings) and the cerebral cortex. Lavender found no response if the stimulated ACL was interrupted and for this reason supposes that broken nerve fibers in the graft after ACL reconstruction cannot regain function [36]. Neuroligamentization of the graft after ACL reconstruction has been demonstrated from a histological point of view (Pacini's corpuscle and free nerve endings in the graft 15 months after reconstruction) [57]. In 1997, Barrack verified that, 6 months after ACL reconstruction in six dogs with patellar tendon, there was evidence of reinnervation of the graft (mechanoreceptors and free nerve endings); moreover, somatosensory evoked potentials were present in all the dogs before ACL lesion, disappeared immediately after ACL reconstruction, and were recorded again 6 months later in two dogs [6]. This study is important because it demonstrates not only histological but also functional reinnervation of the graft after ACL reconstruction. More studies are necessary to verify this evidence also in humans.

In past years, the proprioceptive function of the ACL has probably been seen as only in the knee joint, but instead all the structures contribute to proprioception. A recent paper testing RPP in patients affected by acute isolated ACL lesions found no differences from the contralateral leg in respect to joint position. The authors explain these results with intact afferents from the other parts of the knee joint and the muscles [26]. Other studies testing chronic ACL patients with TTDPM and RPP always found worse results in the injured legs [12, 18]. We do not know the relative importance of the muscles and every part of the joint in the proprioceptive system. In any case, we view that TTDPM and RPP are able to evaluate only limited aspects of the proprioceptive system such as proprioception or kinesthesia; moreover, the validity of the proprioceptive system applies not to knee stability but knee function.

There are contradictory results about the benefit of bandages and braces to proprioceptive function [10, 11, 47, 50]. Muscle fatigue seems to induce proprioceptive deterioration [35, 44, 62]. Hamstring activity is important to avoid anterior tibial displacement, both in ACL-deficient and reconstructed knees. A valid proprioceptive test is the reflex hamstring contraction latency (RHCL) test: this consists of recording latency time between sudden tibial anterior displacement and the consequent hamstring contraction. There is a greater latency of muscle contraction in ACL-deficient knees in comparison not only with control groups of healthy subjects but also with the uninjured contralateral side in the same patient. There is also a correlation between latency and functional instability (frequency of giving way) in ACL-deficient patients [8].

The enhancement of RHCL is important to protect knee joints in the preoperative phase (avoiding giving-way episodes that could provoke chondral and meniscus lesions) and to protect the graft in its healing period soon after ACL reconstruction. It is possible to improve RHCL by performing proprioceptive exercises with the aim of improving speed and facility of hamstring contractions.

A training program with many closed kinetic chain exercises and a progressive reduction in stability (wobble board, eyes open and then closed) and increasing the number of repetitions and rate of contractions is better than a traditional program of muscle strengthening (open kinetic chain and graduated weight-resisted exercises) in improving RHCL and dynamic joint stability [7]. After ACL reconstruction, RHCL improves significantly, but no correlation seems to exist with passive anterior tibial translation performed with the KT1000 arthrometer [9].

A functional exercise program (training of leg muscles in closed kinetic chain and of trunk muscles to improve coordination, postural reactions, and endurance) is also good for normalizing standing balance as measured with force platform in ACL-deficient patients [63].

We sometimes hear during follow-up quantitative evaluation at the end of rehabilitation programs or during the first period of sport activities (for example after ACL reconstruction) athletes expressiving not complete subjective satisfaction, even though stability, range of joint motion, concentric, and eccentric muscle strength are good. In our opinion, this can be attributed to a sport-specific proprioceptive deficit; unfortunately, a device to measure this accurately still does not exist.

In 1999, Shelbourne demonstrated that functional sports agility exercises (based on the individual sport activity) performed early during rehabilitation (starting at a mean of 5 weeks after ACL reconstruction) do not alter joint stability [54]. Due to the described safety of agility exercises, in rehabilitation programs after sports injuries, proprioception must receive the same importance as joint movement and muscle strength.

The Ankle and the Proprioceptive System

Together with the knee, the ankle is where the influence of the proprioceptive system has been more studied. Receptors were found in ankle joint capsules and ankle ligaments by Freeman and Wike in 1967 [23]. An effective proprioceptive system is important to prevent ankle sprains. This injury happens commonly in ankle inversion and plantar flexion, with consequent strain on the lateral compartment (anterior talofibular, posterior talofibular, and calcaneus-fibular ligaments).

The role of some muscles (peroneus brevis and longus, tibialis anterior) as active ankle stabilizers is very important. Ankle sprain is always a high-speed event, so a quick and valid muscle response is necessary to avoid lesions. Muscle contraction latency is an index for testing the proprioceptive system.

Lynch, in 1996, performed tests with a tilt platform in ten uninjured subjects to reproduce quick ankle inversion and plantar flexion (it is difficult to simulate the injury mechanism in laboratory), recording muscle contraction latency with surface EMG [41]. The results showed that increasing the angle of movement lengthens the latency response of peroneus muscles, while with a higher inversion speed there is shorter latency in the same muscles during contraction. A loss of reflex (less protection) has been noted to increase plantar flexion.

Tape is considered to have an influence on neuromuscular activity of the ankle joint. A taped ankle seems more protected from sprains because there is a reduction in range of motion (inversion) and above all in tilting angular velocity; this lower speed of inversion allows active stabilizers to react with a more valid response [40].

Ankle disk exercises are valid injury prevention training because they improve muscle reaction against sprains. Exercises on disk cause quick ankle movement and thus train both kinesthesia (sense of movement) and proprioception (sense of position). Due to capsule and ligament lesions, these fine mechanisms may be altered after injury and seem to predispose to new sprains. For this reason, uninjured as well as previously sprained ankles should be properly trained, especially in athletes. Sheth studied the contraction pattern of ankle muscles in 1997 with surface EMG during simulated ankle sprains before and after proprioceptive training in healthy subjects. Eight weeks of exercises on ankle disk (15 min/day) led to selective modulations in the sequence of muscle contraction: before the exercises there was simultaneous activation of anterior and posterior tibialis, peroneus longus, and flexor digitorum longus muscles, but after training there was a delay in activation of inversion muscles, allowing the peroneals to counteract the sprain [55].

Sprained ankles may differ significantly if the injuries are acute or chronic. Eversion strength can range from 88% of the uninjured side 1 week after sprain to 96% after 12 weeks; RPP error is 190% of the contralateral ankle values at 1 week, with decreases of up to 133% after 12 weeks. The peroneal reaction time to sudden inversion does not differ significantly between healthy and injured ankles. Instability (pathological talar tilt and anterior talar translation) seems to have no adverse effect on eversion strength and RPP [34].

Stabilometric assessment performed with a force platform is another way to test the proprioceptive system after an ankle sprain. In 1996, Leanderson performed a prospective study measuring the postural sway in classical ballet dancers to evaluate the influence of ankle injuries on proprioception [37]. In comparison with preinjury examination and also with the contralateral side, postural stability (one-legged stance, sprained side) was worse for several weeks after spraining; stabilometry showed improvement during and after a rehabilitation program composed of early range of motion exercises in the first period and later with muscle strengthening (weight shoe), proprioceptive exercises on a balance board, and water exercises to diminish weight-bearing.

The Shoulder and the Proprioceptive System

The effectiveness of the proprioceptive system is important in the shoulder joint, especially to prevent instability. Vangsness discovered free nerve endings and mechanoreceptors in the glenoid labrum and ligaments (glenohumeral, coracoclavicular, coracoacromial) [60]. The anatomy of the shoulder joint (especially the glenohumeral joint: ball-and-socket with poor osseous conformity) requires undamaged and well-trained active (muscle and proprioceptive system) and passive (glenoid, ligaments, labrum) elements to assure stability.

From a proprioceptive point of view, the shoulder has been studied less than other joints. Jerosch tried to establish normal values testing healthy volunteers with RPP methods in 1996 [31]. The results showed a low variance in proprioceptive skills among the subjects and an influence of visual aids; better results were obtained above shoulder level than below. This can be explained by hypothesizing an increase in mechanoreceptor activity when the inferior glenohumeral ligament is stretched.

Muscle fatigue induced with isokinetic exercise leads to worse results in TTDPM [14]. When evaluating healthy subjects, RPP and TTDPM on patients with post-traumatic anterior instability and in whom Bankart repair has been performed (open or arthroscopic) show results after surgery that do not differ significantly from those of normal shoulders [61]. However, RPP and TTDPM are low-speed tests and very different if comparing sport activities like swimming or throwing.

Unfortunately, a test to evaluate the proprioceptive system in vivo does not exist; moreover, the upper extremity works mostly in the open kinetic chain while many of the exercises to train the shoulder are in the closed kinetic chain. (Usually we performed exercises for neuromuscular coordination and balance with a ball or an unstable board between the hand and the wall or floor; plyometric exercises are also useful).

Muscle strengthening (especially for the rotator cuff) plays an important role in enhancing the concavity-compression mechanism in athletes and to diminish the risk of muscular fatigue (e.g., in the final phase of a sport event) leading to a loss of proprioception and possible joint lesion. Lephart suggests the following training progression [38] to restore proprioception and neuromuscular control:

1. Joint position sense and kinesthesia: glenohumeral repositioning exercises with and without visual aid, proprioceptive neuromuscular exercises with manual resistance
2. Dynamic joint stabilization: axial loading exercises of the glenohumeral joint (closed kinetic chain with a balance board between hand and floor) to stimulate activation of both glenohumeral and scapulothoracic muscles
3. Reactive neuromuscular control: plyometric exercises throwing (against a wall) and catching a ball
4. Functionally specific activities: according to the athlete's sport and role in the team

Following these guidelines, many other exercises can be planned. It is important to allow good patient compliance by prescribing simple exercises that can be performed also at home.

Training and Prevention

Few studies apply the results of basic research on the proprioceptive system (anatomical and histological identification of mechanoreceptors and free nerve endings, quantitative measurement in laboratory test) in the field of prevention of sport injuries.

Ankle sprain is a frequent lesion in soccer players. A Swedish study [59] demonstrated that coordination training may help to prevent functional instability, reducing the frequency of ankle sprains in athletes with previous ankle injury. The training program was composed of exercises on a disk with a spherical undersurface, with one leg straight and the other raised and flexed at the knee while the arms were placed over the chest. The training time was 10 min five times weekly (10 weeks), then 5 min three times weekly; the length of the study was 6 months. Comparing proprioceptive-trained and control groups (both composed of players with previous ankle problems), the difference in reinjury was significantly lower in the trained group (5% vs. 25%, $p < 0.01$)

It is possible to reduce the incidence of ACL lesions in football players by adding proprioceptive exercises to traditional training programs. In a prospective controlled study [13] of 600 soccer players (semiprofessional or amateur teams), we evaluated the possible preventive effect of gradually increased proprioceptive

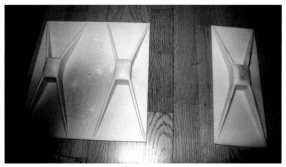

Fig. 4. A simple way to increase the difficulty of proprioceptive exercises by decreasing the stability of the used boards. *Left* bottom view of a board with only one degree of freedom, *right* a smaller, more unstable board

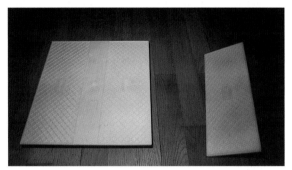

Fig. 5. The same boards described in Fig. 4 seen from above

training (Figs. 4, 5) during three soccer seasons. A control group of 300 players was trained traditionally, without specific balance exercises. The experimental group (300 players) was instructed to train 20 min/day, with five levels of difficulty:

1. Phase 1: balance training without board (single-legged stance on the ground)
2. Phase 2: balance training on a rectangular balance board (each leg alternatively)
3. Phase 3: training on a round board
4. Phase 4: training on a combined round and rectangular board
5. Phase 5: training on a multiplanar board (such as the BAPS biomechanical ankle platform system, CAMP, Jackson, Michigan)

The proprioceptive exercises were performed for 2.5 min four times a day at least three times a week; exercises consisted of anterior and posterior step-ups standing on the board. The subjects were also instructed to follow a neuromuscular facilitation program. During three soccer seasons, ten arthroscopically verified ACL lesions occurred in the proprioception-trained group, while 70 were recorded in the "traditional" group (significant difference, $p < 0.001$). These results show that proprioceptive training should become more important in the training programs of soccer players.

The equipment and sport-specific movements are also important in proprioceptive training: for example, skiers have the ankle fixed by the ski boots, so we must train the knee joint more with them, while for basketball, both knee and ankle proprioception are important due to frequent jumping. The goals of proprioceptive exercises (Fig. 6) are to improve athlete performance, prevent injury and reinjury, and quicken rehabilitation after a lesion.

Unfortunately, there are few studies showing a correlation between proprioceptive training and reduction in sport injuries, while many papers demonstrate improvement only in quantitative laboratory tests (RPP, TTDPM).

Proprioceptive training must be performed throughout the range of joint motion; this is important because the mechanoreceptors seem to be activated selectively at specific angles [35] (Muscle receptors play a primary role in the intermediate range of motion, while joint receptors together with muscle receptors are more important in the extreme ranges of motion). Muscle training focused on building endurance (to delay muscle fatigue and a consequent decline in proprioception) more than on pure strength is important together with proprioceptive programs to prevent sport injuries. When prescribing proprioceptive exercises, we do not forget combined joint lesions (like chondral damage in primary weight-bearing areas or ligament grafts in the healing period) to combine better all the requirements of the rehabilitation program of any patient.

To understand joint biomechanics better, we think that much more effort is necessary to develop tests and perform studies with the single aim of prevention including the influence of the proprioceptive system on sport-specific movements.

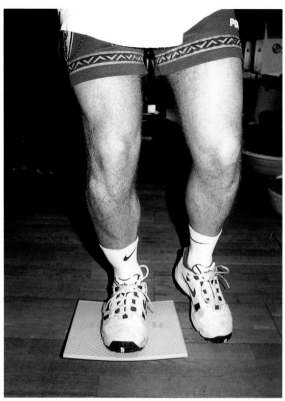

Fig. 6. A simple proprioceptive exercise: one-legged stance on a board with only one degree of freedom

Conclusion

Sport- and role-specific epidemiological studies are necessary to learn the incidence and pathogenesis of lesions and then to develop exercise programs individualized

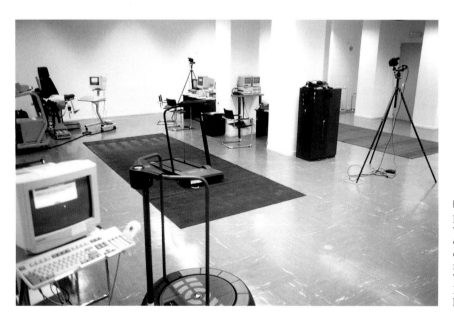

Fig. 7. Evaluations can be properly performed only in well-equipped biomechanical laboratories with a staff experienced in sports traumatology and rehabilitation. The picture shows the "Let People Move" biomechanical laboratory, Perugia, Italy

(according also to anthropometric parameters of athletes). A training program with selective strengthening and proprioceptive and sport- (role-)specific exercises is a valid tool for preventing joint injury and reinjury.

Biomechanical and clinical studies are important to discover correlations between laboratory data and functional results. Quantitative measurement of many parameters such as muscle strength, range of motion, joint stability, motion analysis, gait analysis, reflex muscle contraction latency (on EMG), postural balance (stabilometry with force platform and unstable board), RPP, and TTDPM are fundamental to control functional, neuromuscular, and proprioceptive performance of athletes, allowing rational, individualized, sport-specific training and rehabilitation. These evaluations can be properly performed only in well-equipped biomechanical laboratories with staff experienced in sports traumatology and rehabilitation (Fig. 7).

The RPP and TTDPM are valid systems for measuring proprioception and kinesthesia, but evaluation of the proprioceptive system in its entirety needs the development of better tests to analyze sport activities (high velocity and complexity of movements).

In our opinion, more effort is necessary to let athletes and trainers know that sport-specific proprioceptive exercises have the same importance for improving performance and preventing lesions as warmup, stretching, and strengthening.

References

1. Abbott LC, Saunders JB, Dec M et al (1944) Injuries to the ligament of the knee joint. J Bone Joint Surg 26:503–521
2. Allum JH, Honegger F, Schicks H (1993) Vestibular and proprioceptive modulation of postural synergies in normal subjects. J Vestib Res 3:59–85
3. Allum JH, Honegger F, Acuna H (1995) Differential control of leg and trunk muscle activity by vestibulo-spinal and proprioceptive signals during human balance corrections. Acta Otolaryngol 115:124–129
4. Assimakopoulos AP, Katonis PG, Agapitos MV, Exarchou EI (1992) The innervation of the human meniscus. Clin Orthop 275:232–236
5. Barrack RL, Skinner HB (1990) The sensory function of knee ligaments. In: Daniel D et al (eds) Knee ligaments: Structure, function, injury. Raven Press, pp 95–114
6. Barrack RL, Lund PJ, Munn BG, Wink C, Happel L (1997) Evidence of reinnervation of free patellar tendon autograft used for anterior cruciate ligament reconstruction. Am J Sports Med 25:196–202
7. Beard DJ, Dodd CAF, Trundle HR, Simpson AHRW (1994) Proprioception enhancement for anterior cruciate ligament deficiency. J Bone Joint Surg 76B:654–659
8. Beard DJ, Kyberd PJ, Fergusson CM, Dodd CAF (1993) Proprioception after rupture of the anterior cruciate ligament. J Bone Joint Surg 75B:311–315
9. Beard DJ, Dodd CAF, Simpson AHRW (1996) The effect of reconstruction on proprioception in the anterior cruciate ligament deficient knee. Second World congress on sports trauma. AOSSM, p 749
10. Beynnon BD, Ryder SH, Konradsen L, Johnson RJ, Johnson K, Renstrom P (1999) The effect of anterior cruciate ligament trauma and bracing on knee proprioception. Am J Sports Med 27:150–155
11. Birmingham TB, Kramer JF, Inglis JT, Mooney CA, Murray LJ et al (1998) Effect of a neoprene sleeve on knee joint position sense during sitting OKC and supine CKC tests. Am J Sports Med 26:562–566
12. Borsa PA, Lephart SM, Irrgang JJ, Safran MR, Fu FH (1997) The effects of joint position and direction of joint motion on proprioceptive sensibility in anterior cruciate ligament deficient athletes. Am J Sports Med 25:336–340
13) Caraffa A, Cerulli G, Proietti M, Aisa G, Rizzo A (1996) Prevention of anterior cruciate ligament injuries in soccer. Knee Surg Sports Traum Arthr 4:19–21
14. Carpenter JE, Blasier RB, Pellizzon GG (1998) The effects of muscle fatigue on shoulder joint position sense. Am J Sports Med 26:262–265
15. Cerulli G, Ceccarini A, Alberti PF, Caraffa G (1986) Neuro-morphological studies of the proprioceptivity of the human anterior cruciate ligament. J Sports Traumatol 8:49–52
16. Cerulli G, Caraffa A, Bensi G, Baggiani M, Ragusa F (1997) Studi neurofisiologici sul menisco e ricadute applicative. J Sports Traumatol 19[Suppl]:6–8
17. Conte G, Marcacci M, Spinelli M, Girolami M, Caporali R, Rossi A (1984) Mechanoreceptors in the medial collateral ligament of the human knee. J Sports Traum 6:63–72
18. Corrigan JP, Cashman WF, Brady MP (1992) Proprioception in the cruciate deficient knee. J Bone Joint Surg 74B:247–250
19. Duncan PW, Chandler J, Studenski S, Hughes M, Prescott B (1993) How do physiological components of balance affect mobility in elderly men? Arch Phys Med Rehab 74:1343–1349
20. Ekdahl C, Jarnlo GB, Andersson SI (1989) Standing balance in healthy subjects. Scand J Rehab Med 21:187–195
21. Fitzpatrick R, McCloskey DI (1994) Proprioceptive, visual and vestibular thresolds for the perception of sway during standing in humans. J Physiol 478:173–186
22. Freeman MAR, Wyke B (1964) The innervation of the knee joint. An anatomical and histological study in the cat. J Anat 101:505–532
23. Freeman MAR, Wyke B (1967) The innervation of the ankle joint. An anatomical and histological study in the cat. Acta Anat 68:321–333
24. Friden T, Zatterstrom R, Lindstrand A, Moritz U (1989) A stabilometric technique for evaluation of lower limb instabilities. Am J Sports Med 17:118–122
25. Gillquist J (1996) Knee ligaments and proprioception. Acta Orthop Scand 67:533–545
26. Good L, Roos H, Gottlieb DJ, Renstrom PA, Beynnon BD (1999) Joint position sense is not changed after acute disruption of the anterior cruciate ligament. Acta Orthop Scand 70:194–198
27. Grob KR, Kuster MS, Higgins S, Lloyd D (1998) Comparison of different measurements of proprioception. Eighth ESSKA congress, Nice, p 13
28. Hay L, Bard C, Fleury M, Teasdale N (1996) Availability of visual and proprioceptive afferent messages and postural control in elderly adults. Exp Brain Res 108:129–139
29. Hogervorst T, Brand RA (1998) Mechanoreceptors in joint function. J Bone Joint Surg 80A:1365–1378
30. Jerosch J; Prymka M, Castro WHM (1996) Proprioception of knee joints with a lesion of the medial meniscus. Acta Orthop Belg 62:41–45
31. Jerosch J, Thorvesten L, Steinbeck J, Reer R (1996) Proprioceptive function of the shoulder girdle in healthy volunteers. Knee Surg Sports Traumatol Arthrosc 3:219–225
32. Johansson H, Sjolander P, Sojka P (1991) A sensory role for the cruciate ligaments. Clin Orthop 268:161–175

33. Kennedy JC, Alexander IJ, Hayes KC (1982) Nerve supply of the human knee and its functional importance. Am J Sports Med 10:329–335

34. Konradsen L, Olesen S, Hansen HM (1998) Ankle sensorimotor control and eversion strength after acute ankle inversion injuries. Am J Sports Med 26:72–77

35. Lattanzio PJ, Petrella RJ (1998) Knee proprioception: A review of mechanisms, measurements, and implications of muscular fatigue. Orthop 21:463–471

36. Lavender A, Laurence AS, Bangash IH, Smith RB (1999) Cortical evoked potentials in the ruptured anterior cruciate ligament. Knee Surg Sports Traumatol Arthrosc 7:98–101

37. Leanderson J, Eriksson E, Nilsson C, Wykman A (1996) Proprioception in classical ballet dancers. Am J Sports Med 24:370–374

38. Lephart SM, Pincivero DM, Giraldo JL, Fu FH (1997) The role of proprioception in the management and rehabilitation of athletic injuries. Am J Sports Med 25:130–137

39. Lobenhoffer P, Biedert R, Stauffer E, Lattermann C, Gerich TG, Muller W(1996) Occurrence and distribution of free nerve endings in the distal iliotibial tract system of the knee. Knee Surg Sports Traumatol Arthrosc 4:111–115

40. Lohrer H, Alt W, Gollhofer A (1999) Neuromuscular properties and functional aspects of taped ankles. Am J Sports Med 27:69–75

41. Lynch SA, Eklund U, Gottlieb D, Renstrom PA, Beynnon B (1996) Electromyographic latency changes in the ankle musculature during inversion moments. Am J Sports Med 24:362–369

42. Miyatsu M, Atsuta Y, Watakabe M (1993) The physiology of mechanoreceptors in the anterior cruciate ligament. J Bone Joint Surg 75B:653–657

43. Norrè ME (1993) Sensory interaction testing in platform posturography. J Laryngol Otol 107:496–501

44. Nyland J, Caborn DNM, Johnson DL, Shapiro R (1998) Knee control deficits when crossover cutting during eccentric work induced hamstring fatigue. Eighth ESSKA congress, Nice, p393

45. O'Connor BL (1984) The mechanoreceptors innervation of the posterior attachments of the lateral meniscus of the dog knee joint. J Anat 138:15–26

46. O'Connor BL, McConnaughey JS (1978) The structure and innervation of cat knee menisci and their relation to a "sensory hypothesis" of meniscal function. J Anat 153:431–442

47. Perlau R, Frank C, Fick G (1995) The effect of elastic bandages on human knee proprioception in the uninjured population. Am J Sports Med 23:251–255

48. Petrella RJ, Lattanzio PJ, Nelson MG (1997) Effect of age and activity on knee joint proprioception. Am J Phys Med Rehab 76:235–241

49. Pitman MI, Nainzadeh N, Menche D, Gasalberti R, Song EK (1992) The intraoperative evaluation of the neurosensory function of the anterior cruciate ligament in humans using somatosensory evoked potentials. Arthroscopy 8:442–447

50. Risberg MA, Beynnon BD, Peura GD, Uh BS (1999) Proprioception after anterior cruciate ligament reconstruction with and without bracing. Knee Surg Sports Traumatol Arthrosc 7:303–309

51. Ruffoli R,Augusti A, Giannotti S, Laddaga C, Luppichini N et al (1996) Mechanoreceptors in the posterior cruciate and lateral collateral ligaments of the human knee, and the lateral collateral ligament of the canine knee. J Sports Traum 18:113–122

52. Schultz AR, Miller CD, Kerr CS, Micheli L (1984) Mechanoreceptors in human cruciate ligaments. J Bone Joint Surg 66A:1072–1076

53. Schutte MJ, Dabezies EJ, Zimny ML, Happel LT (1987) Neural anatomy of the human anterior cruciate ligament. J Bone Joint Surg 69A:243–247

54. Shelbourne KD, Davis JT (1999) Evaluation of knee stability before and after participation in a functional sports agility program during rehabilitation after anterior cruciate ligament reconstruction. Am J Sports Med 27:156–161

55. Sheth P, Yu B, Laskowski ER, An K (1997) Ankle disk training influences reaction times of selected muscles in a simulated ankle sprain. Am J Sports Med 25:538–543

56. Skinner HB, Barrack RL, Cook SD (1984) Age related decline in proprioception. Clin Orthop 184:208–211

57. Spinelli M, Laddaga C, Bernicchi G, Candela M, Michelotti M, Giannotti S, Ruffoli R, Conte G, Marchetti N (1998) La neuroligamentizzazione del LCA dopo ricostruzione con PTB. Giorn It Ortop Traumatol 24[Suppl]:361–365

58. Taylor RA, Marshall PH, Dunlap RD, Gable CD, Sizer PS (1998) Knee position error detection in closed and OKC tasks during concurrent cognitive distraction. J Orthop Sports Phys Ther 28:81–87

59. Tropp H, Askling C, Gillquist J (1985) Prevention of ankle sprains. Am J Sports Med 13:259–262

60. Vangsness CT Jr, Ennis M, Taylor JG, Atkinson R (1995) Neural anatomy of the glenohumeral ligaments, labrum and subacromial borsa. Arthroscopy 11:180–184

61. Warner JJP, Lephart S, Fu FH (1996) Role of proprioception in pathoetiology of shoulder instability. Clin Orthop 330:35–39

62. Wojtys EM, Wylie BB, Huston LJ (1996) The effects of muscle fatigue on neuromuscular function and anterior tibial translation in healthy knees. Am J Sports Med 24:615–621

63. Zatterstrom R, Friden T, Linstrand A, Moritz U (1994) The effect of physiotherapy on standing balance in chronic anterior cruciate ligament insufficiency. Am J Sports Med 22:531–536

Chapter 4

Application of Electromyography in Sport Medicine

Mario Lamontagne

The aim of this paper is to provide sound principles of electromyography (EMG) signal acquisition and processing in order to optimize signal quality and therefore lead to better interpretation of mechanical muscle output during sport medicine applications and rehabilitation. Some background information is provided on the source of the EMG signal, factors affecting its quality, recording techniques, signal processing, fidelity and reproducibility of the signal, and some applications in sport medicine and rehabilitation. The descriptions of EMG research applications in rehabilitation are not an exhaustive review of all major areas but only a few examples in the areas of signal reliability, muscle activation and timing, and muscle fatigue.

Introduction

The complexity of the biological system often introduces difficulties into measurement and processing procedures. Unlike physical systems, the biological system cannot be handled in such a way that subsystems can be individually monitored and investigated. The signals produced by the system are thus influenced directly by activity of the surrounding systems. The source of biological signals is the neural or muscular cells. These, however, do not function alone but in large groups. The accumulated effects of all active cells in the vicinity produce an electrical field which propagates in the volume conductor consisting of the various body tissues. Muscle activity can thus be indirectly measured by means of electrodes placed on the skin, conveniently obtained by surface electrodes. This information, however, is more difficult to analyze and results from all neural or muscular activity in unknown locations transmitted through a nonhomogeneous medium.

In spite of these difficulties, electrical signals monitored on the skin surface are of enormous clinical, physiological, and kinesiological importance [6]. The electrical signal associated with muscle contraction is called an electromyogram and the study of electromyograms is called electromyography (EMG) [46].

Electromyography can be a very valuable tool in measuring skeletal muscle electrical output during physical activities. It is important that the EMG is detected correctly and interpreted in light of basic biomedical signal processing, physiological, and biomechanical principles [41]. The usefulness of the EMG signal is greatly dependent on the ability to extract the information contained in it. Electromyography is attractive because it gives easy access to the physiological processes that cause the muscle to generate force and produce movement [10]. Since EMG is easy to use, it might be easily misused to interpret outcomes wrongly. Therefore, it is important to understand the principles of EMG signal detecting and processing to optimize the quality of signal information.

The aim of this chapter is to provide sound principles of EMG signal acquisition and processing to optimize signal quality and lead to better interpretation of mechanical muscle output during movement studies. To achieve this, some background information will be provided on the technical nature of EMG signals and a few applications from sport medicine and rehabilitation presented.

Source of the EMG Signal

Muscle tissue conducts electrical potentials similarly to the way axons transmit action potentials. Muscle unit action potential can be detected by electrodes in the muscle tissue or on the surface of the skin. Several events must occur before a contraction of muscle fibers. Central nervous system activity initiates a depolarization in the motoneuron. This depolarization is conducted along the motoneuron to the muscle fiber's motor end plate. At the end plate, a chemical substance is released that diffuses across the synaptic gap and causes a depolarization of the synaptic membrane (Fig. 1). This phenomenon is called muscle action potential. The depolarization of the membrane transcends along the muscle fibers, producing a depolarization wave that can be detected by recording electrodes. In two-electrode systems over the muscle site, the motor unit action potential (MUAP) waveform is

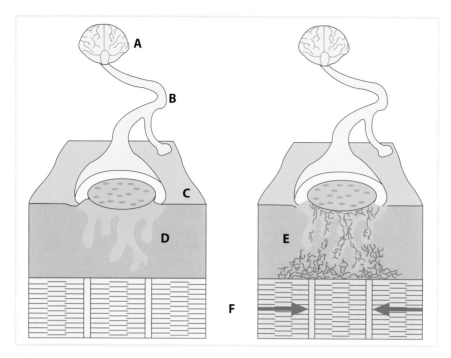

Fig. 1. Schematic diagram of a motor unit illustrating the neuromuscular junction. *A*, brain; *B*, axon, *C*, motor end plate; *D*, synaptic vesicle; *E*, neurotransmitter; *F* muscle fibers

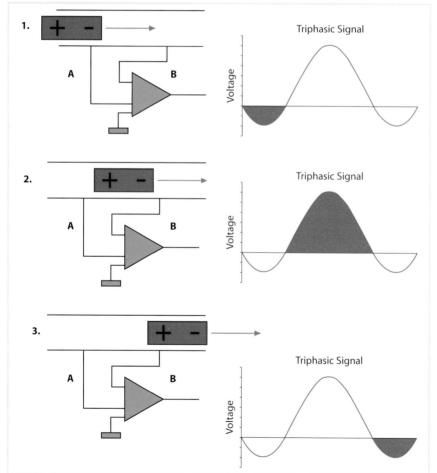

Fig. 2. Schematic diagram of membrane depolarization along the muscle fibers producing a depolarization wave detected by recording electrodes

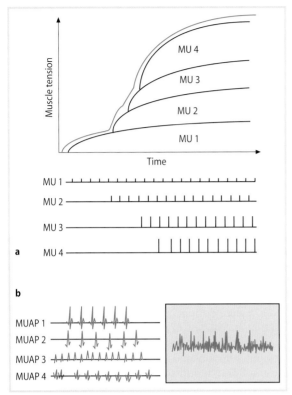

a

b

Fig. 3. Representation of the order of MU recruitment by size (**a**) and algebraic summation of many repetitive sequences of MUAPs for all active motor units in the vicinity of the recording electrodes (**b**)

represented by a triphasic potential, which is the difference in potential between poles A and B (Fig. 2). Once an action potential reaches a muscle fiber, it propagates proximally and distally. A MUAP is the spatiotemporal summation of MUAPs for an entire motor unit (MU). An EMG signal is the algebraic summation of many repetitive sequences of MUAPs for all active motor units in the vicinity of the recording electrodes. The order of MU recruitment is according to their sizes. The smaller ones are active first and the bigger ones are active last [46] (Fig. 3).

Factors Affecting Signal Quality

Many factors may affect the quality of EMG signals. They can be divided into physiological, physical, and electrical types. Some factors can be controlled by the investigator.

The factors over which the investigator has no control contribute to the random component (noise) of the signal, such as the nonhomogeneous medium between the muscle fibers [9] and the electrodes, the nonparallel geometry and nonuniform conduction velocity of the fibers, and the physical and physiological conditions of the muscle. While it is not possible to remove this random component completely from the measurement, the user must be aware of its presence and how to reduce its effects [18]. Other physiological factors not under the control of the investigator that contribute to the signal are the number of active MUs, the MU firing motor, and fiber type and diameter.

The physical factors are those associated with electrode structure and its location on the surface of the skin over the muscle, such as distance between the electrodes, electrode area and shape, location in relation to motor points in the muscle, orientation with respect to muscle fibers, and electrode type (active, surface, or indwelling). The investigator manipulates these factors to improve signal quality.

Electrical factors are related to the recording system used to collect the signal. The fidelity and signal:noise ratio of the signal is based on the quality of the recording unit. The following factors are important for obtaining reliable signals with the highest signal:noise ratio. The differential amplification with a common mode rejection ratio (CMRR) greater than 80 [46] or 120 [10] is used to eliminate noise from power line sources. The CMRR represents the quality of the differential amplifier. An input impedance in the order of $10^9 \Omega$ [42] or $10^{12} \Omega$ [10] is recommended to prevent attenuation and distortion of the signal. According to Perreault, Hunter, and Kearney [37], skin preparation plays an important role in reducing impedance input and therefore signal distortion as well.

The active electrode consists of placing the differential amplifier as close as possible to the recording electrodes and reduces the noise from cable motion [17]. Although, as reported by Nishimura, Tomita, and Horiuchi [34], an active electrode was compared with a conventional one and they ascertained that it could be replaced with a conventional one and was preferable because it required less preparation time and was less affected by environmental noise.

Finally, frequency response of the differential amplifier is an important factor which ensures that the signal is linearly amplified throughout its spectrum. The frequency response of the EMG signal is best between 10 Hz and 1000 Hz, as proposed by Winter [46]. Some experimental data showed that the power frequency spectra were not affected for sampling frequencies as low as 500 Hz [24]. Recommended minimum specifications for surface amplifiers are presented in Table 1. The frequency spectrum can be narrower, which will be shown later in this paper.

Table 1. Minimum requirements for surface EMG amplifier

Variables	Minimum requirements
Input impedance	$>10^{10}$ at DC[a,b]
	$>10^{8}$ at 100 Hz
	$>10^{6}$ [c]
	$>10^{12}$ [d]
CMMRR	>80 dB[a,b]
	>90 dB[c]
Amplifier gain	$200-10,000$[a,b,c]
Frequency response	$1-3000$ Hz[a]
	$1-1000$ Hz[b]
	$1-500$ Hz[d]
Input bias current	<50 mA[a]
Noise	<5 µV RMS with 100 KΩ resistance[a]

[a] Recommended by ISEK.
[b] recommended by Winter (1990).
[c] recommended by De Luca (1993).
[d] recommended by Lamontagne (1992).

Recording Techniques

A wide variety of electrodes are available to measure electrical muscle output. Although micro- and needle electrodes are available, they are not practical for movement studies [41]. Surface electrodes (SE) [11, 14, 22, 28, 29, 32, 37a] and intramuscular wire electrodes (IWE) [1, 2, 8, 15, 16, 19, 30, 31, 36, 38, 44] are commonly used in movement studies (Fig. 4). The former are used mainly in bipolar configuration with differential pre-amplifiers to increase the amplitude of the signals between each detecting electrode and the common ground. The advantage of differential preamplifiers is that they improve signal:noise ratios. Surface electrodes are quick, relatively easy to use, and have fairly good reproducibility [4, 12, 13, 15, 27, 40]. They do detect the average activity of superficial muscles; however, they do not selectively record single MUs [3]. Those lying superficially in a muscle contribute more to the signal than do deeper MUs.

In surface EMG, electrode size and interelectrode distance should be proportional to muscle size. Intramuscular wire electrodes are known to be more selective in detecting MUs than SE. This type of electrode has small leadoff areas between 25 µm and 100 µm and therefore detects fewer MUs. The advantages offered by intramuscular electrodes are: they are much less painful than needle electrodes, rarely interfere with movement, have a low sensitivity to movement artefacts [35], and can be easily implanted and withdrawn [3].

Of course an important question comes to mind: What should we use for sport medicine studies or rehabilitation? The answer depends on specificity needs, reliability, reproducibility, and interpretation of the muscle signal in MU recording.

Signal Processing Techniques

As well explained by Soderberg [41], an analogy can be made between radio or television signals, which are modulated, broadcasted, and demodulated at the destination site, and EMG signals, which undergo similar processes. The detected EMG signal represents a modulation of the alpha motoneuron pool command. The rate of MU firings is frequency modulated by the neural command. The summation of the frequency-modulated MU action potentials produces an amplitude-modulated envelope representative of the recruitment and firing rates of the original neural command. Demodulation refers to processing techniques that extract information related to the neural command.

The demodulation techniques commonly used in the time domain are: full-wave rectification, linear envelope [5, 21, 39, 45], integration of full-wave rectification [46], and root-mean-square processing [7]. Power spectral density (PSD) [22] is the function commonly used for frequency domain analysis of EMG signals (Fig. 5). The parameters used from PSD are median [42] and mean frequency [8, 12, 22] of the EMG signal. The EMG signal processing will provide information on muscle activation timing, estimation of the force produced by the muscle, or to determining an index of the rate at which a muscle fatigues, obtained from the power spectral density.

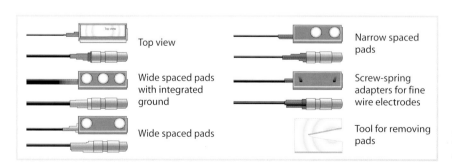

Top view

Wide spaced pads with integrated ground

Wide spaced pads

Narrow spaced pads

Screw-spring adapters for fine wire electrodes

Tool for removing pads

Fig. 4. Illustration of various types of electrodes for recording electromyography

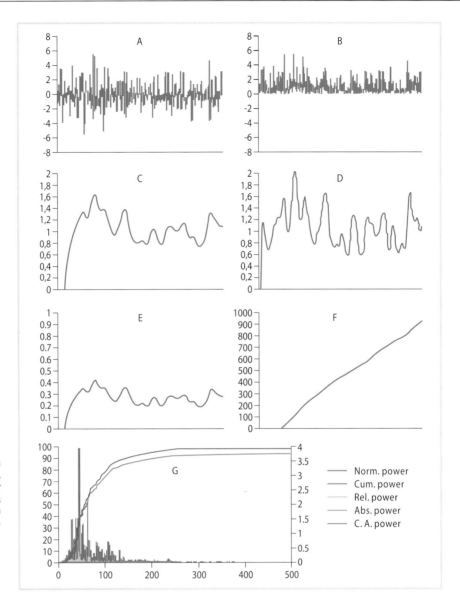

Fig. 5. Example of EMG signal processing as reported in the literature. Raw EMG (*A*), full wave-rectified (*B*), linear envelope EMG filtered with a low-pass filter (Butterworth) at 5 Hz (*C*) and 10 Hz (*D*), linear envelope EMG and peak normalized (0–1) (*E*), integral of the linear envelope EMG (*F*), power spectral density curves (*G*)

Fidelity and Reproducibility of the Signal

The usefulness of the EMG signal is greatly dependent on the ability to extract the information contained in it. Moritani et al. [30] studied different electromechanical changes in the gastrocnemius and soleus muscles with simultaneous recordings using SE and IWE. Bipolar IWEs were inserted in each muscle and SEs were placed over the muscular group. The results demonstrated that, with either a reduced or no EMG signal from the gastrocnemius or soleus, there was still surface EMG activation. This result is acceptable, since the surface EMG is representative of the EMG activity of the whole muscular group. Then, when the EMG signal is very low or when the EMG signal of one muscle is evident and the EMG on another muscle of the group is not,

IWE is preferable over SE. Kadefors and Herberts [20] suggested that surface electrodes be avoided because of the movement between muscle tissue and surface of the skin and the risk of crosstalk from muscles around or near the investigated area. Similar findings have been reported by Giroux and Lamontagne [15] for the use of SE and IWE. More details are provided in the next section of this chapter.

Applications in Sport Medicine and Rehabilitation

Electromyography has been a subject of laboratory research for decades. Only with recent technological developments in electronics and computers has surface

EMG emerged from the laboratory as a subject of intense research, particularly in kinesiology, rehabilitation, and occupational and sports medicine. Most of the applications of surface and intramuscular EMG are based on its use as a measure of signal reliability and muscle activation, timing, contraction profile, strength of contraction (physical load or psychological stress), and fatigue. Again, this paper does not include an exhaustive review of all the various types of EMG applications but only of some applications in sports, rehabilitation, and sport medicine.

Signal Processing and Reliability

One of the important questions in surface EMG consists of finding the optimal sampling rate for dynamic contractions. If you must collect surface EMG for long periods of time or transmit the surface EMG signal by telemetry, the optimal sampling rate becomes an important issue. Lamontagne [25] investigated the effects of different sampling rates on the power surface EMG of the vastus lateralis during concentric and eccentric contractions at constant angular velocities of 30°/s, 60°/s, and 90°/s. Vastus lateralis muscle activity was recorded with surface electrodes connected to a high input impedance differential bioamplifier (Mega Electronics, Kuopio, Finland) with a frequency band width of 3.2 Hz to 32 kHz. The EMG signal and isokinetic device output (torque, angular displacement, and velocity) were synchronously sampled at 4000 Hz and 100 Hz respectively for 4 s. A 1-s window of the EMG signal was selected for processing. This window was digitally filtered with a high-pass filter (according to Butterworth) at 10 Hz and the bias was removed. The PSD was calculated at 500, 300, 250, 225, 200, and 150 harmonics using the fast Fourier transformation. From the PSD processing, median power frequency (MPF) of each trial was recorded and stored for later statistical analysis. The results revealed that the type or velocity of muscle contraction did not significantly affect MPF. The MPF from the PSD calculated with 150 harmonics was significantly different from those calculated at 225, 250, 300, and 500 harmonics. It can be concluded that the raw EMG can be sampled at less than 500 Hz without significantly affecting PSD and ILE EMG (Fig. 6).

Another important question is the level of reliability of EMG signals collected with surface and intramuscular wire electrodes in isometric and dynamic conditions [15]. This study consisted of comparing SE and IWE for isometric and dynamic contractions during an occupational cervicobrachial working task. Six normal adult male subjects were tested on 2 days (two conditions with three trials each). Raw EMG signals from middle deltoid, anterior deltoid, and trapezius muscles were recorded by both IWE and SE for two conditions

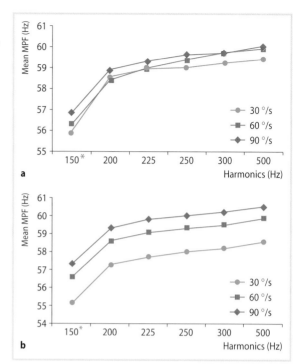

Fig. 6. Median frequency of the power spectrum density calculated with 150, 225, 250, 300, and 500 harmonics at three velocities for concentric (**a**) and eccentric (**b**) contractions

(isometric and dynamic contractions). Full-wave rectified, low-pass filtered, and integrated EMG were processed from raw EMG signals. The statistical analysis performed on the integrated EMG was a factorial analysis model with repeated measurements. The statistical results confirmed that EMG signals from both SE and IWE are reliable between trials on the same day. These statistical results also confirmed that SE is more reliable than IWE in day-to-day investigations. Both electrodes recorded statistically similar signals, although the coefficient of variability between them was very high (STDE 48% and 84% for isometric and dynamic conditions, respectively) (Tables 2, 3).

A major point of interest is the measurement of muscle fatigue using EMG. The change in median frequency of power spectrum density is one of the factors that can be used as an indicator of muscle fatigue [11, 43, 45]. Elfving et al. [13] investigated the reliability of

Table 2. Probability levels for test-retest and day-to-day reliability and electrode comparison (surface vs. intramuscular) in isometric and dynamic contractions

Comparison	Isometric	Dynamic
Test-retest	0.669	0.336
Day-to-day	0.414	0.502
Electrodes (S vs. I)	0.309	0.201

$p < 0.05$.

Table 3. Day-to-day reliability by type of electrode and contraction

Contractions	Isometric		Dynamic	
Electrodes	Surface	Intramuscular	Surface	Intramuscular
P	0.430	0.369	0.806	0.018*
R	0.75	0.79	0.92	0.31
SD (%)	48	30	84	33

P, Probability level; *R*, Pearson correlation; *SD*, standard deviation.
* Significant difference for day-to-day tests.

the median frequency parameters for EMG recording sites at L1 and L5 right and left on the erector spinae. The subjective fatigue ratings of the back muscles (Borg CR-10 scale) and of maximal trunk extension torque (MVC) were also measured as control factors. Eleven subjects with healthy backs performed a 45-s isometric trunk extension at 80% of MVC twice a day on 3 different days. Two-factor analysis of variance was made to obtain the different variances from which the SE and the intraclass correlation coefficient (ICC) were calculated. The SE within a day was somewhat lower than that between days. Both were about the same at all four electrode sites. The 95% confidence interval for the studied variables was: for initial median frequency ±10 Hz, the slope ±0.4%/s – 0.5%/s, for MVC ±36 Nm,

Table 4. Mean values, standard error, and coefficient of variation (in parentheses) for within-subject variation for all six tests (SE_{tot}), between days (SE_{bd}), and within days (SE_{wd}) (Modified from [13])

Variables	Mean values	SE_{tot}^1 (CV)^4	SE_{bd}^2	SE_{wd}^3
Initial MF (Hz)				
L1 right ($n=8$)	53.6	5.5 (10.2)^4	5.5 (10.3)	4.2 (7.9)
L1 left ($n=7$)	54.4	5.3 (9.8)	5.9 (10.8)	2.7 (5.0)
L5 right ($n=8$)	53.3	4.4 (8.2)	4.7 (8.9)	2.6 (5.0)
L5 left ($n=9$)	53.2	4.8 (9.1)	4.8 (9.1)	4.2 (8.0)
Slope of MF (%/s)				
L1 right ($n=8$)	−0.36	0.27 (75)	0.28 (78)	0.24 (67)*
L1 left ($n=7$)	−0.46	0.20 (43)	0.20 (40)	0.17 (37)
L5 right ($n=8$)	−0.58	0.20 (35)	0.22 (38)	0.17 (29)
L5 left ($n=9$)	−0.58	0.27 (46)*	0.30 (52)	0.20 (35)
MVC (Nm)				
Torque ($n=11$)	174	18.6 (10.7)	20.0 (11.5)	17.2 (9.9)
Borg rating (scale of 0–10) (n=8)	5.1	0.8 (16.5)	0.9 (17.3)	0.7 (14.3)

MS_{ws} (mean square within subject), SS_{ws}/df_{ws};
$MS_{ws, wb}$ (mean square between days), $SS_{ws, wb}/df_{ws, wb}$;
$MS_{ws, wa}$ (mean square within days), $SS_{ws, wa}/df_{ws, wa}$.
CV, coefficient of variation.
* Within subject, between conditions $0.01 < p < 0.05$.
^{1} SE_{tot}, $\sqrt{MS_{ws}}$; ^{2} $SE_{bd} = \sqrt{MS_{ws, wb}}$; ^{3} $SE_{wd} = \sqrt{MS_{ws, wa}}$; ^{4} Coefficient of variance = SEM/mean value · 100.

and for the Borg ratings ±1.6. Similar findings by Lamontagne and Sabagh-Yazdi [25] showed that the difference in median frequency of the EMG power spectrum must be large enough to be able to differentiate the state of two conditions. It can be concluded that, with the method presently used, changes or differences within these limits should be regarded as normal variability. The slope may be of limited value because of its large variability. Whether the low intraclass correlation coefficient for the EMG parameters in the test group presently studied implies a low potential in discriminating subjects with back pain cannot be decisively concluded (Table 4).

Muscle Activation and Timing

The following application illustrates the use of surface EMG for measuring muscle activation timing. Mâsse [26] investigated the pattern of propulsion for five male paraplegics in six seated positions. The positions consisted of a combination of three horizontal rear-wheel positions at two seating heights on a single-purpose racing wheelchair. At each trial, the propulsion technique of the subject was filmed at 50 Hz with a high-speed camera for one cycle and the raw EMG signals of the biceps brachii, triceps brachii, pectoralis major, deltoid anterior, and deltoid posterior muscles were simultaneously recorded for three consecutive cycles. The EMG signals were processed to yield the linear envelope (LE) EMG and the integrated EMG (IEMG) of each muscle. Kinematic analysis revealed that the joint motions of the upper limbs were smoother for the low positions than for the high positions, since they reached extension in a sequence (wrist, shoulder, and elbow). Also, elbow angular velocity slopes were found to be less abrupt for the backward-low positions. It was observed that in lowering the seat position, less IEMG was recorded and the degrees of contact were lengthened. Among the seat positions evaluated, the backward-low position had the lowest overall ILE EMG (Fig. 7) and the middle-low position had the lowest pushing frequency. It was found that a change in seat position caused more variation in the IEMG for the triceps brachii, pectoralis major, and the deltoid posterior.

This next application is another good example of surface EMG as a measure of muscle contraction profile. Németh et al. [33] studied six expert downhill skiers with ACL injuries and different degrees of knee instability. The EMG activity was recorded from lower extremity muscles during downhill skiing in a slalom course with and without a custom-made brace applied to the injured knee. Surface electrodes were used with an eight-channel telemetric EMG system to collect recordings from the vastus medialis, biceps femoris, se-

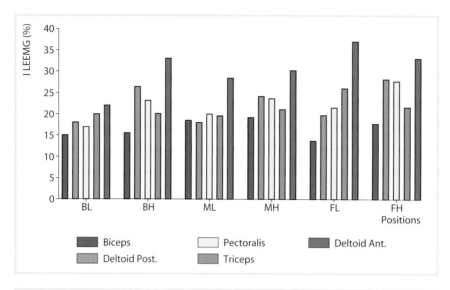

Fig. 7. Mean integrated linear envelope EMG of each muscle for each seating position: backward low (*BL*), backward high (*BH*), middle low (*ML*), middle high (*MH*), forward low (*FL*), and forward high (*FH*)

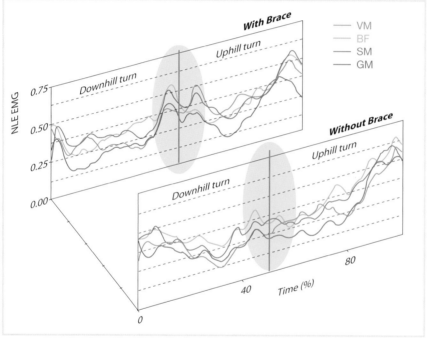

Fig. 8. Normalized linear envelope EMG from the ACL-deficient knee joint with and without brace during slalom race (*n* = 6)

mimembranosus, semitendinosus, and gastrocnemius medialis muscles from both legs. Without the brace, the EMG activity levels of all muscles increased during knee flexion. The biceps femoris was the most activated and reached 50% to 75% of maximal peak amplitude. With the brace, the EMG activity increased in midphase during the upward push for weight transfer and the peak activity occurred closer to knee flexion in midphase. Also, the uninjured knee was influenced by the brace on the injured leg and a decrease in EMG activity was seen during midphase (Fig. 8). Spearman's rank correlation coefficient revealed a significant correlation between an increase in biceps femoris activity

of the injured leg and decreased knee stability. We suggest that the brace caused an increased afferent input from the proprioceptors, resulting in an adaptation of motor control patterns secondarily modifying EMG activity and timing.

Intramuscular and surface EMG can be used to measure activation timing and muscle contraction profile. Lafrenière et al. [23] studied intramuscular EMG of the lateral pterygoid muscles (LPM), surface EMG of the temporalis and masseter muscles, and force measurements of the temporomandibular joint (TMJ) for subjects with internal derangement (ID) of the TMJ (Fig. 9). The analysis of variance results of the ILE EMG

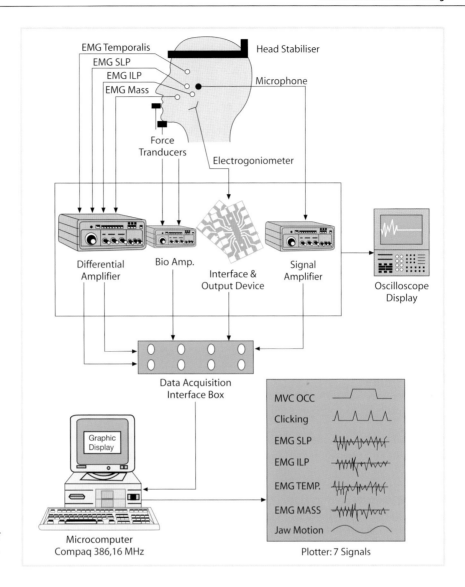

Fig. 9. Schematic diagram of the experimental setup and data acquisition

showed significant differences between the two groups for ILP at rest, resisted protraction, and incisor clench, whereas no significant difference for the masseter and temporalis muscles between both groups (Table 5).

Table 5. Statistical results of ILE EMG for all muscles in each of the five static tasks

TMJ ID vs. controls	Rest	MVC opening	Resisted protrac-tion	MVC molar clench	MVC incisor clench
Masseter	–	–	–	–	–
Temporalis	–	–	–	–	–
ILP	→→	↗	→→	↗	→→
SLP	–	–	–	↗↗	↗

ILP, inferior lateral pterygoid muscle; *SLP*, superior lateral pterygoid muscle.
–, No significant difference ($\alpha \leq 0.05$); → or ↗, tendency; →→ or ↗↗, significant difference ($\alpha \leq 0.05$).

Therefore, there is no apparent reason to believe that the masseter and temporalis are hyperactive in TMJ ID. The ILE EMG of the SLP was significantly lower in the TMJ group during molar clenching. The superior head of the lateral pterygoid muscle (SLP) seemed to have lost its disk-stabilizing function. The ILE EMG signals of the ILP were significantly higher in the TMJ ID group during rest, resisted protraction, and incisor clench (Fig. 10). The ILP muscle probably adapted to control inner joint instability while continuing its own actions, and it seemed to have lost its functional specificity. The results of the isometric force measurements showed that TMJ ID subjects exhibited significantly lower molar bite forces (297.1 N vs. 419 N, $p = 0.042$), confirming that they have less muscle strength and tissue tolerance than subjects with healthy masticator muscle systems. A neuromuscular adaptation could be occurring in the TMJ ID masticator system affecting muscular actions and forces.

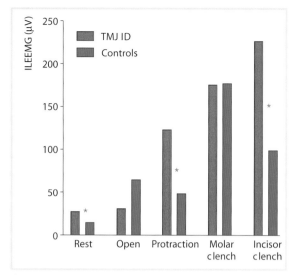

Fig. 10. Integrated linear envelope EMG of the ILP muscle for five static tasks: resting, MVC in opening and resisted protraction, and MVC in molar and incisor clench of TMJ ID and control groups. (*Significant difference $p < 0.05$)

Muscle Fatigue

The surface EMG can also be used as measure of muscle fatigue and recovery. Tho et al. [43] investigated possible differences in muscle fatigue and recovery of knee flexor and extensor muscles in patients with deficient ACL compared with normal patients. Surface EMG of 15 patients with ACL deficiency was performed while the muscles were under 80% of maximum isometric contraction and after 1, 2, 3, and 5 min of rest. During the first 60 s of contraction, all muscles recorded significantly decreased mean power frequency and increased amplitude. The rate of decrease of mean

power frequency was significantly greater in the injured quadriceps and normal hamstrings. All muscles except two recovered to the initial mean power frequency level after 1 min of rest. All but two muscles in the injured and normal limbs recorded an overshoot of mean power frequency during the recovery phase. This overshoot phenomenon was also seen for some muscles in amplitude analysis. The findings confirm the fatigue state in all the muscles, suggest recruitment of more type II fibers as the muscles fatigues, and show the physiological adaptation of the quadriceps and hamstrings to ACL insufficiency (Table 6). The current study indirectly shows dissociation between low intramuscular pH and mean power frequency during the recovery phase. It also indirectly suggests that atrophied thigh muscles have fiber-type composition similar to that of the normal side.

Lamontagne and Sabagh-Yazdi [25] investigated the possible influence of functional knee braces on various factors of muscle fatigue. They measured isometric, isokinetic, and muscle fatigue parameters such as MVC, peak velocity (PK), power, and number of repetitions to muscle fatigue during isokinetic exercise and muscle fatigue during 50-s isometric contraction. For 50-s isometric exercise at 80% MVC, muscle fatigue was measured by the decrease in median frequency (MF) of EMG signals.

Two groups of healthy and ACL-deficient knee joint subjects with an average age of 28.8 years and 26.6 years, respectively, volunteered for this study. Each group was composed of six males and two females. Two separate sessions were necessary to measure isometric, isokinetic, and muscle fatigue parameters for braced and unbraced conditions. For the brace condition, the subjects wore a functional knee brace. All tests were performed on an isokinetic device (Kin-Com 500H,

Muscle	Injured Knee Coefficient of MF (SD)	Amplitude (SD)	Change (%)	Normal Knee Coefficient of MF (SD)	Amplitude (SD)	Change (%)
Vastus medialis	−0.096 (0.073)	125 (172)	42	−0.069 (0.064)	132 (95)	76
Rectus femoris	−0.136 (0.086)	64 (119)	20	−0.100* (0.046)	60 (112)	23
Vastus lateralis	−0.105 (0.087)	89 (141)	29	−0.054* (0.073)	165 (184)	67
Medial hamstrings	−0.207 (0.124)	125 (132)	58	−0.266* (0.112)	119 (149)	49
Lateral hamstrings	−0.159 (0.155)	204 (178)	80	−0.222 (0.152)	228 (269)	71
Medial gastrocnemius	−0.105 (0.132)	62 (63)	40	−0.208** (0.146)	52 (53)	33
Lateral gastrocnemius	−0.151 (0.118)	88 (72)	63	−0.187 (0.139)	54 (61)	28

Table 6. Coefficient of MF change and amplitude increase during 80% MVC for 60 s (Modified from [43])

* $p < 0.05$ (paired t-test); ** $p < 0.01$ (paired t-test).

Table 7. Average percentage of decline of the median frequency

Muscles	ACL-deficient						Healthy					
	VL	RF	VM	G°	MH	LH	VL	RF	VM	G°	MH	LM
Braced	9.1	27.6	14.8	1.8	35.0	27.3	18.4	24.9	12.3	1.7	39.3	34.5
Unbraced	12.0	22.4	9.0*	10.6*	43.4	24.0	8.9*	21.2	16.4	9.5*	48.0	28.5

* Significant difference between conditions ($p < 0.05$); ° significant difference between groups ($p < 0.05$).

Chattanooga, USA) while the EMG signal was collected at 1000 Hz for six muscles: rectus femoris (RF), vastus lateralis (VL), vastus medialis (VM), gastrocnemius (G), medial hamstring (MH), and lateral hamstring (LH).

Analysis of EMG data revealed no significant differences in EMG amplitude or the integral of the LE EMG between the groups and conditions. During the 50-s isometric exercise at 80% MVC, the fatigue state is represented by decline in the MF values of EMG signals greater than 10 Hz. A muscle fatigue state was obtained in all muscles. Percentage of decline of MF in the gastrocnemius differed significantly between groups ($p < 0.05$). Percentages of decline of MF in VM and G of the ACL group and VL and G of the healthy group were found to be statistically significant ($p < 0.05$) between conditions (Table 7). In subjective assessment of muscle fatigue using the Borge scale (0 – 10) at 10-s intervals during the 50-s isometric exercise at 80% MVC, outcomes showed a high correlation between the subjective perception of fatigue and percentage of decline of the MF ($r = 0.64$) for VL and RF muscles during the brace condition. All other muscles showed very low correlation.

In conclusion, muscle fatigue was measured in both brace and unbraced conditions; however, wearing functional knee braces did not induce more muscle fatigue.

Conclusion

In clinical setting and especially in rehabilitation, it is very important that the EMG acquired is based on sound principles of signal acquisition and processing in order to optimize signal quality. This leads to better interpretation of mechanical muscle output during rehabilitation or sport medicine studies. General trends can be stated from the applications to muscle activation and timing, contraction profile, strength of contraction, and fatigue. In signal processing and reliability, the raw EMG can be sampled at less than 500 Hz without significantly affecting the power spectrum density and the linear envelope of the EMG signal. In comparison between surface and intramuscular electrodes, it was confirmed that SE is more reliable than IWE in day-to-day investigations. Both electrodes recorded statistically similar signals, although the coefficient of variability between the two types was very high. As for signal reliability, we demonstrated that the

difference in MF of the EMG power spectrum must be large enough to be able to differentiate the two conditions. In muscle activation and timing, it has been shown that, for the most effective performance, muscles must work in synergy. In muscle fatigue, findings confirmed the fatigue state in all the muscles, suggesting recruitment of more type II fibers as the muscles fatigues, and show the physiological adaptation of the quadriceps and hamstrings to ACL insufficiency.

From all these applications, it is clear that few directive lines can be drawn and applied to rehabilitation programs. Factors like signal reliability, muscle synergy, proprioception mechanisms, and muscle fatigue mechanisms have been of great interest in rehabilitation, but these topics certainly need more research in order to understand muscle rehabilitation for ordinary people as well as elite athletes.

References

1. Andersson EA, Nilsson J, Thorstensson A (1997) Intramuscular EMG from the hip flexor muscles during human locomotion. Acta Physiol Scand 161(3)361–370
2. Arokoski JP, Kankaanpaa M, Valta T, Juvonen I, Partanen J, Taimela S, Lindgren KA, Airaksinen O (1999). Back and hip extensor muscle function during therapeutic exercises. Arch Phys Med Rehabil 80(7)842–850
3. Basmajian J, De Luca C (1985) Muscle alive. Their function revealed by electromyography. Fifth edn. Williams and Wilkins, Baltimore
4. Bilodeau M, Arsenault AB, Gravel D, Bourbonnais D (1994) EMG power spectrum of elbow extensors: A reliability study. Electromyogr Clin Neurophysiol 34(3)149–158
5. Chen J-J, Shiavi RG, Zhang L-Q (1992) A quantitative and qualitative description of electromyographic linear envelopes for synergy analysis. IEEE Trans Biomed Eng 39(1)9–18
6. Cohen A (1986) Biomedical signal processing. Vol 1. Time and frequency domain analysis. CRC Press, Boca Raton, USA
7. Cook TM, Zimmermann CL, Lux KM, Neubrand CM, Nicholson TD (1992) EMG comparison of lateral step-up and stepping machine exercise. J Orthop Sports Phys Ther 16(3)108–113
8. Davis BA, Krivickas LS, Maniar R, Newandee DA, Feinberg JH (1998) The reliability of monopolar and bipolar fine-wire electromyographic measurement of muscle fatigue. Med Sci Sports Exerc 30(8)1328–335
9. De la Barrera EJ, Milner TE (1994) The effects of skinfold thickness on the selectivity of surface EMG. Electroencephalogr Clin Neurophysiol 93(2)91–99
10. De Luca C (1993a) The use of surface electromyography in biomechanics. Paper presented at the the 14th ISB Congress, Paris
11. De Luca CJ (1993b) Use of the surface EMG signal for performance evaluation of back muscles. Muscle Nerve 16(2)210–216

12. Elert J, Karlsson S, Gerdle B (1998) One-year reproducibility and stability of the signal amplitude ratio and other variables of the electromyogram: Test-retest of a shoulder forward flexion test in female workers with neck and shoulder problems. Clin Physiol 18(6)529–538

13. Elfving B, Nemeth G, Arvidsson I, Lamontagne M (1999) Reliability of EMG spectral parameters in repeated measurements of back muscle fatigue. J Electromyogr Kinesiol 9(4)235–243

14. Ferdjallah M, Wertsch JJ (1998) Anatomical and technical considerations in surface electromyography. Phys Med Rehabil Clin N Am 9(4)925–931

15. Giroux B, Lamontagne M (1990) Comparisons between surface electrodes and intramuscular wire electrodes in isometric and dynamic conditions. Electromyogr Clin Neurophysiol 30(7)397–405

16. Hagberg M, Kvarnstrom S (1984). Muscular endurance and electromyographic fatigue in myofascial shoulder pain. Arch Phys Med Rehabil 65(9)522–525

17. Hagemann B, Luhede G, Luczak H (1985). Improved "active" electrodes for recording bioelectric signals in work physiology. Eur J Appl Physiol 54(1)95–98

18. Harba MI, Teng LY (1999) Reliability of measurement of muscle fiber conduction velocity using surface EMG. Front Med Biol Eng 9(1)31–47

19. Kadaba MP, Wootten ME, Gainey J, Cochran GV (1985) Repeatability of phasic muscle activity: Performance of surface and intramuscular wire electrodes in gait analysis. J Orthop Res 3(3)350–359

20. Kadefors R, Herberts P (1977) Single fine wire electrodes: Properties in quantitative studies of muscle function. In: Asmussen E, Jorgenssen K (eds) Biomechanics VI-A. University Park Press, Baltimore

21. Kuster M, Wood GA, Sakurai S, Blatter G (1994) Downhill walking: A stressful task for the anterior cruciate ligament? A biomechanical study with clinical implications. 1994 Nicola Cerulli Young Researchers Award. Knee Surg Sports Traumatol Arthrosc 2(1)2–7

22. Kwatny E, Thomas DH, Kwatny HG (1970). An application of signal processing techniques to the study of myoelectric signals. IEEE Trans Biomed Eng 17(4)303–313

23. Lafrenière CM, Lamontagne M, Elsawy R (1997) The role of the lateral pterygoid muscles in TMJ disorders during static conditions. J Craniomandib Prac 15(1)38–52

24. Lamontagne M, Coulombe V (1992) The effects of EMG sampling rate on the power spectral density under eccentric contractions of the vastus lateralis. Paper presented at the the second North American Conference of Biomechanics, Chicago

25. Lamontagne M, Sabagh-Yazdi F (1999) The influence of functional knee braces on muscle fatigue. Paper presented at the 26th International Society of Biomechanics, Calgary, Canada

26. Mâsse L, Lamontagne M, O'Riain M (1992) Biomechanical analysis of wheelchair propulsion for various seating positions. J of Rehab Research and Development 29(3)12–28

27. Mathieu PA, Aubin CE (1999) Back muscle activity during flexions/extensions in a second group of normal subjects. Ann Chir 53(8) 761–772

28. McGill S, Juker D, Kropf P (1996) Appropriately placed surface EMG electrodes reflect deep muscle activity (psoas, quadratus lumborum, abdominal wall) in the lumbar spine. J Biomech 29(11)1503–1507

29. Merletti R, Knaflitz M, Deluca CJ (1992) Electrically evoked myoelectric signals. Crit Rev Biomed Eng 19(4)293–340

30. Moritani T, Muro M, Kijima A (1985). Electromechanical changes during electrically induced and maximal voluntary contractions: Electrophysiologic responses of different muscle fiber types during stimulated contractions. Exp Neurol 88(3)471–483

31. Morris AD, Kemp GJ, Lees A, Frostick SP (1998) A study of the reproducibility of three different normalisation methods in intramuscular dual fine wire electromyography of the shoulder. J Electromyogr Kinesiol 8(5)317–322

32. Németh G, Kronberg M, Brostrom LA (1990) Electromyogram (EMG) recordings from the subscapularis muscle: Description of a technique. J Orthop Res 8(1)151–153

33. Németh G, Lamontagne M, Tho KS, Eriksson E (1997) Electromyographic activity in expert downhill skiers using functional knee braces after anterior cruciate ligament injuries. Am J Sports Med 25(5)635–641

34. Nishimura S, Tomita Y, Horiuchi T (1992). Clinical application of an active electrode using an operational amplifier. IEEE Trans Biomed Eng 39(10)1096–1099

35. Notermans S (1984) Current practice of clinical electromyography. Elsevier, New York

36. Park TA, Harris GF (1996) "Guided" intramuscular fine wire electrode placement. A new technique. Am J Phys Med Rehabil 75(3)232–234

37. Perreault EJ, Hunter IW, Kearney RE (1993) Quantitative analysis of four EMG amplifiers. J Biomed Eng 15(5)413–419

37a Preece AW, Wimalaratna HS, Green JL, Churchill E, Morgan HM (1994) Noninvasive quantitative EMG. Electromyogr Clin Neurophysiol 34(2)81–86

38. Shiavi R (1974) A wire multielectrode for intramuscular recording. Med Biol Eng 12(5)721–723

39. Shiavi R, Zhang LQ, Limbird T, Edmondstone MA (1992) Pattern analysis of electromyographic linear envelopes exhibited by subjects with uninjured and injured knees during free and fast speed walking. J Orthop Res 10(2)226–236

40. Sinderby C, Lindstrom L, Grassino AE (1995) Automatic assessment of electromyogram quality. J Appl Physiol 79 (5)1803–1815

41. Soderberg G (1992) Selected topics in surface electromyography for use in the occupational setting: Expert perspectives. DHHS National Institute for Occupational Safety and Health, Publ. No. 91–100, pp. 179

42. Sparto PJ, Parnianpour M, Reinsel TE, Simon S (1997) Spectral and temporal responses of trunk extensor electromyography to an isometric endurance test. Spine 22(4)418–425

43. Tho K, Németh G, Lamontagne M, Eriksson E (1997) Electromyographic analysis of muscle fatigue in anterior cruciate ligament deficient knees. Clin Orthop (340)142–151

44. Thorstensson A, Carlson H, Zomlefer MR, Nilsson J (1982) Lumbar back muscle activity in relation to trunk movements during locomotion in man. Acta Physiol Scand 116(1)13–20

45. Van Lent ME, Drost MR, v d Wildenberg FA (1994) EMG profiles of ACL-deficient patients during walking: The influence of mild fatigue. Int J Sports Med 15(8)508–514

46. Winter D (1990) Biomechanics and motor control of human motion. 2nd edn. John Wiley Sons Inc, Toronto

CHAPTER 5

Rehabilitation of Rotator Cuff Injuries   5

Alberto Selvanetti, Arrigo Giombini, Ignazio Caruso

Introduction

The shoulder complex is particularly susceptible to injury, as it maintains a precarious interplay between stability and motion and is repetitively stressed in occupational and sporting activities. Rotator cuff disorders are among the most common causes of pain and impaired performance in athletes, mainly those involved in repetitive overhead throwing activities and contact sports [1]. In athletes, cuff disease represents a possibly coexistent spectrum of pathologies progressing from tendon strain and edema through inflammation and microscopic failure of fibers after repetitive wear, the final stages being gross cuff fraying and tear. According to some authors [2–4], rotator cuff lesions may be classified based on the etiological mechanism of injury proposed by the following scheme:

1. Primary or secondary compressive cuff lesion: external or subacromial impingement syndrome, posterosuperior or internal impingement syndrome
2. Primary or secondary tensile cuff lesion
3. Macrotraumatic cuff failure resulting from a single direct or indirect traumatic accident or from repetitive microtrauma displayed by a single event

Athletes involved in contact sports are more likely to sustain traumatic cuff tears because of the arms being forcefully abducted or violently pulled away from the body or by a fall or blow to the outstretched arm in a forced elevated position.

The etiology of rotator cuff disease may not be due to a single cause but is most likely multifactorial, with a combination of both extrinsic and intrinsic factors (age-related tendon degeneration, tensile overloading, trauma, precarious tendon vascularity, glenohumeral instability, scapulothoracic dysfunction, and congenital abnormalities).

Basic Principles of Shoulder Reeducation

In any nonoperative and postoperative rehabilitation program of a cuff-injured athlete, the main objectives are the resolution of symptoms and a return to the athlete's preinjury levels of performance with respect to the specific individual demands while also reducing the risks of reinjury. That implies addressing all components of the rehabilitation plan such as control of inflammation, pain relief, restoration of normal range of motion (ROM), strength, endurance, power, speed, neuromuscular coordination and proprioception of the upper limb, postural correction, reprogramming of correct sport-specific patterns, and maintenance of total body conditioning.

When designing a rehabilitation program, the most important factor for a successful outcome is thorough and accurate evaluation to address the exact diagnosis, since more than one cause of cuff pathology can be present at any one time. That implies a clear understanding of shoulder anatomy, biomechanics, and pathophysiology to define and treat local anatomical lesions as well as acquaintance with the specific physiological requirements and adaptations of the particular sport to be able to evaluate and possibly correct any biomechanical and/or functional deficits and subclinical maladaptations of the whole body.

Patient education is also important for successful outcome and promotes compliance: athletes must be given easy-to-understand instructions on the etiopathogenesis of pathology and how to manage it, including treatment options and practical advice about the proper execution of exercises.

The principles to be integrated when planning rehabilitation of a cuff-injured athlete are shown in Table 1 [5].

Table 1. Objectives of the rehabilitation program for rotator cuff injuries in athletes

1. Control of pain and inflammation
2. Reestablishment of the normal activation patterns of the kinetic chain
3. Restoration of the shoulder range of motion
4. Dynamic scapulothoracic and glenohumeral stabilization
5. Restoration of the humeral control and the shoulder neuromuscular coordination
6. Taking the "SAID" principle into account
7. Cardiovascular conditioning

Pain and Inflammation Control

Pain should be controlled in the early stages of rehabilitation because it induces muscle inhibition that alters muscle firing patterns and shoulder joint function. Strategies for decreasing pain and inflammation include:

1. Relative rest with avoidance of aggravating positions, arcs of motion, and activities
2. Short-term shoulder immobilization when required (sling, abduction brace)
3. Modalities: cryotherapy [6, 7], transcutaneous electrical nerve stimulation (TENS), interferential currents, high-voltage galvanic stimulation, ultrasound, low-level laser, hyperthermia, microwave diathermy
4. Drugs: analgesics, nonsteroidal anti-inflammatory medications, and occasionally subacromial injections of corticosteroids [8, 9]
5. Soft-tissue massage
6. Inactivation of cervical and shoulder active trigger points

For the time being, no firm conclusion is possible to support or refute the efficacy of common interventions (nonsteroidal anti-inflammatory drugs, corticosteroid injections, physiotherapy) in managing shoulder pain. As outlined in recent reviews, the methodological scores for most studies are low, there is lack of concordance in the labeling and definition of shoulder disorders, and careful consideration of selection criteria and outcome measures is often disregarded. So it is surely erroneous to conclude that these treatments do not work at all. Medications and physical modalities are used adjunctively to exercise therapy in treating enthesopathies, and there is not yet evidence that they have a statistically significant clinical effect on the natural history of rotator cuff disorders [10 – 19].

Reestablishment of Normal Activation Patterns of the Shoulder

As most shoulder activities in land-based sports work from orderly sequences of motion from the ground through the trunk, the entire kinetic chain should be integrated into the rehabilitation process to minimize overload on the shoulder. It is necessary to evaluate and possibly correct any breakdowns and improper sequencing along the kinetic chain: poor shoulder and body stance posture, inflexibilities, muscular weakness, and strength imbalances of the upper limbs, neck, trunk, hip, and lower limbs, abnormalities of the scapular position and dyskinesia of the scapulothoracic joint, and disorders of the acromioclavicular and sternoclavicular joints. Restoring normal activation of kinetic chain patterns should be addressed in the early stages of shoulder rehabilitation to allow for recovery of the most efficient sequences of force and velocity generation and transfer from the proximal links to the hand through the shoulder.

Restoration of Range of Motion

Shoulder ROM is paramount for overhead-throwing athletes. These athletes often exhibit tightness of the posterior shoulder capsule and musculature with limitation of horizontal adduction and internal rotation: this can cause abnormal glenohumeral kinematics by forcing the humeral head anteriorly and superiorly into the acromial arch, and it can lead to increased stress to the posterior shoulder structures during the follow-through phases of throwing and serving [20, 21]. Then, any deficit of shoulder complex ROM and flexibility should be corrected early to allow normal motor patterns to be recreated. Techniques or exercises to improve and maintain mobility and provide gentle stress to the healing collagen tissue include passive and active-assisted ROM exercises in pain-free ranges [22, 23], gentle joint mobilization provided there is no excessive shoulder capsular laxity or generalized joint hypermobility [24], passive and proprioceptive neuromuscular facilitation (PNF) stretching, myofascial release techniques, and swimming pool exercises [25 – 27].

Passive and active-assisted ROM exercises include Codman's pendulums, elevation and forward flexion with opposite arm cradle while leading with the thumb, supine modified elevation/external rotation, T-bar- or stick-assisted motions (extension, flexion in the sagittal plane with the arm externally rotated and supinated and in the scapular plane or POS, that is 30° – 45° anteriorly to the coronal plane, combined adduction/internal rotation behind the back, external/internal rotation in increasing POS abduction), rope and pulleys (flexion, abduction in the POS).

Grade I or II glenohumeral mobilizations and gentle long arm distractions may be used in the early stages of healing for pain relief and to regain motion limited by pain, while grade III or IV mobilizations can be added in later rehabilitation phases to improve ROM limited by capsuloligamentous tightness. The presence of anterior capsular laxity and underlying instability of the glenohumeral joint contraindicates joint mobilizations that attenuate the anterior capsule.

Increasing internal rotation and eliminating posterior shoulder tightness can increase the performance of overhead athletes [28], so painless posterior capsular mobilizations and posterior shoulder stretches with static or PNF methods should be done. Examples include external rotation stretch below 90° of abduction (Fig. 1) and supine horizontal adduction stretch with

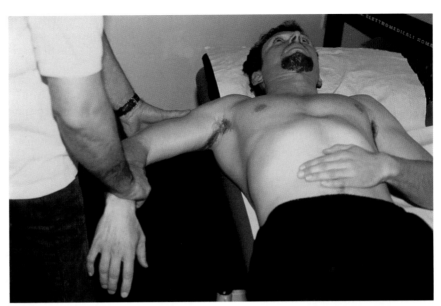

Fig. 1. Assisted stretching of the external rotators muscles below the level of the shoulder in supine position

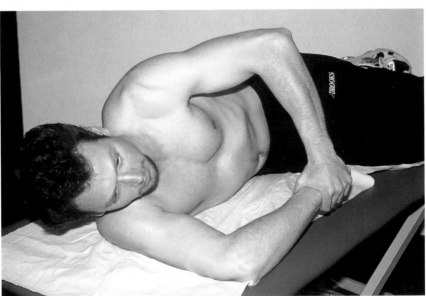

Fig. 2. Posterior shoulder capsular stretching with scapular stabilization

scapular stabilization (Fig. 2). Posterior and inferior glides in the POS can also contribute to improve internal rotation [29–31]. Furthermore, stretching of a shortened pectoralis minor decreases the posterior tilting of the scapula in the sagittal plane in subjects with impingement, avoiding impinging of the rotator cuff against the acromion during arm elevation [32].

Scapulothoracic and Glenohumeral Stabilization

The goal is to increase the efficiency of the mechanisms of compression and depression of the humeral head to maintain dynamic stability of the shoulder.

In shoulder activities, the rotator cuff muscles (supraspinatus, infraspinatus, teres minor, subscapularis) contribute to the dynamic stability of the glenohumeral joint through the passive tension of the muscle bulk and acting as humeral head depressor and stabilizer by compressing the joint surfaces and tightening the static constraints. They do this while participating with the deltoid in the abduction force couple and with themselves in a rotation force couple. The most efficient activity of the cuff is between 70° and 100° of abduction [33–35]. In normal shoulder function, the scapula has several interrelated roles [36, 37]:

1. Firm socket for the glenohumeral joint. When coordinated with the moving humerus, scapular motion is able to maintain the glenohumeral in-

stant center of rotation constrained in the physiological normal path throughout the full shoulder ROM [38] and accomplish proper orientation of the glenoid fossa with the humeral head, keeping the glenohumeral angle within a "safe zone" of 30° of angulation from the neutral position in the POS to decrease shear and translatory forces [39]. These actions allow an optimal "concavity-compression" effect of the glenohumeral joint: the proper alignment of the glenoid allows adequate function of the bony constraints to glenohumeral motion and maintains efficient position and correct length-tension relationships of the rotator cuff muscles, thus ensuring maximal compression into the glenoid socket.

2. Stable base for function of many muscular groups:
   a. Scapulothoracic stabilizers (trapezius, rhomboids, levator scapulae, serratus anterior, pectoralis minor) that contribute to normal joint arthrokinematics by controlling position and motion of the scapula along the thoracic wall. Acting as force couples, they stabilize the scapula (upper and lower portion of the trapezius and rhomboids, both paired with the serratus anterior muscle) and elevate the acromion to avoid impinging the rotator cuff during arm elevation (lower trapezius and serratus anterior both paired with the upper trapezius and rhomboids). They also play a key role in sports activities like swimming recovery and in the different phases of throwing and serving motions by facilitating the cocking position of arm (scapular retraction) and contributing to dissipate the deceleration forces during follow-through (scapular protraction).
   b. Extrinsic muscles of the shoulder complex (deltoid, biceps brachii, triceps brachii): they work in synergy to enhance both strength and power to perform gross motor activities of the glenohumeral joint. The biceps brachii plays an important role in throwing and serving activities, acting as depressor of the humeral head during the late cocking phases and as decelerator during the follow-through [39 – 42].
   c. Rotator cuff muscles.
3. Link in the kinetic chain for transferring energy and force from legs and trunk to the hand.

Abnormal scapular position and motion, alteration of the scapulohumeral rhythm, thoracic spine alignment, and muscular imbalance are thought to contribute to impairment of normal shoulder function. The pathologic process may cause a disorganization of firing patterns of the scapular stabilizing muscles, usually by reflex inhibition, that leads to loss of proximal stability,

increased demands on the rotator cuff musculature and biceps, poor performance, and augmented risk of shoulder dysfunction such as impingement or instability [32, 43 – 45].

The goals of reeducation of scapular dyskinesia and muscle imbalance are to restore normal motor patterns and force couples to improve scapular position and motion, trunk posture, rotator cuff efficiency, and shoulder neuromuscular control [46]. Exercises to rehabilitate the scapular muscles include [37]:

1. Isometric drills. Shoulder pinches with emphasis on upright posture and full scapular retraction and depression and punches with resistance applied to the hand and the lateral border of the scapula (Fig. 3). In early stages, the control of proper scapular position may be enhanced by biofeedback or scapular taping in a retracted position [47, 48]. The latter serves both to control cervicobrachial and upper trapezius pain and to normalize disorganized or inhibited scapular motor firing patterns mechanically assisting the scapular stabilizers and avoiding substitution scapulothoracic patterns for glenohumeral motion.

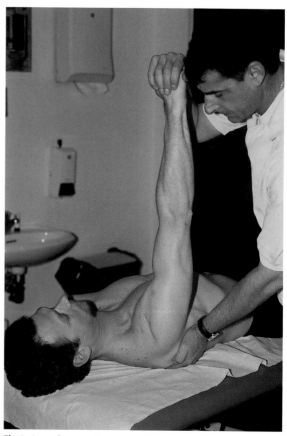

Fig. 3. Scapular punching against manual resistance applied to the hand and the lateral border of the scapula

2. Closed-chain activities. They can be started as early as 5 weeks after rotator cuff repairs [49]. In the early phases of rehabilitation, exercises should first be performed below the shoulder level at less than 45° abduction and 60° flexion of the arm and then proceed up to 90° abduction, as tolerated. Usually they are first done with axial limb compression against fixed resistance, such as stabilizing the involved hand in sideways position on a table or wall while standing and by performing specific scapular patterns, first in straight planes of retraction/protraction and elevation/depression, then in diagonal and circular movement patterns with or without rhythmic stabilization. Exercises should also include weight shifts on a table and progressive weight-bearing drills (quadruped, tripod, and unilateral balancing). Further advancements include weight bearing over unstable bases such as foam mats and proceeding from large to smaller Swiss balls on the wall and on the ground, uni- and multidirectional balance boards and slide boards, and the Fitter (Fig. 4). Exercises may further progress from hand placement on the sides of the devices to their top or the middle, to one hand on top of the other, and finally to a single-arm stance (Fig. 5). Other drills include push-up progression (wall, table, floor in knee-assisted position, regular push-ups, and push-ups on unstable surfaces), push-ups with a plus [50], step-ups in a push-up position, stepping in a sideways direction, inclined press with narrow grip, press-ups, dips [51–53], and upper body ergometer (UBE).

3. Open-chain activities. These should be initiated on the basis established by both exercise groups outlined above and include PNF scapular patterns and rhythmic stabilizations with the shoulder in varying degrees of flexion and/or abduction, prone horizontal abduction in external rotation with scapular retraction, dynamic hug [54], forward punch [50, 55], pull-downs, rowing progression (prone, bent, seated) [42], push-up plus [56], prone 110° abduction in neutral rotation [56], and plyometrics (Fig. 6) [51, 56–58].

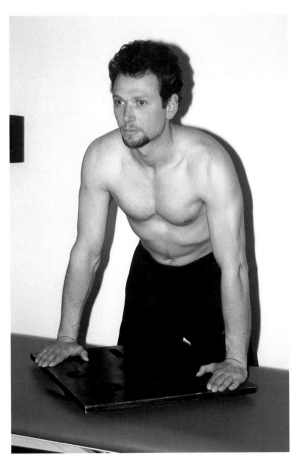

Fig. 4. Closed-chain weight shift

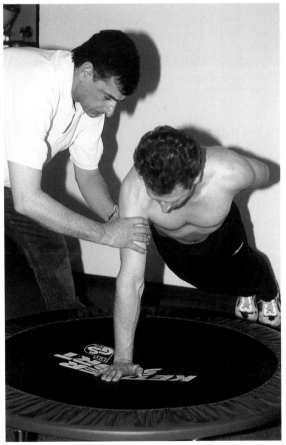

Fig. 5. Closed-chain balancing on a minitrampoline in push-up position with rhythmic stabilization

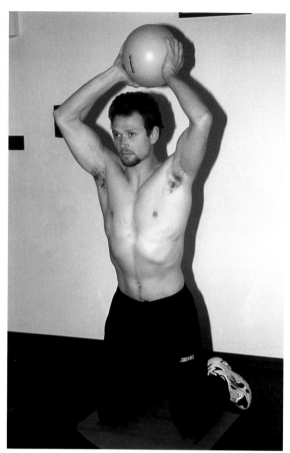

Fig. 6. Overhead two-handed pass with a plyoball performed on an unstable surface

Most of the scapular rehabilitation exercises should be done before an emphasis on rotator cuff strengthening. According to Kibler [37, 59], criteria for initiating advanced rotator cuff and open-chain arm activities should include a lateral slide asymmetry of less than 1 cm in the third position of the lateral scapular slide test and smooth motion of the scapula on the injured and uninjured side with both ascent and descent.

Early rotator cuff exercises should be done in a closed-chain fashion: examples are isometric standing or kneeling weight-bearing and weight shifts, isometric push-ups, and axial compressions against a wall or table with resisted arm flexion/extension and adduction/abduction and circles. In more advanced phases, increasingly challenging activities should be implemented, such as resisted lateral hand slides on a slide board, resisted PNF-type movements (such as quadruped exercise with D2 upper extremity and D1 lower extremity patterns applied to the contralateral limb), push-ups on unstable platforms, lateral step-ups, plyometric push-ups onto a Swiss ball, and upper extremity crawls (straight, retrograde or lateral walking on the floor or a treadmill).

Open-chain strengthening exercises for the rotator cuff initially should include pain-free submaximal isometrics with the arm passively positioned in 30°–45° of POS abduction in neutral rotation to reduce passive supraspinatus tension. Then the exercises are progressed with emphasis on scapulothoracic muscular function to implement multiangled rotational isometrics and isotonics with free weights or tubing in the POS from 30°–45° to 90° of abduction in supported and unsupported positions, supine internal and external rotation, side-lying abduction 0°–45° in neutral rotation [60], prone shoulder extension in external rotation, prone 100° horizontal abduction in external rotation, scaption with internal rotation ("empty can" position) [61] or external rotation ("full can" position), 90°/90° prone external rotation [62–65], PNF diagonals, and seated rowing progression (narrow, middle, wide grip) [58].

Due to the importance of the biceps brachii to glenohumeral stabilization and deceleration of the throwing arm, exercises to strengthen this muscle concentrically and eccentrically should be implemented early. Once scapular and rotator cuff muscle balancing has been achieved, analytic strengthening is directed toward the propellor muscles (pectoralis major, latissimus dorsi) [66].

Reestablishment of Humeral Control and Neuromuscular Coordination

Control of the moving humerus is required for functional activities of the shoulder in overhead athletes. Deficits in proprioception and normal muscular coordination in the shoulder may impair functional stability and performance of complex activities by interfering with normal recruitment patterns and the timing of muscular contraction. Then, after injury or surgery, neuromuscular control and coordination around the shoulder complex should be reestablished early through integrated use of closed- and open-chain exercises, PNF patterns, proprioceptive activities, and plyometrics.

Closed-chain activities [59, 67, 68] provide for:

1. Enhanced dynamic stabilization at the scapulothoracic and glenohumeral joints by cocontraction of force couples of both the scapular and cuff muscles and reflex stimulation of the joint mechanoceptors and proprioceptive pathways as well as congruency of the glenohumeral joint surfaces with low shear and high compressive forces
2. Early strengthening that allows open-chain activities. These involve agonist-antagonist force couples, require large ROM, allow increased mobility of the proximal and distal joints, generate high

forces and acceleration-deceleration, and are useful to address strength deficits of a weakened muscle in the later phases of rehabilitation and as part of a preparticipation conditioning program. They should be performed in a pain-free ROM, avoiding long levers around the shoulder and rotator cuff impingement and reducing strain of capsuloligamentous structures. Progression should include gravity-minimized, gravity-assisted, and gravity-resisted positions, moving from below horizontal to near and above shoulder level, choosing the POS in early exercises because torsional stresses to the glenohumeral joint capsule are minimized, rotator cuff vascularity is improved, and subacromial cuff impingement is decreased when the arm is elevated because there is a more direct line of pull for the deltoid and supraspinatus, and greater glenohumeral joint congruity and stability is allowed by optimizing length/tension relationships for the deltoid and cuff muscles [69–71]. Exercises should advance from submaximal isometrics in a pain-free range to isotonics performed with low resistance and high repetition to emphasize muscular endurance, important because it affords fatigue resistance and long-term dynamic stabilization for the glenohumeral joint during repetitive overhead activities.

Elastic tubing is a versatile tool that provides constant resistance allowing both concentric and eccentric stimulation throughout the ROM independently of position. Resistance can easily be adjusted in small increments to match the patient's progress by modifying the stretch of the tubing or using a more resistive elastic device. Upper body ergometry is useful to improve muscular strength and endurance; both the forward and backward directions are done.

Proprioceptive neuromuscular facilitation adopts spiral/diagonal movement patterns that closely simulate the normal functional planes of motion [72, 73]. This rehabilitative method is useful to enhance neuromuscular control of the shoulder girdle by promoting cocontractions and facilitating the efficiency of muscle synergies, and to develop kinesthetic awareness. Proprioceptive neuromuscular facilitation patterns can be performed in various positions (such as supine, on the side, seated, or standing) against manual resistance, incorporating rhythmic stabilization and slow reversal hold techniques applied to the arm at various points in the range, or with rubber tubing, pulley, or free weights, or isokinetically. In the rehabilitation of injured overhead athletes, PNF D2 flexion and extension patterns and their modifications are useful to replicate overhead activities.

Proprioceptive nerve endings and free nerve endings are found in the glenohumeral ligaments, joint capsule, glenoid labrum, coracoacromial ligament, rotator cuff, and subacromial bursa [74–79]. In healthy persons, shoulder joint position sense significantly worsens with muscle fatigue [80], and this as well as kinesthesia are diminished in patients with injured shoulders [81, 82]. Proprioceptive training restores the synergy and synchrony of muscular firing patterns necessary for functional activities. Exercises of shoulder proprioceptive reprogramming should be integrated early in the rehabilitation by activities encouraging reflex joint stabilization in closed and open kinetic modes as well as joint position sensibility exercises and kinesthetic exercises [83, 84]. Examples are passive and active glenohumeral positioning and repositioning with/without visual input and manual resistance and isometric holding in resting position progressing to end ranges of the sport-specific patterns of motion. Initially, low forces can be applied slowly, advancing to high forces applied rapidly and unexpectedly.

Plyometrics (stretch shortening drills) are among the more appropriate exercises for functional shoulder rehabilitation and enhancement of the neuromuscular coordination by combining strength with speed of movements. The concept is to use the myotatic stretch reflex and proprioceptive stimulus to produce a large amount of muscular momentum and force through a stretching-shortening cycle [85], that is, an eccentric contraction followed by a rapid concentric contraction. Furthermore, by reproducing these cycles at functional positions, plyometrics also stimulate proprioceptive feedback to fine-tune muscular activity patterns. Upper extremity (UE) plyometrics should be implemented in the advanced phases of reeducation after tissue healing has occurred, full ROM is obtained, closed-chain exercises have stabilized the joint, and neurologic retraining has been implemented. Plyometrics should be performed only two or three times weekly because of the risk of additional microtrauma to the healing shoulder [67, 86].

An upper extremity plyometric program is usually organized in four exercise groups [87–90]: warm-up drills, throwing movements, trunk drills, and wall drills. It may be initiated with wall and corner push-ups, progressing to Swiss balls and tubing drills and 2-lb to 10-lb medicine ball throws (chest pass, underhand, and soccer pass with or without trunk rotation, side-to-side pass, and one-hand softball and baseball throws) as tolerated.

The SAID Principle

When planning a program to return a cuff-injured athlete to preinjury performance levels, it is important to apply the principle of "specific adaptation to imposed demands" (SAID). That means specifically tailoring the late stages of rehabilitation to duplicate the sport-specific dynamics and match individual needs by restoring the complex neuromuscular and conditioning patterns required by the sport to be performed.

Cardiovascular Conditioning

Total body aerobic conditioning is initiated as early as possible after injury or surgical intervention if it does not aggravate pain or impair healing. Goals are to minimize effects of disuse and provide psychological benefits. Activities include walking, stationary biking, stepping, treadmill, UBE, and deep-water running.

Function-Based Sequential Progression of a Shoulder Reeducation Program

A general comprehensive protocol of rehabilitation for cuff-injured athletes is outlined, but activities and speed of progression must be individualized as they depend on many factors including patient age, personality, expected functional requirements, reactivity to treatment, type and severity of pathology, biological healing times, surgical procedure performed, and complications.

Four stages of rehabilitation with specific goals are described, each containing exercises and techniques to accomplish the objectives, and progression from one phase to another should be based on criteria that must be fulfilled rather than on time alone, as healing times may vary from individual to individual [91, 92].

Phase 1: Acute or Protected

Goals and Treatment

1. Decrease pain and inflammation and allow safe tissue healing using rest from painful activities, medications, modalities, soft-tissue massage, grade I–II joint mobilizations, and short-term immobilization by sling or abduction pillow (if strictly necessary).
2. Improve painless shoulder motion and flexibility with passive and active-assisted ROM exercises in pain-free arcs below 90° abduction (pendulum swings, opposite arm cradling, T-bar, rope and pulley), joint mobilizations, static and PNF stretching, transverse friction massage, hydrotherapy, and myofascial release.
3. Enhance early scapular stabilization and control with isometric scapular protraction, retraction and depression, scapular PNF straight patterns, early UE closed-chain activities with shoulder abducted < 45° and flexed < 60° (weight bearing and weight shifts).

4. Prevent disuse muscular ipotonotrophy with isometrics and light isotonics (1-lb to 3-lb free weights, rubber tubing) at hand, wrist, and elbow and submaximal pain-free isometrics for rotator cuff with coactivation of scapular muscles with arm in POS below 90° abduction and 90° flexion.
5. Postural exercises.
6. Cardiovascular and general conditioning: treadmill, stationary biking, stepping, UBE, deep-water running, minitrampoline, agility drills (with running and jumping, slider or Fitter boards), lower extremity and trunk stretching and strengthening, leg and trunk stabilization exercises.

Criteria for the next phase: minimal pain and tenderness on clinical examination, tissue sufficiently healed for active motion and tissue loading, pain-free passive range of motion (PROM) 75% of opposite side ROM, manual muscle strength grading 4 of 5 in respect to the noninjured shoulder, scapular control in neutral glenohumeral position (dominant and nondominant side scapular asymmetry < 1.5 cm).

Phase 2: Intermediate or Recovery

Goals and Treatment

1. Normalize and maintain pain-free shoulder motion and flexibility: progress to active-assisted, then active ROM to and above 90° abduction with scapula stabilized, increase intensity of stretching to end range, and restore posterior shoulder flexibility, joint mobilizations (if any stiffness persists).
2. Improve scapular control: scapular PNF patterns in diagonals, closed-chain exercises at 90° flexion and 90° abduction, push-up progression, push-ups with a plus, step-ups, medicine ball catch and push, dips.
3. Improve upper limb strength balance, endurance, and glenohumeral dynamic stabilization: isolated open-chain isotonic (tubing, dumbbell) scapulothoracic, rotator cuff, elbow, and wrist exercises; glenohumeral PNF patterns, closed-chain exercises at 90° flexion, then 90° abduction for glenohumeral depressors and internal/external rotators, and light plyometric exercises (push-ups and chest, soccer, underhand throws).
4. Restore kinetic chain and force generation patterns: normalization of all inflexibilities throughout the chain, normal agonist/antagonist force couples in legs (squats, plyometric depth jumps, lunges, hip extensions), trunk rotation exercises with medicine ball or tubing, leg and trunk stabilization integrated exercises (rotational/diagonal patterns from hip to shoulder,

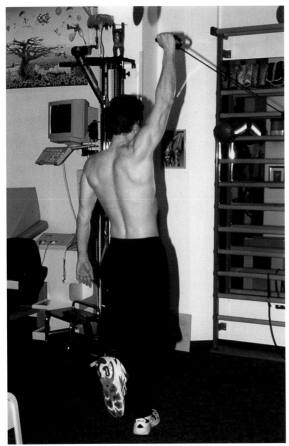

Fig. 7. Association of hip and trunk stabilization and scapular retraction in a diagonal pattern

medicine ball throws) (Fig. 7), and normal throwing and serving motion without resistance.
5. Address proprioception deficits: joint reposition-ing and kinesthetic drills.
6. Cardiovascular and general conditioning.

Criteria to progress to the next phase: no pain or ten-derness on clinical examination, full functional pain-less scapulothoracic and glenohumeral PROM, manual cuff strength grading 4+ or 5 of 5 with respect to the noninjured shoulder, scapular control in glenohumeral neutral position (dominant and nondominant side scapular asymmetry <1 cm), normal kinetic chain function.

Phase 3: Advanced or Functional

The focus of this phase is the SAID principle. Goals and treatment are:

1. Maintain shoulder mobility with self-stretches and ROM exercises.

2. Maintain and increase muscular strength, power, speed, and endurance of the upper extremity with continuation of scapulothoracic neuromus-cular control drills, tubing and dumbbell exer-cises with increasing loads and emphasis on high speed, eccentrics, diagonal and multiplanar pat-terns progressing to provocative functional posi-tions and UE closed-chain exercises on unstable surfaces, advanced plyometrics, and isokinetics (velocity spectrum training 180 by 300°/sec).
3. Continue proprioceptive exercises.
4. Establish correct motor patterns of sport-specif-ic motions: visual feedback with videotape or mirror, technical assistance from coach.
5. Initiate sport-specific training.

Criteria for the next phase: no pain or tenderness on clinical examination, full functional painless active range of motion (AROM), strength deficit less than 20% of the noninjured shoulder, normal kinetic chain function.

Phase 4: Return to Activity

Goals: gradual return to full recreational activities or sport. This is introduced with:

1. Continuation of specific exercises to address any remaining deficits and improve performance re-lated to functional requirements.
2. Development of a sport-specific controlled maintenance program to improve the athlete's ability to withstand sports demands and prevent further overload injuries: exercises for flexibility, strength, endurance, power, and proprioception should be implemented [93, 94].
3. Athlete education to correct weight-training technique for prevention of subsequent shoulder injuries [94–96].

Criteria for a gradual return to sports include no pain or tenderness on clinical examination, full painless ROM, adequate scapular and glenohumeral stability, strength within 10% of the contralateral limb, power and endurance based on functional demands, normal shoulder arthrokinetics, regaining of proprioceptive abilities, satisfactory kinetic chain integration, and ability to perform athletic activity confidently at a competitive level.

Treatment of Rotator Cuff Injuries by Etiology

Reeducation protocols for some of the most common rotator cuff disorders are proposed in Tables 2–5.

Table 2. Conservative rehabilitation of rotator cuff tendinopathy or impingement syndrome

I. Phase 1: acute or protected (1–2 weeks)
A. Goals
  1. Reduce pain and inflammation and allow safe tissue healing
  2. Improve painless shoulder motion and flexibility
  3. Enhance early scapular stabilization and control in neutral glenohumeral position
  4. Prevent muscle ipotonotrophy of the upper limb
  5. Maintain general conditioning and strength of noninjured body parts

B. Rest from painful activities, avoiding active use of the arm below 90° abduction and flexion in a pain-free motion during activities of daily living, medications, modalities, grade I–II joint mobilizations, massage of cervicoscapular district and upper limb

C. Passive and active-assisted ROM exercises in pain-free arcs below 90° abduction (pendulums, opposite arm cradling, T-bar, rope and pulleys with the palm supinated and the humerus externally rotated), joint mobilizations (glenohumeral, sternoclavicular, scapulothoracic), gentle static and PNF stretching (especially for posterior shoulder capsule and musculature, avoiding cross-arm adduction), transverse friction massage, hydrotherapy, myofascial release

D. Scapular submaximal isometrics (retraction, depression, punch), self or manual scapular PNF patterns, early UE closed-chain activities (weight bearing and weight shifts)

E. Submaximal pain-free isometrics for biceps, deltoid, and rotator cuff with coactivation of scapular muscles with arm below 90° abduction and 90° flexion in the POS

F. Isometrics and light isotonics (free weights, rubber tubing) at hand, wrist, and elbow

G. Arthrokinematic training (scapular taping, biofeedback)

H. Postural reeducation

I. General aerobic and anaerobic exercises

J. Criteria to progress to the next phase
  1. Minimal pain and tenderness on clinical examination
  2. Pain-free PROM 75% of opposite side (painless arc in abduction)
  3. Manual muscle strength grading 4 of 5 in respect to the noninjured shoulder
  4. Scapular control in neutral glenohumeral position (dominant side/nondominant side scapular asymmetry <1.5 cm)

II. Phase 2: intermediate or recovery (2–4 weeks)
A. Goals
  1. Normalize and maintain pain-free shoulder motion and flexibility
  2. Improve scapular neuromuscular control and glenohumeral dynamic stabilization
  3. Restore and improve upper limb strength, balance, and endurance
  4. Normalize kinetic chain movement patterns of shoulder complex
  5. Continue total body conditioning and strengthening of noninjured body parts

B. Continue modalities, as needed, and postural reeducation

C. Progress pain-free active-assisted then active ROM exercises to and above 90° abduction in POS, increase intensity of self-stretching to end range, grade I–III joint mobilizations (if stiffness persists)

D. Scapular and glenohumeral PNF patterns (avoid cross-body adduction in PNF D1), closed chain exercises at 90° flexion and 90° abduction for scapular stabilizers, glenohumeral depressors and internal/external rotators, push-up progression, push-up with a plus, step-ups, dips

E. Continue isometrics, initiate isolated open-chain isotonic elbow and wrist exercises, scapulothoracic, rotator cuff with emphasis on the POS (tubing, dumbbells)

F. Light plyometric exercises: medicine ball catch and push (chest, soccer, and underhand pass)

G. Joint repositioning and kinesthetic drills

H. Normalization of all inflexibilities throughout chain, normal agonist-antagonist force couples in legs (squats, plyometric depth jumps, lunges, hip extensions), trunk rotation exercises with medicine ball or tubing, integrated exercises with rotational/diagonal patterns from leg to shoulder

I. General aerobic and anaerobic exercises

J. Criteria to progress to the next phase
  1. No pain or tenderness on clinical examination
  2. Full functional painless PROM
  3. Manual muscle strength grading 4+/5 compared to noninjured shoulder
  4. Scapular control in glenohumeral neutral position (dominant side and nondominant side scapular asymmetry <1 cm)
  5. Normal kinetic chain function
  6. Ability to perform ADL pain-free

III. Phase 3: advanced or functional (4–6 weeks)
A. Goals
  1. Maintain and increase upper extremity flexibility, strength, power, speed, and endurance
  2. Increase neuromuscular control and establish correct motor patterns
  3. Initiate sport-specific training

B. Self-stretches and ROM exercises from the previous phase

C. Continuation of scapulothoracic neuromuscular control drills, tubing and dumbbell exercises, increasing loads and emphasis to high speeds, eccentrics, diagonal and multiplanar patterns progressing to provocative functional positions

D. Continuation of proprioceptive exercises

E. UBE for endurance

F. Advanced plyometrics

G. Isokinetics: internal and external rotation training in neutral position (180–300°/sec)

H. Sport-specific functional progression with correction of the remaining biomechanical deficits

I. Criteria to progress to the next phase
  1. No pain or tenderness on clinical examination
  2. Full functional painless AROM
  3. Satisfactory strength (equal to about 90% of the noninjured shoulder) and neuromuscular control
  4. Normal kinetic chain function
  5. Pain-free ADLs

IV. Phase 4: return to activity (7 – 10 weeks)
A. Goal: gradual return to full recreational activities or sport

B. Continuation of above protocol

C. Sport reentry and maintenance programs

D. Criteria for a gradual return to sports
1. No pain or tenderness on clinical examination
2. Full painless ROM
3. Adequate scapular and glenohumeral stability
4. Strength within 10% of contralateral levels
5. Power and endurance based on functional demands
6. Normal shoulder arthrokinetics
7. Regaining of proprioceptive abilities
8. Satisfactory kinetic chain integration
9. Ability to perform athletic activity confidently at a competitive level

Table 3. Rehabilitation protocol after arthroscopic acromioplasty (subacromial decompression) with intact rotator cuff. NB: An open surgery acromioplasty, which involves the deltoid, should be protected with PROM for at least 3 weeks, and full functional painless ROM should be usually achieved 4 – 6 weeks after surgery

I. Preoperative measures
Instruction in use of sling or abduction pillow, cryotherapy, therapeutic exercise (gentle early P/AAROM exercises for shoulder, AROM and strengthening exercises for elbow, wrist, hand)

II. Phase 1: acute or protected phase (weeks 1 – 4)
A. Goals
1. Control of pain and inflammation
2. Allow healing
3. Gradually regain painless ROM
4. Increase strength
5. Maintain general body fitness and strength of noninjured body parts

B. 1 – 2 weeks
1. Immobilization in sling for up to 2 weeks unless showering or doing exercises. Sutures are removed 14 days postop
2. Modalities for relief of pain and inflammation: cryotherapy, TENS, interferential currents, high-voltage galvanic stimulation, massage of cervicoscapular district and upper limb, NSAID as needed
3. ROM and flexibility exercises in painless arcs: pendulums, supine P/AA "full can" scaption and forward elevation opposite arm cradle below 90°, T-bar exercises at 0° abduction for all motions with deemphasized internal rotation past neutral and extension, pulley exercises for flexion below 90°
4. Active scapular pinches, nonweight-bearing depression, and punches
5. AROM and strengthening exercises for hand, wrist, and elbow (biceps curls and triceps extensions with elbow supported)
6. Cervical ROM and flexibility exercises
7. May need Coban wrapping or isotonic glove for finger or hand swelling
8. Trunk stabilization exercises and postural exercises as tolerated
9. General conditioning program (as medical conditions permit): walking, stationary biking, stair machine, lower limb strengthening

C. 3 – 4 weeks
1. Continuation and progression of all the above exercises
2. Addition of P/AA internal/external rotation in POS abduction below painful arc, cross-body adduction, extension, overhead pulley, and contract-relax stretch procedures with emphasis on posterior shoulder stretches. Trying to get 90° P/AA abduction by 3 – 4 weeks
3. Joint mobilizations. grade I – II without restrictions, grade III cautiously until 6 weeks (if stiffness persists)
4. AROM exercises below shoulder level discouraging scapular compensation: shoulder forward flexion, gravity eliminated internal/external rotation, abduction in POS and extension
5. Strengthening exercises
a. Submaximal multiangled nonpainful isometrics with the arm in a modified neutral position: supraspinatus at 30° and 60° in "full can" position, external/internal rotation, flexion/extension, abduction, biceps and triceps with elbow supported, scapular patterns
b. Short-arc to full-arc isotonics (tubing and light dumbbells beginning with 1 – 2 lb): scapular patterns, arm in POS for extension/flexion below 90°, external/internal rotation, supraspinatus in external rotation to 60°, elbow flexion/extension
6. Pool therapy
7. No lifting of heavy objects causing axial traction

D. Criteria to progress to the next phase
1. Minimal pain and tenderness on clinical examination
2. Pain-free PROM in most planes of at least 75% of opposite side
3. Fair strength (3 of 5) as graded by manual muscle test evaluation
4. Scapular control (dominant /nondominant side scapular asymmetry < 1.5 cm)

III. Phase 2: intermediate or recovery phase (weeks 5 – 6)
A. Goals
1. Full pain-free PROM
2. Regain and improve strength, power, and neuromuscular control of the shoulder complex
3. Normalize arthrokinematics
4. Maintenance of cardiovascular fitness and strength of noninjured body parts

B. Modalities and joint mobilizations as needed

C. Continuation of all above exercises

D. ROM and flexibility exercises: addition of P/AAROM extension and modified elevation/external rotation

E. Progress as tolerated with multiangled isometrics and isotonic strengthening for scapulothoracic, rotator cuff, deltoid, biceps, and triceps muscles with emphasis on scapular muscle integration and discouraging scapular compensation

F. Neuromuscular control exercises for scapular and cuff muscles: modified weight-bearing stabilization drills and weight shifts, PNF patterns (D2 flexion RS at 30°, 60°, 90°, and 120° and tubing D2 flexion with isometric holds)

G. UBE for ROM, endurance and strengthening

H. Swimming in protected ROM

I. Trunk stabilization exercises and postural exercises as tolerated

J. General conditioning program: walking, biking, stair machine, deep water running

K. Criteria to progress to the next phase
  1. No pain or tenderness on clinical examination
  2. Full painless PROM
  3. Good manual muscle strength (4+ to 5 of 5 for scapula and rotator cuff)
  4. Adequate joint stabilization and neuromuscular coordination
  5. Normal kinetic chain function

IV. Phase 3: advanced or functional phase (weeks 7–12)
A. Goals
  1. Maintain full painless ROM
  2. Enhance strength, power, speed, and endurance
  3. Optimize neuromuscular control, gradual return to functional activities

B. Continuation of the previous program

C. Stretching for cervical spine, shoulder, elbow, and wrist

D. Strengthening exercises with emphasis on high speed and eccentrics, progress external/internal rotation strengthening into POS abduction toward and above shoulder level

E. Advanced reactive neuromuscular training: plyometrics

F. Protected range weight lifting

G. General conditioning program

H. Initiation of sport-specific program

I. Criteria to progress to the next phase
  1. No pain or tenderness on clinical examination
  2. Full functional painless AROM
  3. Strength 90% of noninjured shoulder level
  4. Normal kinetic chain function

V. Phase 4: return to activity (weeks 13–16)
A. Goals
  1. Gradual return to recreational activities and sport
  2. Prevention of reinjury

B. Continue flexibility and strengthening exercises

C. Functional progression through sport-specific exercises

D. Maintenance program

E. Criteria for a gradual return to sports
  1. No pain or tenderness on clinical examination
  2. Full painless ROM
  3. Adequate scapular and glenohumeral stability
  4. Strength within 10% of contralateral extremity
  5. Power and endurance based on functional demands
  6. Normal shoulder arthrokinetics
  7. Recovered proprioceptive abilities
  8. Satisfactory kinetic chain integration
  9. Ability to perform athletic activity confidently at a competitive level

Table 4. Rehabilitation protocol after repair of small rotator cuff tears (<1 cm)

I. Preoperative measures
Instruction in use of sling or abduction pillow, cryotherapy, therapeutic exercise (gentle early P/AAROM exercises for shoulder, AROM and strengthening exercises for elbow, wrist, and hand)

II. Phase 1: acute or protected phase (weeks 1–6)
A. Goals
  1. Control pain and inflammation
  2. Allow healing

  3. Gradually regain painless ROM
  4. Increase strength, maintenance of general body fitness, and strength of noninjured body parts

B. 1–3 weeks
  1. Immobilization in sling plus abduction pillow for up to 2–3 weeks unless showering or doing exercises. Sutures are removed 14 days postop
  2. Modalities for relief of pain and inflammation: cryotherapy, TENS, interferential currents, massage of cervicoscapular district and upper limb, NSAID as needed
  3. ROM and flexibility exercises in painless arcs: pendulums, supine P/AA "full can" scaption and forward elevation opposite arm cradle below 90°, P/AA in POS at 0° abduction with T-bar for all motions with deemphasized internal rotation past neutral, pulley exercises for flexion below 90°
  4. Active scapular pinches, nonweight-bearing depression, and punches
  5. AROM exercises for hand, wrist, and elbow (biceps curls and triceps extensions with elbow supported)
  6. Cervical ROM and flexibility exercises
  7. May need Coban wrapping or isotoner glove for finger or hand swelling
  8. Trunk stabilization exercises and postural exercises as tolerated
  9. General conditioning program (as medical condition permits): walking, leg strengthening, stationary biking, stair machine

C. 4–6 weeks
  1. Continuation and progression of all the above exercises
  2. Progress P/AAROM exercises to and over 45° POS abduction, addition of internal rotation below painful arc, extension, overhead pulley, and contract-relax stretch procedures in POS
  3. Joint mobilizations – grade I–II without restrictions, grade III cautiously until 6 weeks
  4. AROM exercises below 90° discouraging scapular compensation: gravity-eliminated shoulder forward flexion, internal/external rotation, abduction in POS and extension
  5. Strengthening exercises
  a. Submaximal nonpainful isometrics with the arm in modified neutral position: supraspinatus at 30° and 60° in "full can" position, external/internal rotation, flexion/extension, abduction, biceps and triceps with elbow supported, scapular patterns
  b. Short-arc isotonics (late phase): scapular patterns, tubing with arm in POS for extension/flexion below 90°, external/internal rotation, supraspinatus in external rotation to 60°, elbow flexion/extension
  6. Pool therapy
  7. No lifting of heavy objects causing axial traction

D. Criteria to progress to the next phase
  1. Minimal pain and tenderness on clinical examination
  2. Pain-free PROM in most planes at least 75% of contralateral levels
  3. Fair manual muscle strength of scapular and cuff muscles (3 of a grading of 5)
  4. Scapular control (dominant/nondominant side scapular asymmetry <1.5 cm)

III. Phase 2: intermediate or recovery phase (weeks 7–12)
A. Goals
  1. Full pain-free ROM

2. Regain and improve strength, power, and neuromuscular control of the shoulder complex
3. Normalize arthrokinematics
4. Maintenance of cardiovascular fitness and strength of noninjured body parts

B. Modalities and joint mobilizations as needed

C. Continuation of all above exercises

D. ROM and flexibility exercises: gradual increase of P/AA flexion to 180° and external/internal rotation to 90° POS abduction, addition of cross-body adduction and modified elevation plus external rotation. AROM exercises: against gravity extension, external/internal rotation, abduction

E. Strengthening exercises: multiangled submaximal non-painful isometrics and light isotonics (tubing, dumbbells) for scapulothoracic, rotator cuff, deltoid, biceps, and triceps muscles, with the arm in POS and emphasis on scapular muscle integration and discouraging scapular compensation

F. Neuromuscular control exercises for scapular and cuff muscles: modified weight-bearing stabilization drills and weight shifts, PNF patterns (D2 flexion RS at 30°, 60°, 90°, 120° and tubing D2 flexion with isometric holds)

G. UBE for ROM and endurance (8–10 weeks)

H. Swimming in protected ROM

I. Trunk stabilization exercises and postural exercises as tolerated

J. General conditioning program: walking, biking, stair machine, deep water running

K. Criteria to progress to the next phase
1. No pain or tenderness on clinical examination
2. Full functional painless PROM
3. Rotator cuff strength rating 4 of 5
4. Normal kinetic chain function
5. Performance of pain-free ADLs

IV. Phase 3: advanced or functional phase (weeks 13–20)
A. Goals
1. Maintain full painless ROM
2. Enhance strength, power, speed, and endurance
3. Optimize neuromuscular control of the shoulder complex
4. Gradual return to functional activities

B. Continuation of previous program

C. Stretching for cervical spine, shoulder, elbow, and wrist

D. Aggressive strengthening for scapular, rotator cuff, deltoid, biceps, and triceps muscles, progressing in resistance and position into POS abduction to near and above shoulder level

E. Advanced reactive neuromuscular training: plyometrics

F. UBE for strengthening

G. Protected range weight lifting

H. General conditioning program

I. Initiation of sport-specific program

J. Criteria to progress to the next phase
1. No pain or tenderness on clinical examination
2. Full functional painless AROM

3. Rotator cuff strength rating at about 90% of level of the noninjured shoulder
4. Normal kinetic chain function

V. Phase 4: return to activity (weeks 21–26)
A. Goals
1. Gradual return to recreational activities and sport
2. Prevention of reinjury

B. Continue all flexibility and strengthening exercises

C. Functional progression through sport-specific exercises

D. Maintenance program

E. Criteria for a gradual return to sports
1. No pain or tenderness on clinical examination
2. Full painless ROM
3. Adequate scapular and glenohumeral stability
4. Strength within 10% of contralateral levels
5. Power and endurance based on functional demands
6. Normal shoulder arthrokinetics
7. Regaining of proprioceptive abilities
8. Satisfactory kinetic chain integration
9. Ability to perform athletic activity confidently at a competitive level

Table 5. Rehabilitation protocol after repair of medium-large rotator cuff tears (1 cm – 5 cm)

I. Preoperative measures
Instruction in use of sling or abduction pillow, cryotherapy, therapeutic exercise (gentle early P/AAROM exercises for shoulder, AROM and strengthening exercises for elbow, wrist, hand)

II. Phase 1: acute or protected phase (weeks 1–6)
A. Goals
1. Control of pain and inflammation
2. Allow healing
3. Gradual regain painless ROM
4. Increase strength to prevent muscle atrophy
5. Maintain general body fitness and strength of noninjured body parts

B. 1–2 weeks
1. Immobilization in sling or abduction brace at 45° of abduction and 0° of rotation unless doing exercises for 2–3 weeks
2. Modalities for relief of pain and inflammation: cryotherapy, TENS, interferential currents, massage of cervicoscapular district and upper limb, NSAID as needed
3. ROM and flexibility exercises in painless arcs: pendulums, supine P/AA "full can" scaption and forward elevation opposite arm cradle below 90°, P/AA at 45° POS abduction with T-bar for all motions with external rotation to 30° deemphasized internal rotation past neutral and extension, pulley exercises for flexion below 90°
4. Active scapular pinches, nonweight-bearing depression, and punches
5. AROM exercises for hand, wrist, and elbow (biceps curls and triceps extensions with elbow supported)
6. Cervical ROM and flexibility exercises
7. Observe for finger swelling: may need Coban wrapping or isotoner glove
8. Trunk stabilization exercises and postural exercises as tolerated
9. General conditioning program as medical condition permits: walking, stationary biking, stair machine, lower limb strengthening

C. 3–6 weeks
1. Discontinue sling or brace
2. Continuation of all above exercises
3. Progress P/AAROM flexion to 145° and external rotation at 60° POS abduction, addition of internal rotation below painful arc, extension, and overhead pulley
4. Joint mobilizations. grade I–II without restrictions, grade III cautiously until 6 weeks
5. AROM exercises discouraging scapular compensation: gravity-eliminated shoulder forward flexion below 90°, external rotation to 30°, internal rotation to neutral, abduction in POS and extension
6. Submaximal pain-free isometrics for scapular, rotator cuff (POS position), elbow, triceps, deltoid muscles
7. Pool therapy
8. No lifting of heavy objects causing axial traction

D. Criteria to progress to the next phase
1. Minimal pain and tenderness on clinical examination
2. Pain-free PROM 75% of opposite side (excluding internal rotation)
3. Fair manual muscle strength of internal/external rotation and flexion (manual muscle test evaluation score 3 of 5)
4. Scapular control (dominant/nondominant side scapular asymmetry < 1.5 cm)

III. Phase 2: intermediate or recovery phase (weeks 7–14)
A. Goals
1. Full pain-free ROM (at weeks 10–12)
2. Regain and improve strength, power, and neuromuscular control of the shoulder complex
3. Normalize arthrokinematics

B. Modalities and gentle joint mobilizations as needed

C. Continuation of all the above exercises

D. ROM and flexibility exercises: gradual increasing of P/AA flexion to 160° and P/AA external/internal rotation above 45° of POS abduction to 90° or tolerance, addition of cross-body adduction, extension, and modified elevation and external rotation

E. Strengthening exercises: multiangled submaximal nonpainful isometrics and light isotonics (tubing, dumbbells) for scapulothoracic, rotator cuff, deltoid, biceps, and triceps muscles, with the arm in POS and emphasis on scapular muscle integration and discouraging scapular compensation

F. Neuromuscular control exercises for scapular and cuff muscles

G. UBE for ROM and endurance (8–10 weeks)

H. Swimming in protected ROM

I. Trunk stabilization exercises and postural exercises as tolerated

J. General conditioning program: walking, biking, stair machine

K. Criteria for progression to next phase
1. No pain or tenderness on clinical examination
2. Full functional painless PROM
3. Rotator cuff strength equal to 70% of contralateral level
4. Normal kinetic chain function
5. Performance of ADLs with arm at side

IV. Phase 3: advanced or functional phase (weeks 15–26)
A. Goals
1. Maintain full painless ROM
2. Enhance strength, power, speed, and endurance
3. Optimize neuromuscular control of the shoulder complex
4. Gradual return to functional activities

B. Continuation of previous program

C. Stretching for cervical spine, shoulder, elbow, and wrist

D. Aggressive strengthening for scapular, rotator cuff, deltoid, biceps, and triceps, progressing in resistance and position into POS abduction to near and above shoulder level. Begin PNF patterns

E. Advanced reactive neuromuscular training: plyometrics

F. UBE for strengthening

G. Protected range weight lifting

H. General conditioning program

I. Initiation of sport-specific program

J. Criteria to progress to the next phase
1. No pain or tenderness on clinical examination
2. Full functional painless AROM
3. Shoulder muscle strength at about 90% of contralateral level
4. Normal kinetic chain function
5. Resumption of pain-free ADLs

V. Phase 4: return to activity (weeks 27–32)
A. Goals
1. Gradual return to recreational activities and sport
2. Prevention of reinjury

B. Continue all flexibility and strengthening exercises

C. Functional progression through sport-specific exercises

D. Maintenance program

E. Criteria for a gradual return to sports
1. No pain or tenderness on clinical examination
2. Full painless ROM
3. Adequate scapular and glenohumeral stability
4. Strength within 10% of contralateral level
5. Power and endurance based on functional demands
6. Normal shoulder arthrokinetics
7. Regaining of proprioceptive abilities
8. Satisfactory kinetic chain integration
9. Ability to perform athletic activity confidently at a competitive level

Rehabilitation techniques and progressions are outlined for the athletic population. In sedentary or nonathletic individuals, the progression may be slower, and some methods may not be utilized at all or only in later phases of rehabilitation.

External Impingement Syndrome

External impingement syndromes result from mechanical compression of the rotator cuff tendons and subacromial bursa against the overlying coracoacromial arch, especially during elevation of the arm. It can be primary [97] or secondary to subtle underlying glenohumeral instability or to scapulothoracic muscle fatigue and weakness or chronic tendinopathy of rotator cuff muscles [98, 99]. Patients usually respond to a nonoperative rehabilitation program centered on decreasing pain and inflammation, normalizing range of motion, and strengthening scapular stabilizers, rotator cuff, and humeral depressors. Depending on the degree of cuff pathology, arthroscopic subacromial decompression, debridement of partial cuff tears, and repair of full thickness tears are usually successful in those who fail a conservative program. If instability is the main problem, then surgical stabilization of the shoulder capsule is warranted.

Internal Impingement Syndrome

The internal impingement syndrome is produced by the repeated pinching of the undersurface of the supraspinatus and/or infraspinatus tendon between the greater humeral tuberosity and the posterosuperior border of the glenoid when the shoulder is in abduction, extension, and maximal external rotation in susceptible persons (overhead-throwing sports, workers) [100 – 113]. Another acute mechanism of injury is a violent active elevation of the arm by a fall or a blow to the outstretched arm. Predisposing factors are thought to be decreased humeral retroversion, scapulothoracic dysfunction, and poor throwing technique. Glenohumeral capsular laxity or instability should not be thought a prerequisite of this syndrome [114, 115]. Associated injuries include partial tears of the undersurface of the supraspinatus tendon, posterosuperior glenoid labral damage, and posterosuperior osteochondral impaction lesions of the humeral head. Anterior labral fraying, superior labrum anterior-to-posterior (SLAP) lesion, and damage of the biceps tendon anchor may coexist. Nonoperative treatment concentrates on posterior musculotendinous and capsular stretching programs and improvement of dynamic stability of the glenohumeral joint to prevent excessive anterior humeral displacement. If conservative treatment is unsuccessful, operative treatment of the posterior pathology includes arthroscopic debridement of the undersurface of the involved tendon(s) and glenoid labral fraying. Biceps/labral stabilization may be advocated.

Tensile Overload

Fatigue failure of the rotator cuff may result from the repetitive microtrauma of tensile stresses, primarily by eccentric muscle contractions incurred in overhead activities by the posterior cuff to decelerate the arm (primary tensile overload) [116, 117]. The resulting cuff dysfunction leads to increased glenohumeral translations and secondary impingement. The presence of congenital or acquired glenohumeral capsular laxity, labral insufficiency, muscle weakness, or a tight posterior glenohumeral capsule can increase tensile loads on the musculotendinous cuff units that must withstand the simultaneous functions of deceleration and stabilization of the humeral head on the glenoid (secondary tensile overload) [118, 119]. Nonoperative treatment is focused on the eccentric strengthening of the shoulder girdle musculature without exacerbating the problem, dynamic stabilization by neuromuscular and proprioceptive conditioning, and addressing any sport-related technical faults. Failure of the conservative regimen may result in surgical debridement of the rotator cuff tear, eventually associated with proper evaluation and treatment of coexistent labral tears and/or the capsular laxity. Complete tears should be treated with mini-open repair.

Macrotraumatic Failure

Injury of the rotator cuff results from a single traumatic event (i.e., anterior dislocation of the glenohumeral joint), sometimes occurring to a weakened tendon secondary to aging or accumulation of microtraumas [120]. A conservative symptomatic treatment consisting of rest, analgesic medications, modalities, gentle ROM, and progressive scapular and cuff strengthening exercises is advocated. If this fails to return the athlete to the desired level of competition, surgery is warranted. Cuff tears are usually treated by debridement or repair, and subacromial decompression may be necessary in case of marked subacromial soft tissue thickening and fibrosis. Any coexistent lesion (i.e., labrum) should be evaluated and properly addressed. The rehabilitation program and its rate of progression are dictated by the size of the cuff tear and integrity of surrounding tissue.

Acknowledgements. We wish to thank Eli Berger, PT, and Antonio Pontecorvi, PT, for their technical collaboration.

References

1. Glousman R (1993) Electromyographic analysis and its role in the athletic shoulder. Clin Orthop Rel Res 288:27–34
2. Meister K, Andrews JR (1993) Classification and treatment of rotator cuff injuries in the overhead athlete. J Orthop Sports Phys Ther 18:413–421
3. Morrison DS (1996) Conservative management of partial-thickness rotator cuff lesions. In: Burkhead WZ Jr (ed) Rotator cuff disorders. Williams and Wilkins, Baltimore, pp 249–257
4. Blevins FT (1997) Rotator cuff pathology in athletes. Sports Med 24:205–220
5. Kelley MJ (1995) Anatomic and biomechanical rationale for rehabilitation of the athlete's shoulder. J Sports Rehabil 4:122–154

6. Speer KP, Warren RF, Horowitz L (1996) The efficacy of cryotherapy in the postoperative shoulder. J Shoulder Elbow Surg 5:62–68

7. Levy AS, Kelly B, Lintner S, Speer K (1997) Penetration of cryotherapy in treatment after shoulder arthroscopy. Arthroscopy 13:461–464

8. Goupille P, Sibilia J (1996) Local corticosteroid injections in the treatment of rotator cuff tendinitis (except for frozen shoulder and calcific tendinitis). Groupe Rhumatologique Francais de l'Epaule (GREP). Clin Exp Rheumatol 14:561–566

9. Tillander B, Franzen LE, Karlsson MH, Norlin R (1999) Effect of steroid injections on the rotator cuff: An experimental study in rats. J Shoulder Elbow Surg 8:271–274

10. Van der Windt DAWM, Van der Heijden GJMG, Scholten RJPM, Koes BW, Bouter LM (1995) The efficacy of nonsteroidal anti-inflammatory drugs (NSAIDs) for shoulder complaints: A systematic review. J Clin Epidemiol 48:691–704

11. Simunovic Z (1996) Low level laser therapy with trigger points technique: A clinical study on 243 patients. J Clin Laser Med Surg 14:163–167

12. Ginn KA, Herbert RD, Khouw W, Lee R (1997) A randomized, controlled clinical trial of a treatment for shoulder pain. Phys Ther 77:802–809

13. Winters JC, Sobel JS, Groenier KH, Arendzen JH, Meyboom de Jong B (1997) Comparison of physiotherapy, manipulation, and corticosteroid injection for treating shoulder complaints in general practice: Randomised, single blind study. BMJ 314:1320–1325

14. Van der Heijden GJMG, Van der Windt DAWM, Kleijnen J, Koes BW, Bouter LM (1996) Steroid injections for shoulder disorders: A systematic review of randomised clinical trials. Br J Gen Pract 46:309–316

15. Van der Heijden GJMG, Van der Windt DA, De Winter AF (1997) Physiotherapy for patients with soft tissue shoulder disorders: A systematic review of randomised clinical trials. BMJ 315:25–30

16. Van der Heijden GJMG, Leffers P, Wolters PJ, Verheijden JJ, Van Mameren H, Houben JP, Bouter LM, Knipschild PG (1999) No effect of bipolar interferential electrotherapy and pulsed ultrasound for soft tissue shoulder disorders: A randomised controlled trial. Ann Rheum Dis 58:530–540

17. Green S, Buchbinder R, Glazier R, Forbes A (1998) Systematic review of randomised controlled trials of interventions for painful shoulder: Selection criteria, outcome assessment, and efficacy. BMJ 316:354–360

18. Van der Windt DA, Van der Heijden GJ, Van den Berg SG, Ter Riet G, De Winter AF, Bouter LM (1999) Ultrasound therapy for musculoskeletal disorders: A systematic review. Pain 81:257–271

19. Winters JC, Jorritsma W, Groenier KH, Sobel JS, De Jong MB, Arendzen HJ (1999) Treatment of shoulder complaints in general practice: Long term results of a randomised, single blind study comparing physiotherapy, manipulation, and corticosteroid injection. BMJ 318:1395–1396

20. Harryman D, Sidles J, Clark J, McQuade K, Gibb T, Matsen F (1990) Translation of the humeral head on the glenoid with passive glenohumeral motion. J Bone Joint Surg Am 72:1334–1343

21. Tyler TT, Roy T, Nicholas SJ, Gleim GW (1999) Reliability and validity of a new method of measuring posterior shoulder tightness. J Orthop Sports Phys Ther 29:262–274

22. Dockery ML, Wright TW, LaStayo PC (1998) Electromyography of the shoulder: An analysis of passive modes of exercise. Orthopedics 21:1181–1184

23. Lastayo PC, Wright T, Jaffe R, Hartzel J (1998) Continuous passive motion after repair of the rotator cuff. A prospective outcome study. J Bone Joint Surg Am 80:1002–1011

24. Maitland GD. Peripheral manipulation (third edn). Butterworth, London, 1991

25. Speer KP, Cavanaugh JT, Warren RF, Day L, Wickiewicz TL (1993) A role for hydrotherapy in shoulder rehabilitation. Am J Sports Med 21:850–853

26. Kelly BT, Kirkendall DT, Speer KP (1996) The rationale for aquatic physical therapy in the shoulder. Med Sci Sports Exerc 28:S180

27. Fujisawa H, Suenaga N, Minami A (1998) Electromyographic study during isometric exercise of the shoulder in head-out water immersion. J Shoulder Elbow Surg 7:491–494

28. Kibler BW, McQueen C, Uhl T (1988) Fitness evaluation and fitness findings in competitive junior tennis players. Clin Sports Med 7:403–418

29. Johanson RL, Callis M, Potts J, Shall LM (1995) A modified internal rotation stretching technique for overhead and throwing athletes. J Orthop Sports Phys Ther 21:216–219

30. Donatelli RA, McMahon TJ (1997) Manual therapy techniques. In: Donatelli RA (ed) Physical therapy of the shoulder (third edn). Churchill Livingstone, New York, pp 335–364

31. Conroy DE, Hayes KW (1998) The effect of joint mobilization as a component of comprehensive treatment for primary shoulder impingement syndrome. J Orthop Sports Phys Ther 28:3–14

32. Lukasiewicz AC, McClure P, Michener L, Pratt N, Sennett B (1999) Comparison of 3-dimensional scapular position and orientation between subjects with and without shoulder impingement. J Orthop Sports Phys Ther 29:574–586

33. Pink MM, Perry J (1996) Biomechanics. In: Jobe FW (ed) Operative techniques in upper extremity sports injuries. Mosby, St Louis, pp 109–123

34. Payne LZ, Deng XH, Craig EV, Torzilli PA, Warren RF (1997) The combined dynamic and static contributions to subacromial impingement. A biomechanical analysis. Am J Sports Med 25:801–808

35. Morrey BF, Itoi E, Kai-Nan An (1998) Biomechanics of the shoulder. In: Rockwood CA Jr, Matsen III FA (eds) The shoulder (second edn). W.B. Saunders Co, Philadelphia, pp 233–276

36. Paine RM, Voight M (1993) The role of the scapula. J Orthop Sports Phys Ther 18:386–391

37. Kibler WB (1998) The role of the scapula in athletic shoulder function. Am J Sports Med 26:325–337

38. Matsen FA III, Harryman DT II, Sidles JA (1991) Mechanics of glenohumeral instability. Clin Sports Med 10:783–788

39. Glousman RE, Jobe FW, Tibone J, Moynes D, Antonelli D, Perry J (1988) Dynamic electromyographic analysis of the throwing shoulder with glenohumeral instability. J Bone Joint Surg 70A:220–226

40. Rodosky MW, Harner CD, Fu F (1994) The role of the long head of the biceps muscle and superior glenoid labrum in anterior stability of the shoulder. Am J Sports Med 22:121–130

41. Warner JJP, McMahon PJ (1995) The role of the long head of the biceps brachii in superior stability of the glenohumeral joint. J Bone Joint Surg Am 77:366–372

42. Litchfield R, Hawkins R, Dillman CJ, Atkins J, Hagerman G (1993) Rehabilitation of the overhead athletes. J Orthop Sports Phys Ther 18:433–441

43. Jobe FW, Pink M (1993) Classification and treatment of shoulder dysfunction in the overhead athlete. J Orthop Sports Phys Ther 18:427–432

44. Ludewig PM, Cook TM, Nawoczenski DA (1996) Three-dimensional scapular orientation and muscle activity at selected positions of humeral elevation. J Orthop Sports Phys Ther 24:57–65

45. Kebaetse M, McClure P, Pratt NE (1999) Thoracic position effct on shoulder range of motion, strength, and three-dimensional scapular kinematics. Arch Phys Med Rehabil 80:945–950

46. Wang C-H, McClure P, Pratt NE, Nobilini R (1999) Stretching and strengthening exercises: their effect on three-dimensional scapular kinematics. Arch Phys Med Rehabil 80:923–929

47. Host H (1995) Scapular taping in the treatment of anterior shoulder impingement. Phys Ther 75:803–812

48. Morin GE, Tiberio D, Austin G (1997) The effect of upper trapezius taping on electromyographic activity in the upper and middle trapezius region. J Sport Rehabil 6:309–318

49. Kibler WB, Livingston BK, Bruce RB (1995) Current concepts in shoulder rehabilitation. Adv Oper Orthop 3:249–300

50. Kamkar A, Irrgang JJ, Whitney SL (1993) Nonoperative management of secondary shoulder impingement syndrome. J Orthop Sports Phys Ther 17:212–224

51. Townsend H, Jobe FW, Pink M, Perry J (1991) Electromyographic analysis of the glenohumeral muscles during a baseball rehabilitation program. Am J Sports Med 19:264–272

52. Wilk KE, Arrigo C, Andrews JR (1994) Current concepts in the rehabilitation of the athlete's shoulder. J South Orthop Assoc 3:216–231

53. Pink MM, Screnar PM, Tollefson KD et al (1996) Injury prevention and rehabilitation in the upper extremity. In: Jobe FW, Pink MM, Glousman RE et al (eds) Operative techniques in upper extremity sports injuries. Mosby, St Louis, pp 3–14

54. Decker MJ, Hintermeister RA, Faber KJ, Hawkins RJ (1999) Serratus anterior muscle activity during selected rehabilitation exercises. Am J Sports Med 27:784–791

55. Dickoff-Hoffman SA (1994) Neuromuscular control exercises for shoulder instability. In: Andrews JR, Wilk KE (eds) The athlete's shoulder. Churchill Livingstone, New York, pp 435–450

56. Moseley JB, Jobe FW, Pink M, Perry J, Tibone J (1992) EMG analysis of the scapular muscles during a shoulder rehabilitation program. Am J Sports Med 20:128–134

57. McCann PD, Wootten ME, Kadaba MP, Bigliani LU (1993) A kinematic and electromyographic study of shoulder rehabilitation exercises. Clin Orthop 288:179–188

58. Hintermeister RA, Lange GW, Schultheis JM, Bey MJ, Hawkins RJ (1998) Electromyographic activity and applied load during shoulder rehabilitation exercises using elastic resistance. Am J Sports Med 26:210–220

59. Kibler WB. Shoulder rehabilitation: Principles and practice (1998) Med Sci Sports Exerc 30[Suppl]:S40–S50

60. Horrigan JM, Shellock FG, Mink JH, Deutsch AL (1999) Magnetic resonance imaging evaluation of muscle usage associated with three exercises for rotator cuff rehabilitation. Med Sci Sports Exerc 31:1361–1366

61. Jobe FW, Moynes DR (1982) Delineation of diagnostic criteria and a rehabilitation program for rotator cuff injuries. Am J Sports Med 10:336–339

62. Blackburn TA, McLeod WD, White B, Wofford L (1990) EMG analysis of posterior rotator cuff exercises. Athl Train 25:40–45

63. Ballantyne BT, O'Hare SJ, Paschall JL, Pavia-Smith MM, Pitz AM, Gillon JF, Soderberg GL (1993) Electromyographic activity of selected shoulder muscles in commonly used therapeutic exercises. Phys Ther 73:668–682

64. Kelly BT, Kadman WR, Speer KP (1996) The manual muscle examination for rotator cuff strength: An electromyographic investigation. Am J Sports Med 24:581–588

65. Malanga GA, Jenp YN, Grownwy EC, An KN (1996) EMG analysis of shoulder positioning in testing and strengthening the supraspinatus. Med Sci Sports Exerc 28:661–664

66. Jobe FW, Pink M (1993) Classification and treatment of shoulder dysfunction in the overhead athlete. J Orthop Sports Phys Ther 18:427–432

67. Wilk KE, Arrigo CA, Andrews JR (1996) Closed and open kinetic chain exercises for the upper extremity. J Sport Rehabil 5:88–102

68. Kibler WB, Livingston BK, Chandler TJ (1997) Shoulder rehabilitation: Clinical application, evaluation and rehabilitation. In: Springfield DS (ed) Instructional course lectures 46. American Academy of Orthopaedic Surgeons, Rosemont USA, pp 43–51

69. Johnston TB (1937) The movements of the shoulder joints: A plea for the use of the "plane of the scapula" as the plane of the reference for movements occurring at the humeroscapular joint. J Bone Joint Surg Br 25:252–260

70. Poppen NK, Walker PS (1976) Normal and abnormal motion of the shoulder. J Bone Joint Surg Am 58:195–201

71. Wilk KE, Arrigo C (1993) Current concepts in the rehabilitation of the athletic shoulder. J Orthop Sports Phys Ther 18:365–375

72. Kabat H (1965) Proprioceptive facilitation in therapeutic exercise. In: Lichts E (ed) Therapeutic exercise. Elizabeth Licht, New Haven, pp 327–343

73. Voss DE, Ionfa MK, Myers BJ (1986) Proprioceptive neuromuscular facilitation. Harper and Row, New York

74. Jerosch J, Steinbeck J, Clahsen H, Schmitz-Nahrath M, Grosse-Hackmann A (1993) Function of the glenohumeral ligaments in active stabilisation of the shoulder joint. Knee Surg Sports Traumatol Arthrosc 1:152–158

75. Vangsness CT Jr, Ennis M, Taylor JG, Atkinson R (1995) Neural anatomy of the glenohumeral ligaments, labrum and subacromial bursa. Arthroscopy 11:180–184

76. Ide K, Shirai Y, Ito H, Ito H (1996) Sensory nerve supply in the human subacromial bursa. J Shoulder Elbow Surg 5:371–382

77. Lephart SM, Pincivero DM, Giraldo JL, Fu FH (1997) The role of proprioception in the management and rehabilitation of athletic injuries. Am J Sports Med 25:130–137

78. Gohlke F, Janssen E, Leidel J, Heppelmann B, Eulert J (1998) Histopathological findings in the proprioception of the shoulder joint. Orthopade 27:510–517

79. Morisawa Y (1998) Morphological study of mechanoreceptors on the coracoacromial ligament. J Orthop Sci 3:102–110

80. Carpenter JE, Blasier RB, Pellizzon GG (1998) The effects of muscle fatigue on shoulder joint position sense. Am J Sports Med 26:262–265

81. Smith RL, Brunolli J (1989) Shoulder kinesthesia after shoulder dislocation. Phys Ther 69:106–112

82. Forwell LA, Carnahan H (1996) Proprioception during manual aiming in individual with shoulder instability and controls. J Orthop Sports Phys Ther 23:111–119

83. Borsa PA, Lephart SM, Kocher MS, Lephart SP (1994) Functional assessment and rehabilitation of shoulder proprioception for glenohumeral instability. J Sports Rehabil 3:84–104

84. Slobounov SM, Poole ST, Simon RF, Slobounov ES, Bush JA, Sebastianelli W, Kraemer W (1999) The efficacy of modern technology to improve healthy and injured shoulder joint position sense. J Sports Rehabil 8:10–23

85. Voight ML. Stretch-strengthening: An introduction to plyometrics (1992) Orthop Phys Ther Clin North Am 1:243–252

86. Cordasco FA, Wolfe IN, Wooten ME, Bigliani LU (1996) An electromyographic analysis of the shoulder during a medicine ball rehabilitation program. Am J Sports Med 24:386–392

87. Chu D (1989) Plyometrics exercises with a medicine ball. Bittersweet Publishing Co, Livermore, USA

88. Gambetta V, Odgers S (1991) The complete guide to medicine ball training. Optimum Sports Training, Sarasota, USA

89. Wilk KE, Voight M, Keirns MA, Gambetta V, Andrews JR, Dillman CJ (1993) Stretch-shortening drills for the upper extremity: Theory and clinical application. J Orthop Sports Phys Ther 17:225–239

90. Wilk KE (1996) Conditioning and training techniques. In: Hawkins RJ, Misamore GW (eds) Shoulder injuries in athletes. Churchill Livingstone, New York, pp 339–364

91. Wilk KE, Arrigo C (1992) An integrated approach to upper extremity exercises. Orthop Phys Ther Clin North Am 1:337–360

92. Wilk KE, Harrelson GL, Arrigo C, Chmielewski T (1998) Shoulder rehabilitation In: Andrews JR, Harrelson GL, Wilk KE (eds) Physical rehabilitation of the injured athlete (second edn) W.B. Saunders Co, Philadelphia, pp 478–553

93. Wilk KE, Andrews JR, Arrigo CA et al (1997) Preventive and rehabilitative exercises for the shoulder and elbow (fifth edn). American Sports Medicine Institute, Birmingham, USA

94. Powers ME (1998) Rotor cuff training for pitchers. J Sports Rehabil 7:285–299

95. Hawkins R, Litchfield R, Atkins G, Hagerman G, Dillman CJ (1996) Rehabilitation of the shoulder. Ann Chir et Gyn 85:173–184

96. Fees M, Decker T, Snyder-Mackler L, Axe MJ (1998) Upper extremity weight-training modifications for the injured athlete: A clinical perspective. Am J Sports Med 26:732–742

97. Neer CS, Walsh RP (1977) The shoulder in sports. Orthop Clin North Am 8:583–591

98. Nirschl RP (1988) Prevention and treatment of elbow and shoulder injuries in the tennis player. Clin Sports Med 7:289–308

99. Jobe FW, Tibone JE, Jobe CM et al (1990) The shoulders in sports. In: Rockwood CA Jr, Matsen FA III (eds) The shoulder. W.B. Saunders Co, Philadelphia, pp 961–990

100. Walch G, Liotard JP, Boileau P, Noel E (1991) Un autre conflit de l'épaule: Le "conflit glénoïdien postéro-superieur". Rev Chir Orthop Reparatrice Appar Mot 77:571–574

101. Walch G, Boileau P, Noël E, Donell ST (1992) Impingement of the deep surface of the supraspinatus tendon on the posterosuperior glenoid rim: An arthroscopic study. J Shoulder Elbow Surg 1:238–245

102. Walch G, Liotard JP, Boileau P, Noël E 1993) Le conflit glénoïdien postéro-supérieur: un autre conflit de l'épaule. J Radiol 74:47–50

103. Jobe CM, Sidles J (1993) Evidence for a superior glenoid impingement upon the rotator cuff (abstract). J Shoulder Elbow Surg 2:S19

104. Liu SH, Boynton E (1993) Posterior superior impingement of the rotator cuff on the glenoid rim as a cause of shoulder pain in the overhead athlete. Arthroscopy 9:697–699

105. Davidson PA, Elattrache NS, Jobe CM, Jobe FW (1995) Rotator cuff and posterior-superior glenoid labrum injury associated with increased glenohumeral motion: A new site of impingement. J Shoulder Elbow Surg 4:384–390

106. Rossi R, Ternamain PJ, Cerciello G, Walch G (1994) Il conflitto glenoideo postero-superiore dell'atleta: valore diagnostico della radiologia tradizionale e della risonanza magnetica. Radiol Med 87:22–27

107. Tirman PF, Bost FW, Steinbach LS, Mall JC, Peterfy CG, Sampson TG, Sheenan WE, Forbes JR, Genant HK (1994) MR arthrographic depiction of tears of the rotator cuff: Benefit of abduction and external rotation of the arm. Radiology 192:851–856

108. Tirman PF, Bost FW, Garvin GJ, Peterfy CG, Mall JC, Steinbach LS, Feller JF, Crues III JV (1994) Posterosuperior glenoid impingement of the shoulder: Findings at MR imaging and MR arthrography with arthroscopic correlation. Radiology 193:431–436

109. Jobe CM (1995) Posterior superior glenoid impingement: Expanded spectrum. Arthroscopy 11:530–536

110. Jobe CM (1996) Superior glenoid impingement: Current concepts. Clin Orthop Rel Res 330:98–107

111. Giombini A, Rossi F, Pettrone FA, Dragoni S (1997) Posterosuperior glenoid rim impingement as a cause of shoulder pain in top level waterpolo players. J Sports Med Phys Fitness 37:273–278

112. Halbrecht JL, Tirman P, Atkin D (1999) Internal impingement of the shoulder: Comparison of findings between the throwing and nonthrowing shoulders of college baseball players. Arthroscopy 15:253–258

113. Paley KJ, Jobe FW, Pink MM, Kvitne RS, ElAttrache NS (2000) Arthroscopic findings in the overhand throwing athlete: Evidence for posterior internal impingement of the rotator cuff. Arthroscopy 16:35–40

114. MacFarland EG, Hsu CY, Neira C, O'Neil O (1999) Internal impingement of the shoulder: A clinical and arthroscopic analysis. J Shoulder Elbow Surg 8:458–460

115. Barber FA, Morgan CD, Burkhart SS, Jobe CM (1999) Labrum/biceps/cuff dysfunction in the throwing athlete. Arthroscopy 15: 852–857

116. Lombardo SJ, Jobe FW, Kerlan RK, Carter VS, Shields CL Jr (1977) Posterior shoulder lesions in throwing athletes. Am J Sports Med 5:106–110

117. Andrews JR, Broussard TS, Carson WG (1985) Arthroscopy of the shoulder in the management of partial tears of the rotator cuff: A preliminary report. Arthroscopy 1:117–122

118. Jobe FW, Kvitne RS, Giangarra CE (1989) Shoulder pain in the overhand or throwing athlete: The relationship of anterior instability and rotator cuff impingement. Orthop Rev 18:963–975

119. Andrews JR, Alexander EJ (1995) Rotator cuff injury in throwing and racquet sports. Sports Med Arthroscopy Rev 3:30–38

120. Blevins FT, Hayes WM, Warren RF (1996) Rotator cuff injury in contact athletes. Am J Sports Med 24:263–267

CHAPTER 6

Rehabilitation of the Unstable Shoulder

6

Jean-Pierre Liotard, Gilles Walch

Introduction

In 1985, in collaboration with Gilles Walch, I opened a rehabilitation unit entirely devoted to immediate postoperative management of the shoulder. Later on, this unit became a department of 40 inpatient beds which I ran up to 1997. During that period, I treated a total of 3682 patients. I then saw shoulder rehabilitation in a different light, with priority being given to the restoration of range of motion and particularly elevation of the arm necessarily passing by the zero position of the shoulder. Two methods proved particularly efficient: swimming for immediate postoperative rehabilitation and self-directed overhead stretching of the arms with clasped hands.

Regarding shoulder instability, I personally followed up 135 patients who had had their shoulders stabilized surgically and then designed a simple postoperative rehabilitation protocol focused on the above priority, that is, early restoration of range of motion based on gentle movements and above all avoiding active contraction of the muscles. This is now being carried out on an outpatient basis.

The conservatively treated unstable shoulder requires a different approach. Since 1986, I had found that eccentric exercises according to the simple protocol described by Stanish yielded interesting results on knee pain (quadriceps mechanism) in athletes. I adapted these eccentric exercises to the surgically treated shoulder and used them conjointly with a method of proprioceptive rehabilitation allowing correct centering of the humeral head. Then I designed a modification of this method (based on eccentric exercises) for throwing athletes using a special pendulum exercise (ballistic movement with a brief stabilization overhead) and derived plyometric exercises.

Indications and Principles of Rehabilitation of the Unstable Shoulder

After reporting on our own experience, I shall briefly present a type of rehabilitation that can be proposed based on a different approach to the unstable shoulder.

The Diagnostic Approach to the Unstable Shoulder Assists in Placing Indications for Rehabilitation

Recognition of the lesions leads to analysis of the involved mechanisms and selection of the appropriate treatment methods. Then rehabilitation depends on whether or not the lesion has been repaired: (1) the lesion causing the instability has been repaired and the postoperative regimen is that for a stabilized shoulder, where rehabilitation is governed by healing time, a known parameter or (2) the lesion has not been repaired and the postoperative regimen is that of an unstable shoulder, where rehabilitation is based on recognition of the lesions and evaluation of their duration and severity, which are highly variable.

Anterior Instability

Anterior instability is the most common type of instability. Anteromedial dislocation is a typical injury which may be either a first episode or a relapse. It is easily identified: the dislocating motion in abduction/retropulsion/external rotation is identified during the interview; clinical examination reveals apprehension during the passive cocking phase of throwing, as readily recognized by the patient; the radiographic assessment shows one or several lesions (posterior indentation in the superolateral aspect of the humeral head, fracture of the anterior-inferior glenoid rim). A stabilizing surgical operation is proposed if physical therapy has failed after at least one relapse. Then the solution of choice is the screwed coracoid bone block. Anteromedial dislocation is a well-known event for which rehabilitation protocols have been clearly established: (1) anterior instability treated by anterior screwed coracoid bone block, (2) following a recent first episode of anteromedial dislocation, and (3) following a longstanding or recurrent anteromedial dislocation.

Posterior Instability

Posterior instability is much less common than the anterior form. It is found in athletes and results from high-energy trauma, falls onto the arm, or direct trauma to the stump of the shoulder. Posterior dislocation is more difficult to identify. In the patient history it is sometimes referred to as an episode of anterior instability. During clinical examination, the physician will test for apprehension in abduction/forward elevation/internal rotation; roentgenograms will be used for detection of anterior indentation in the inferomedial aspect of the humeral head and fracture of the posterior-inferior glenoid rim. After the stabilizing procedures (screwed iliac bone block and posterior capsular tightening), a well-defined rehabilitation protocol is used. In contrast, rehabilitation for conservatively treated posterior instability is very uncommon.

Other Types of Instability

Anterior or posterior subluxation cannot actually be classified as instability in the absence of radiological evidence of repetitive damage, even on arthro-CT scans. These minor events should be differentiated from other clinical pictures that may be seen in the throwing athlete and whose causes are posterosuperior glenoid impingement, structural or acquired hyperlaxity, or muscular deficiency resulting from injury to specific peripheral nerves. However, during sports activities, subluxation is a common sensation; the athlete feels a discomfort that is neither localized nor systematic. It may be recent and not be severe. In this situation, using arthro-CT for assessment of lesions is out of the question. A simple rehabilitation program over a limited period of time is advisable, whether it be for instability, glenoid impingement, hyperlaxity, or muscular deficiency. In my experience, the same postoperative regimen has been used in any of these cases. Should rehabilitation prove ineffective, a more accurate diagnosis is necessary.

The Principles of Rehabilitation of the Unstable Shoulder Are Based on Experience

Since 1985, all my observations have confirmed that whenever it was possible to restore about 150° of elevation, physical therapy could be continued, whereas when this was not possible, further exercises were precluded because of the pain caused by persistent capsular stiffness or unresolved subacromial impingement. Regarding shoulder instability, Saha demonstrated that immobilization in 150° of elevation is the optimal position for reduction of unstable fractures of the tuberosities, as this so-called zero position provides optimal balance of the glenohumeral joint. The zero position can actually be observed in the throwing motion: during the cocking phase, the arm is brought into retropulsion/external rotation past the zero position; then, during the acceleration phase, the arm is brought into forward elevation/internal rotation past the zero position again. In each sport, the arm is brought into specific positions during back and forth motion through this zero position. Rehabilitation aims at restoring the zero position and then controlling motion beyond that position during throwing. Practically, rehabilitation consists of two stages: progressive restoration of full range of motion and restoration of proprioceptive and plyometric control of the throwing motion.

Progressive Restoration of Full Range of Motion

Restoration of range of motion depends on healing time. The mean healing time for capsuloligamentous lesions in the unstable shoulder is 6 weeks. When managed surgically, an additional 3 months are necessary for healing of the bone block. Healing should be controlled in terms of both time and space, which means control of the forces applied to the scar tissue. To achieve optimal healing, one must respect the permissible tensioning threshold value for the collagen fibers that form the mechanical frame of this scar tissue. In practice, to achieve a well-controlled healing while avoiding microtears in the scar tissue, motion is started immediately but progresses slowly until healing is completed, that is, between 6 weeks and 3 months after surgery. One considers that full range of motion is restored when ranges of passive elevation and internal/external rotation are symmetrical and painless as measured at the beginning of a session of gentle passive exercises.

Restoration of Proprioceptive and Plyometric Control of the Throwing Motion

This is the most specific phase of the rehabilitation protocol for the unstable shoulder. In our approach to anterior instability, proprioceptive and plyometric control involves the anterior capsuloligamentous system and the internal rotators, particularly the subscapularis. This avoids the risk of anterior stretching injury during the cocking motion. We see no pathogenicity in the acceleration phase of throwing, but this will be discussed later on. During the cocking phase, the internal rotators have a very intense eccentric activity, whereas during the acceleration phase, they have an intense concentric activity. This cycle consisting of a stretching phase followed by a contraction phase is a plyometric cycle controlled by proprioception. Proprioceptive control involves a double mechanism: immediate and delayed. The immediate control is sensible to the slightest stretch and involves the neuromuscular spindles and capsuloligamentous mechanical receptors. This immediate control allows initiation of the muscle activity and setting this activity to a reflex mode, particularly the subscapularis, which acts in an eccentric fashion during the cocking phase. The delayed control involves the tendinous mechanical receptors; it is sensitive to excessive tendon tensioning (e.g., subscapularis). The delayed control allows inhibition of the muscle activity; it comes into play ideally before the tendon gets damaged. It is an inhibitor and protective reflex.

It should be pointed out that pain is a significant threshold between these two modes of control of the throwing motion. Passing this threshold during the cocking phase causes damage which results in an anterior instability lesion. In this case, pain must be analyzed as a cause of discomfort during the acceleration phase of throwing. This is the reason why one may be inclined to attribute the functional impairment to an assumed painful injury occurring during the acceleration phase rather than by an actual one during the cocking phase. Chronologically, during a plyometric cycle, the cocking phase does precede the acceleration phase: that is why the first injury is occuring during the late cocking phase. I shall return to this later on.

In rehabilitation, analysis is much more simple: any pain should represent the maximum permissible load level for a shoulder, and one should never exceed this subjective threshold value. Trying to force the motion beyond pain may also cause damage: in the conservatively treated unstable shoulder, this will result in poor healing due to overstretching of the capsuloligamentous lesions, thus increasing the potential for recurrent instability. In postoperative rehabilitation, pain may induce reflex stiffness as in adhesive capsulitis, which slows down progression. Extremely high muscular forces may result in nonunion or even loosening of the bone block.

Postoperative Rehabilitation of the Unstable Shoulder

One must bear in mind that a shoulder which has been treated surgically is no longer unstable. Rehabilitation aims at restoring progressively a full range of motion. In this respect, the simple self-directed exercise called overhead triple locking is most efficient. Forty-five days after operation, the capsuloligamentous structures have completely healed and a functional range of motion has been restored; at 90 days, bone has united and a full range of motion has been restored. There may be slight variations in healing time, whether an anterior or posterior bone block has been used. Thereafter, with progressive resumption of athletic activities, the patient will generally regain full control of his throwing motion.

Overhead Triple Locking

The self-directed overhead triple locking (OTL) stretching exercise is very simple indeed. In practice, the hands are folded (Fig. 1a) and placed behind the head at the occiput, with elbows back in the so-called siesta position (Fig. 1b). Then the arms are stretched

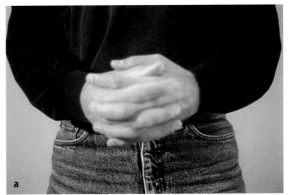
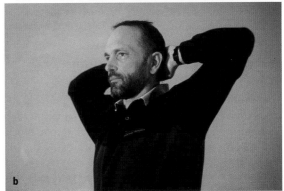
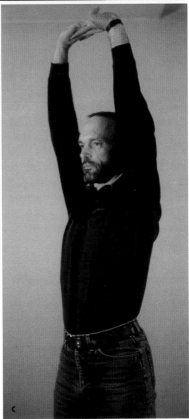

Fig. 1. Overhead triple locking (OTL). **a** Proprioceptive contact, hands folded. **b** Siesta position, external rotations (ER). **c** Stretching in full elevation

overhead until the elbows are fully extended with the palms of the hands facing upwards (fingers still interlocked) (Fig. 1c). In triple locking, the fingers are interlocked, the elbows are locked in full extension, and the shoulders are locked in full elevation. In the beginning, OTL can be performed with the patient sitting in a beach chair position to avoid any spinal compensation. Later on, the OTL can be performed in the standing position wherever and whenever desired. As it only takes 10 s to perform this exercise properly, it can be repeated several times each day. In the early rehabilitation period, the OTL is meant to limber the shoulder joint; once this has been achieved, it is used to stretch the thoracic muscles; eventually, it simply becomes a method of neurophysiological relaxation for the patient.

Overhead Triple Locking as a Limbering Exercise for the Shoulder Joint

The position with the hands clasped behind the head, elbows backwards, has an effect on the anterior capsule. According to the progression of the bone block healing process, a variant consists in moving the elbows forward until they meet: this has an effect on the posterior capsule. Stretching the arms overhead with the palms of the hands facing upwards affects the inferior pole of the capsule. Therefore, OTL limbers the entire capsule and covers 95% of the glenohumeral range of motion in the three directions; the remaining 5% corresponding to the final degrees of internal rotation are dealt with by placing hands in the back. Regarding the rotator cuff, OTL, which is performed entirely with clasped hands, is an ergonomic passive self-motion cycle that protects the patient against forced maneuvers. With the hands exactly behind the occiput and not behind the nucha, the humerus is elevated almost 150°, which corresponds to the zero position with its attached advantages: elimination of the detrimental deltoid elevating force, no subacromial impingement since the greater tuberosity passes under the acromial arch, and relaxation of the rotator cuff, which is subjected to balanced tensions.

Overhead Triple Locking as a Complete Stretching Exercise

In the late phase of limbering up, the OTL gradually involves all the muscles of the shoulder girdle and thorax from the center to the periphery of the glenohumeral joint: forward displacement and adduction of the scapulae with concentric activation of the stabilizers, trapezius, and rhomboidei; lengthening of the pectoralis major and latissimus dorsi with eccentric activation of the serratus anterior; straightening and extension of the spine with isometric activation of the paravertebral muscles; and gradual activation of abdominal and intercostales muscles. This diffuse muscle activation involving the whole thorax (all contraction modes) is maximal in the standing position, where all the pelvic and lower limb muscles come into play. Overhead triple locking provides complete stretching, similar to what is achieved with the famous "sun salutation" yoga posture.

Overhead Triple Locking as a Neurophysiological Relaxation Exercise

The OTL can be compared to a deep yawn, which is often accompanied by stretching. When complete, it provides for a few seconds a nice, relaxed feeling which often makes the patient close his eyes. Relaxation is followed (as with deep yawning) by a refractory period which eliminates the need for immediate repetition of the exercise. This relaxing effect is cumulative over 1 day or more and becomes optimal when the patient has made a habit of doing it. This relaxing effect is very strong during the postoperative period because during stretching, the operated shoulder is completely forgotten (from a nociceptive point of view). This gate-control effect is easy to understand: when the hands are folded, contact is established with the distal pulps. This simple contact (which is interrupted when a stick is used) activates the sensorimotor cortical area to which the hands are applied (cf. Penfield homunculus); the proprioceptive impulses generated by the finger interlocking and all the above mentioned muscle activations largely override the nociceptive impulses received from the operated shoulder, which explains this gate-control type of analgesic effect. In rehabilitation, pain is a signal for maximum permissible stretching with respect to the ongoing healing process. Stretching becomes more complete and the proprioceptive relaxing effect increases as the nociceptive impulses progressively decrease with time and healing.

Rehabilitation Protocol After an Anterior Screwed Coracoid Bone Block Procedure

Except in special cases (high-performance athletes, revision surgery, or bilateral surgery performed with a 15-day interval between the two operations), rehabilitation is always performed on an outpatient basis. The length of hospital stay is 2 days, after which the patient returns home with his arm in a simple sling. Sutures are removed 10 days after the operation. Forty-five days after surgery, the patient returns for a control visit in the presence of the physical therapist. A total of 20 sessions of physical therapy are prescribed and an individualized rehabilitation program is established for a period of 45 days (detailed information is provided to the patient).

From 3 to 45 Days Postoperatively: Restoration of a Functional Range of Motion

After the operation, the involved limb is kept at rest in a sling for 10 days. Then sutures are removed, the patient gets rid of the sling and, up to 45 days postoperatively, passive exercises are performed under the supervision of the therapist for restoration of a passive range of motion. Function is gradually restored for activities of daily living: 150° of elevation, 30° of external (ER) and internal rotation allowing the hand to reach the back. Passive and self-directed passive exercises are associated with hydrotherapy. The patient is encouraged to swim breast stroke, doing smooth and painless movements, and neither requested nor authorized to make any muscular effort.

From 45 to 90 Days Postoperatively: Restoration of Full Range of Motion

Forty-five days after the operation, the physiatrist examines the scar, evaluates range of motion, and checks for neuromuscular complications. At this stage, the spontaneous active motion pattern has been restored and the patient is fit for activities of daily living. The therapist teaches the OTL exercise that will have to be done at home each day, at first occasionally and then more and more often as stretching gets easier and more complete. Of course swimming is encouraged; activities of daily living require limited efforts. The patient is not allowed to resume sports requiring use of the arms; he can still do basic exercises as long as these do not actively involve the shoulder muscles. The last visit is scheduled 90 days after surgery; anteroposterior views are taken with three rotations of the humerus and one lateral view of the glenoid (Bernageau view to assess incorporation of the bone block).

After 90 Days: Resumption of Athletic Activities

Ninety days after the operation, the physician assesses the range of motion. The patient should have recovered a full range of painless movement. The control x-ray should confirm complete incorporation of the bone block. Strength is evaluated in elevation and rotation against manual resistance; it should be back to normal (although no specific strengthening exercises have been done). It is then considered that sound union has been achieved and normal range of motion and strength have been restored: the signal for the patient to resume athletic activities, knowing that it will take him 1 or 2 months of gradual efforts to return to the previous level of sport. No specific muscle strengthening is recommended, since there is no instability; resumption of the previous basic and specific training will suffice.

Rehabilitation Protocol After a Posterior Screwed Iliac Bone Block Procedure

The patient is discharged from hospital 3 days after the operation. His shoulder is immobilized in a splint with the arm at the side in 0° of external rotation so as to prevent internal rotation and allow the posterior capsule to heal after the tightening procedure associated with the bone block. After 30 days, he returns for assessment. From the 30th to 90th day postoperatively, the patient should perform passive and self-directed passive exercises to recover range of motion using (when possible) the therapy pool, as hydrotherapy promotes restoration of motion. A short stay in our shoulder rehabilitation department may also be indicated. A visit is scheduled at 90 days for clinical and radiographic assessment to make sure that the bone block is fully incorporated. A last visit is usually scheduled at 135 days for evaluation of the final outcome. The use of a splint during the first postoperative month accounts for this longer healing time.

Nonoperative Rehabilitation for Anterior Instability

In case the unstable shoulder has been treated conservatively, everything should be attempted to avoid operation which, in addition to the nuisance inherent in any type of surgery, spoils part of the patient's athletic season. In this respect, rehabilitation should not be more penalizing than surgery or last more than 3 months. Rehabilitation is focused mainly on muscle strengthening (to be discussed later). We have adopted our own simple method using a protocol with a limited duration of a few weeks and which meets both time and muscular requirements: weighted pendulum exercise and derived plyometric exercises.

Weighted Pendulum Exercise

Weighted pendulum exercise (WPE) is a complete pendulum exercise with progressive loading. In practice, the arm is extended overhead in a stable position with a light weight in the hand (Fig. 2a). Then the pendular cycle consists in letting the weight follow the descending ballistic impulse (Fig. 2b), bringing the arm into retropulsion (Fig. 2c). The movement does not stop and the patient's arm should immediately swing back to the initial position using the ascending ballistic impulse (Fig. 2d), which should be sufficient to stabilize the weight again in the overhead position without any effort (Fig. 2e). After the weight has been stabilized overhead and allowing the shoulder to relax for a very short lapse, a new pendular cycle begins. The patient is in ipsilateral single leg stance with the knee flexed to break

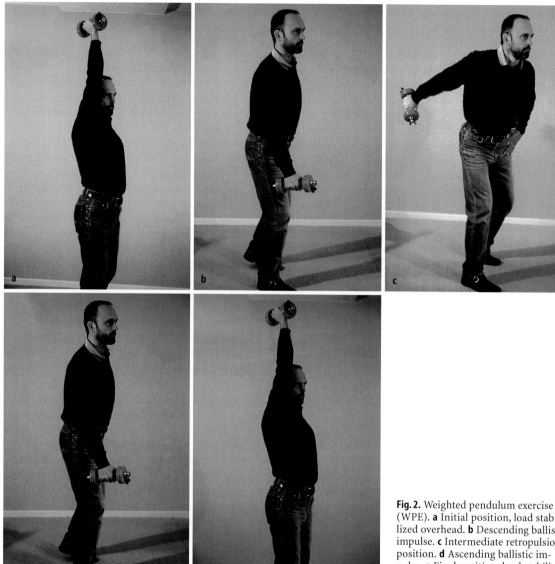

Fig. 2. Weighted pendulum exercise (WPE). **a** Initial position, load stabilized overhead. **b** Descending ballistic impulse. **c** Intermediate retropulsion position. **d** Ascending ballistic impulse. **e** Final position, load stabilized overhead

and accompany the movement; the contralateral foot is used as a stabilizing guy and the contralateral hand rests on the hip to prevent any spurious motion of the arm. The elbow should remain fully extended to avoid any whipping effect during the movement. The weight should be smoothly stabilized overhead, avoiding any posterior jerk when it reaches the vertical position. This exercise is best performed with the patient standing in front of a mirror for self-monitoring of the movement and acquisition of automatisms.

The Weighted Pendulum Exercise Is Harmless

The ballistic effect generates a centrifugal force within the glenohumeral joint which is proportional to the load, with a so-called decoaptation component that

tends to move the humeral head away from the glenoid and the coracoacromial arch. This component protects from anterosuperior impingement. The weight is smoothly stabilized overhead and not brought posteriorly: the arm is never ranged in full elevation/retropulsion/external rotation to avoid the risk of potential impingement, whether anterosuperior or posterosuperior. Therefore, WPE does not cause any trauma to the rotator cuff. As it does not generate retropulsion/external rotation forces, WPE also does not result in tensioning of the lesion, nor does it stir up instability-related pain. As a matter of fact, even though patients first hesitate to do the exercise with this weight in their hand through a range of motion of this magnitude, none of them has experienced any apprehension or pain during the movement, even with heavy weights.

Weighted Pendulum Exercise Teaches Multijoint Control

Control of the load intensifies as the load increases. It gradually involves all the ipsilateral articular chains, from hand closing to weight bearing. The glenohumeral joint is the rotation center of the whole system between the pendulous arm and the trunk and lower limb unit. Between the center of rotation of the shoulder and its periphery, several muscle masses and systems are progressively involved: capsuloligamentous system of the glenohumeral joint and rotator cuff, beyond the shoulder the deltoid, trapezius, and major depressors, beyond the shoulder girdle the paravertebral, abdominal, and intercostales muscles, and beyond the thorax the whole weight-bearing lower limb. The patient performs the exercise alternately with the right and left arms using gradually increasing loads. The WPE is an exhaustive multijoint exercise.

Weighted Pendulum Exercise Induces a Control Load-Related Muscle Activity

At the initial load level, WPE is a simple active-assistive exercise in elevation in which load is controlled by the hand. As in the overhead triple locking exercise, a gate-control type of neurophysiological effect is induced, especially since WPE is performed with the healthy arm first, is harmless to the rotator cuff, and does not involve the causative lesion. Control from all the involved muscles intensifies as the load increases. In no case is it a concentric exercise against resistance. It is an eccentric control reflex exercise that is performed during the descending and ascending ballistic phases. Due to the lack of experimental work, it is indeed difficult to appreciate objectively the intensity of the scapulothoracic muscle activity, even though it is a fact: typical delayed pain from eccentric training (e.g., sore trapezius after a session performed under maximum loading conditions).

Protocol of the Weighted Pendulum Exercise

Standard Protocol: Test Session Performed at Threshold Loads (Plus or Minus)

The therapist shows the WPE exercise to the patient, beginning with the unaffected side. Every detail of the exercise must be memorized: correct weight bearing, elbow fully extended, weight stabilized overhead with a brief relaxation of the shoulder. Throwing athletes are quick to memorize the exercise while others will need prolonged assistance. The initial threshold load corresponds to 10% of the body weight rounded off to the next full kilogram. An experienced athlete will start at the threshold load and a less experienced one may start at the threshold load minus 1 kg. The proto-

col is as follows: ten repetitions of the exercise performed at the selected initial load beginning with the healthy arm comprises one set; five sets performed alternately with the healthy and affected arm, that is 100 repetitions altogether (2×50), comprise one session. The patient is requested to perform one session per day 5 days a week (no exercises during the weekend). During the second week, the load is increased by 1 kg and the protocol is unchanged. In the third week, the load is further increased by 1 kg. This ends the 3-week cycle. Thereafter, if response to the treatment is satisfactory, the therapist suggests continuing with three sessions under maximum loading conditions at intervals of 2 days to allow for some rest (for instance on Monday, Wednesday, and Friday). For these three sessions, the initial load is set to 10% of body weight. The protocol of the first session consists of: one set of ten repetitions with each arm. Then the load is increased by 1 kg and the patient does another set of ten repetitions with each arm. The load is gradually increased in 1 kg increments up to the maximum load that the patient can stand – generally the nondominant side fails first because the hand is weaker. During the second session 2 days later, the load is increased in 1 kg increments but with two sets of ten repetitions performed alternately with each arm at each increment. During the third session 2 days later, three sets are performed at each 1-kg increment. In all, the WPE is carried out over a period of 4 weeks.

Advanced Protocol: Plyometric Exercises Derived from Weighted Pendulum Exercise

Plyometric exercises focus on dynamic control of the cocking phase of throwing by the internal rotators, particularly the subscapularis. The patient is requested to move his arm in a ballistic manner from internal rotation to external rotation with a weight in his hand while controlling the load eccentrically at the end of the movement and then to bring the arm back into internal rotation. This plyometric exercise uses the plyometric cycle of the throwing motion. It is intended to achieve control of the cocking phase under power/speed conditions as realistically as possible. The plyometric training mainly involves the subscapularis; it is performed in all three planes of space through a gradually increasing range of abduction to approximate progressively the real motion. The first exercise is done in standing position with the arm along the side and the elbow flexed at 90° (Fig. 3): ballistic movement in the horizontal plane from internal rotation (Fig. 3a) to external rotation (Fig. 3b), and then plyometric swing back to internal rotation (Fig. 3c). The second exercise is done in the standing position, with the patient bent over and his arm hanging toward the floor (Fig. 4): ballistic movement in the coronal plane from adduction and in-

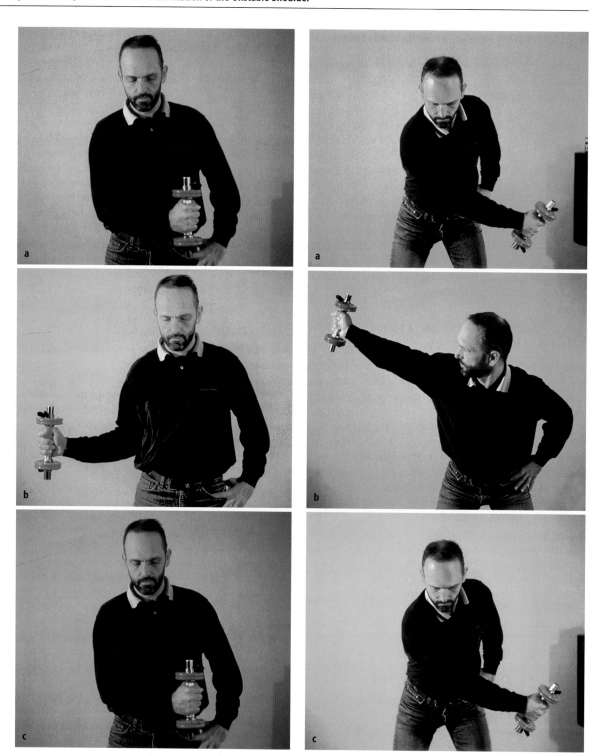

Fig. 3. Plyometric training of the subscapularis in the horizontal plane. **a** Initial position, static internal rotation (IR). **b** Control in external rotation, eccentric training of the subscapularis and plyometric swing back. **c** Final position, static IR

Fig. 4. Plyometric training of the subscapularis in the coronal plane. **a** Initial position, static adduction/internal rotation (ADD/IR). **b** Control in abduction/external rotation (ABD/ER), eccentric training of the subscapularis and plyometric swing back. **c** Final position, static ADD/IR

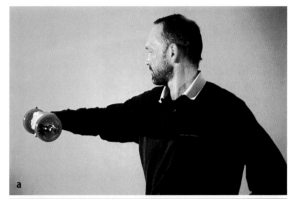

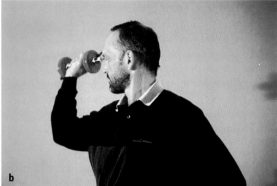

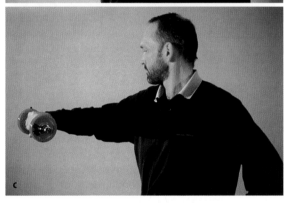

Fig. 5. Plyometric training of the subscapularis in the sagittal plane. **a** Initial position, static abduction/internal rotation (ABD/IR). **b** Control in abduction/external rotation (ABD/ER), eccentric training of the subscapularis and plyometric swing back. **c** Final position, static ABD/IR

ternal rotation (Fig. 4a) to abduction and external rotation (Fig. 4b), and then plyometric swing back again. The third exercise is performed in the standing position with the arm in 90° of abduction and the elbow flexed 90° (slightly forward) (Fig. 5): ballistic movement in the sagittal plane from internal rotation (Fig. 5a) to ER (Fig. 5b) and then a plyometric swing back into internal rotation (Fig. 5c). By increasing abduction of the arm (over 90°) and placing the elbow more or less anteriorly or posteriorly, the patient replicates his own throwing position. The common rule to

all the exercises is to increase gradually the load up to the maximum the patient can stand without pain or instability. He has then reached his tolerated stress level, with a maximum load at low speed. By decreasing load while increasing speed (as in racquetball), one reaches the same stress level: the goal is to restore painless movement and a feeling of stability. In all the above exercises, the initial load is low (2–3 kg), then gradually increased up to about 10% of body weight. The approach is less standardized than in the pendulum exercise; the patient's own feelings are determinant, since the motion is very close to his personal throwing motion. The ultimate exercise consists in replicating the true, complete, throwing motion with a weight: weighted racket for tennis, weighted ball for handball.

Rehabilitation After a First Episode of Anteromedial Dislocation

After a first episode of anteromedial dislocation, plain roentgenograms are taken: views of the dislocated shoulder and repaired shoulder, AP views with three rotations of the humerus for detection of a fracture of the greater tuberosity, Garth views for clear identification of the fracture of the anterior-inferior glenoid rim and indentation in the posterolateral aspect of the humeral head. One also checks for the absence of any acromiosternoclavicular lesion and neural injury (circumflex nerve). Immobilization in a sling and rehabilitation are then scheduled.

Healing with Use of a Sling

A sling is used for healing of post-traumatic and unstable shoulders. Immobilization is scheduled according to age. The older the patient, the shorter the immobilization: 45 days in a sling for a fresh capsuloligamentous lesion in a patient aged 20 years, 1 month in a patient aged 30 years, 15 days in a patient aged 40 years. Above the age of 40 years, one should check for a concomitant rotator cuff tear. The patient is allowed to take his arm out of the sling and let it hang along the body for self-care, to remove numbness from the arm from time to time, and to avoid ankylosis. No exercises, including isometric exercises, should be performed because they may cause pain, which will be more prejudicial to the muscle trophicity than immobilization in a sling.

Restoration of Functional and Full Range of Motion

Range of motion (ROM) exercises are started after full healing with the sling has been achieved, preferably in a swimming pool to benefit from the buoyancy of water, which facilitates painless movements. Passive and self-directed passive exercises are performed avoiding muscular efforts apart from those required for swimming, which is authorized as soon as a functional range of motion of 150°/30°/L5 has been restored. For 20-year-old patients, this phase of the rehabilitation program lasts about 15 days after 45 days of immobilization; the older the patient, the longer the passive motion phase. The risk of post-traumatic stiffness also increases with the age of the patient. Sixty days after the initial trauma, healing of the capsuloligamentous lesions is complete and the patient is fit for a sedentary lifestyle with routine activities.

Proprioceptive Rehabilitation

Weighted pendulum exercises are performed during 4 weeks, at the end of which the patient has acquired satisfactory control of maximum loads without stressing the freshly healed capsuloligamentous system. At this stage, one considers that there is no abnormal residual laxity of the anterior capsuloligamentous system and therefore no need for plyometric exercises. The patient is encouraged to return progressively (1–2 months) and carefully to his preinjury level of activities. This "running in" period is mandatory for a first episode of dislocation, as healing must not be disturbed. Should the patient experience pain at resumption of activities, it is better to progress more slowly than to intensify the efforts as, again, only time can guarantee positive healing.

Rehabilitation for Recurrent Anteromedial Dislocation

Generally, lesions resulting from repetitive damage do not heal and there is a residual laxity of the anterior capsuloligamentous structures. After a few days' rest, restoration of range of motion is quicker and of course much easier. Proprioceptive rehabilitation follows, with a complete 4-week program of pendulum exercises. If this phase is uneventful, that is, pain-free, the derived plyometric exercises are performed concomitantly. The goal is to achieve control of the maximum load as early as possible so that the athlete can return to his sport while remaining on the alert against recurrence of instability. Consciously or not, the athlete will temporarily restrain his movements. To achieve positive results, the athlete should get into the habit of including plyometric exercises in his warmup and regularly keeping them up.

Prophylactic Rehabilitation for Shoulder Instability

According to our approach to shoulder instability, the cocking phase of throwing is, at all stages, the cause of this instability. Will the athlete benefit from an efficient prophylactic method of treatment which minimizes detrimental effects of the forced cocking motion? This question links up with that of patients who experience discomfort during throwing but whose roentgenograms reveal no evidence of repetitive damage. The primary condition is that the prophylactic treatment should be simple and easy to perform. Our approach will vary depending on whether the shoulder is supple or stiff.

Prophylactic Rehabilitation for Supple Shoulders

This is the most common case. The goal is to improve control of the shoulder in the final degrees of external rotation. Prevention consists of incorporating WPE and derived plyometric exercises into normal training. In practice, the athlete who knows his useful load in WPE can gain time either by training at the same load level for varying durations or by doing a special session periodically with loads progressively increasing up to the maximum load. The same applies to the derived plyometric exercises by selecting the most efficient exercise and load. It is recommended to make a rule of performing the whole athletic motion under adequate loading conditions during warmup.

Prophylactic Rehabilitation for Stiff Shoulders

This is a less common case. Comparative evaluation of both shoulders is necessary in elevation and rotation (internal/external) to determine whether stiffness is structural (bilateral) or acquired (unilateral): a discrepancy of 10° is meaningful. The goal is to limber the shoulder in order to decrease its overall stresses: the OTL is of course the method of choice and should be used as often as necessary. Limbering up of the capsule should be supplemented by the usual stretching of the shoulder girdle, including the pectoralis major and triceps. If this yields good results as confirmed by rating of the shoulder, stretching should be done routinely. Should the patient still feel discomfort in spite of the limbering up, then proprioceptive exercises, pendulum, and derived exercises are necessary (as previously described). Any residual stiffness should be managed accordingly: hydrotherapy and extra-articular injections under fluoroscopic guidance.

Discussion

The principles and protocols described above are what we currently use for rehabilitation of unstable shoulders. They are based on our approach to this instability, the type of stabilizing procedures that have been performed, and the means available for rehabilitation. Three issues will be discussed: the cocking phase of throwing, which is the cause of pathologies other than anterior instability; the acceleration phase of throwing, which causes a specific pathology different from instability; and other methods of rehabilitation for the throwing motion.

The Cocking Phase of the Throwing Motion Is the Cause of Pathologies Other than Anterior Instability

Shoulder instability as presently recognized is only part of the instability felt by many throwing athletes. We also believe that the potential pathogenicity of the throwing motion is not limited to anterior instability. The cocking phase may cause posterosuperior glenoid impingement or reveal hyperlaxity, which will disable the throwing athlete. We propose the same proprioceptive rehabilitation protocol for the cocking motion, which aims at abolishing the pain from impingement and addresses hyperlaxity by increasing muscle tone progressively. Regarding impingement, the rehabilitation should yield results rapidly, in only a few weeks, and may be enhanced by injections under fluoroscopic guidance. In contrast, regarding hyperlaxity, the rehabilitation should be progressive over several months. To guarantee long-lasting results: in case of posterosuperior glenoid impingement, the cocking motion should be permanently modified and restrained; in case of hyperlaxity, proprioceptive exercises should be included in normal training.

The Acceleration Phase of Throwing is the Cause of a Specific Pathology Different from Instability

The acceleration phase of throwing is probably responsible for peripheral neuropathies from stretching (suprascapular and Bell's nerves). If treated after the onset period and if there is no indication for neurolysis, our protocol consists of appropriate exercises aimed at restoring better proprioceptive control, avoiding the high ranges of motion which cause the symptoms. In my experience, only one patient had a negative neurological response (immediately) to the pendulum exercise. Several months earlier, she had had axillary nerve palsy due to nerve compression in the quadrilateral space. The day after the first session of weighted pendulum exercises, she had diffuse, painful impairment of her shoulder motion which, although it was regressive, led to the discontinuation of rehabilitation. As to whether the cocking motion may be responsible for injuries from eccentric stretching of the external rotators or proximal injuries such as detachment of the long head of the biceps, I have noted that during the weighted pendulum exercise the descending ballistic impulse generates a normal amount of stresses in the shoulder. Our protocol allows for progressive loading up to the maximum, without any overstretching. A tennis player performing at a national level presented with a SLAP (Superior Labrum, An-

terior and Posterior) lesion evidenced by arthroscopy. She had been unable to play at her level for 2 years. After completing the protocol of pendulum exercises and without any additional rehabilitation or injections, she resumed training and later participated in competitions at her previous level of athletic performance.

Other Methods of Rehabilitation for the Throwing Motion

Some will hold either the cocking phase or the acceleration phase of the throwing motion responsible for instability or other disabling conditions, but in practice these two phases cannot be dissociated. However, obviously the cocking phase precedes the acceleration phase, and any injury occurring during the cocking phase has an effect on acceleration and follow-through phases. Finally, the plyometric aspect of the throwing motion concerns both agonist and antagonist muscles. Although we privilege the internal rotators, our rehabilitation protocol necessarily involves also the external rotators. This applies both to the pendulum exercise and the derived plyometric exercises. When doing this type of exercise, the athlete may insist more on a specific group of muscles without the therapist being aware of it. Other methods provide this type of exercise: manual resistance with the proprioceptive neuromuscular facilitation (Kabat), which requires a third person and therefore cannot be easily incorporated in the basic training, and closed loop proprioceptive and plyometric exercises, which are quite far from real throwing motion. Plyometric exercises performed with a medicine ball and a trampoline for optimization of the plyometric effect are the most appropriate for throwing sports such as baseball, whereas exercises performed with weights are more appropriate for racket sports such as tennis. Both types of exercise replicate the real motion. Exercises performed against elastic resistance are concentric and do not include a true plyometric phase. Although they are very convenient and easy to perform, we have found that they are neither very efficient nor well tolerated. Multidirectional and polyarticular bodybuilding including isokinetic exercises require special equipment and other habits than those we are in.

Conclusion

This approach to rehabilitation is based on documented results and a wealth of experience. Biomechanical, anatomical, and functional rationales are only used a posteriori as support to communication and argumentation with other colleagues. The athlete and physical training instructor, the physical therapist and physiatrist, the surgeon and sports physician must have a common language. We have chosen to perform exclusively proprioceptive and plyometric exercises. All the arguing about different or complementary technical options advocated by other teams should not make one overlook reality: the quality of the ongoing healing process and the cumulative stresses sustained by the patient during daily living and athletic activities have biomechanical consequences which are much more critical to the patient's progression than such-or-such specific point in the rehabilitation protocol. Finally, considering the social coverage of rehabilitation provided by health care systems, we propose specially designed rehabilitation protocols of limited duration. These may require significant means – for instance in the immediate postoperative course – but rapidly involve the patient, who is instructed how to perform the exercises and treated early on an outpatient basis.

References

1. Stanish WD, Rubinovich MR, Curwin S (1986) Eccentric exercise in chronic tendinitis. Clin Orthop 208:65–68
2. Saha AK (1950) Mechanism of shoulder movements and a plea for the recognition of "zero position" of glenohumeral joint. Indian J Surg 12:153–165
3. Saha AK (1971) Dynamic stability of the glenohumeral joint. Acta Orthop Scand 42:491–505
4. Matsen F, Harryman DT, Sidles J (1991) Mechanics of glenohumeral instability. Clin Sports Med 10:783–788
5. Johnson T (1937) Movements of the shoulder joint: plea for use of the "plane of the scapula" as plane of reference for movements occurring at the humero-scapula joint. Br J Surg 25:252–257
6. Maitland GD (1983) Treatment of glenohumeral joint by passive movement. Physiotherapy 69:3–7
7. Harryman DT, Sidles JA, Clark JM (1990) Translation of the humeral head on the glenoid with passive glenohumeral motion. J Bone Joint Surg AM 72:1334–1338
8. Burkhead W, Rockwood C (1992) Treatment of instability of the shoulder with an exercise program. J Bone Joint Surg 74A:890–896

Chapter 7

Rehabilitation of Elbow Injuries

7

Kevin E. Wilk, James R. Andrews

Introduction

Injuries to the elbow joint occur often in athletes. Although less common than injuries to the knee, shoulder, and ankle joints, those to the elbow can present a significant challenge to the sports medicine clinician. Often they are difficult to rehabilitate due to athletes' unique anatomy and the often excessively high stresses applied to the elbow joint during specific sport movements. Elbow injuries can occur due to microtraumatic repetitive stresses or macrotraumatic force. Overhead athletes experience sports-specific patterns of injury to the elbow. The repetitive overhead motion involved in throwing or tennis service is responsible for unique specific injuries. These may be caused by chronic stress overload or repetitive traumatic stress. Conversely, injuries to the elbow can occur due to large magnitude stresses during sports such as football, hockey, wrestling, or soccer. In these contact sports, falls onto an extended arm, blows to the arm, or abnormal movements can result in elbow dislocations, fractures, or muscular strains.

The purpose of this chapter is to discuss nonoperative and postoperative rehabilitation programs for a variety of elbow maladies. A rationale for each treatment protocol will be presented with an emphasis on multiphased, progressive rehabilitative regimens that are based on scientific research and clinical experience. The ultimate goal of therapy is to return athletes to their sports as safely and quickly as possible. Certain criteria must be met first: painless full range of motion (ROM) with sufficient strength, power, and endurance. These are accomplished by implementation of isometric, isotonic, and isokinetic exercises. Flexibility is gained by means of static and dynamic stretching in addition to proprioceptive neuromuscular facilitation techniques. A gradual return to sport is then allowed.

Injuries to the Overhead Athlete

The overhead athlete is susceptible to specific elbow injuries. Most of these injuries are seen in baseball pitchers but can also occur in javelin throwers and tennis players [1]. A number of forces act on the elbow during the act of throwing [2, 3], including valgus stress with tension across the medial aspect of the elbow. These forces are maximal during the acceleration phase (Fig. 1). Compression forces are applied to the lateral aspect of the elbow during the throwing motion. The posterior compartment is subjected to tensile, compressive, and torsional forces during acceleration and

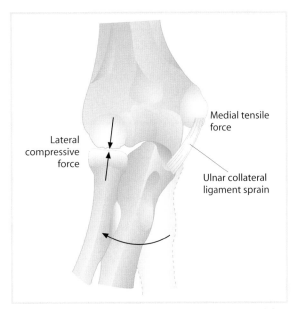

Fig. 1. Anterior view of the elbow with valgus load applied during throwing. Tensile load is placed on the medial side, particularly on the UCL. On the lateral side, there is a compressive force across the radiocapitellar joint

Table 1. Classification of elbow injuries in the overhead athlete

Medial Pathology
  Ulnar neuropathy
  Medial Epicondylitis/flexor-pronator tendinitis
  Ulnar collateral ligament sprains

Lateral Pathology
  Lateral epicondylitis/extensor tendinitis
  Osteochondritis dissecans

Posterior Pathology
  Valgus extension overload
  Olecranon stress fracture
  Triceps tendinitis

deceleration phases. This may result in valgus extension overload within the posterior compartment leading to osteophyte formation, stress fractures of the olecranon, or physeal injury [4, 5]. Table 1 classifies common injuries seen in the overhead athlete based on anatomic location.

Rehabilitation Program Overview

Rehabilitation programs for athletes must utilize the principles of training- and sport-specificity. Several principles of rehabilitation should be recognized and instituted: (1) the effects of immobilization must be minimized, (2) healing tissue must not be overstressed, (3) the patient must fulfill certain criteria throughout the phases, (4) the program must be based on current scientific and clinical research, (5) the process must be adaptable to each patient and his/her specific goals, and (6) the rehabilitation program must be a team effort with the physician, therapist, athletic trainer, and patient all working together toward a common goal. Ongoing communication with all involved is essential to expedite successful outcomes. Compliance with the rehabilitation program is enhanced by proper patient education.

Medial Pathology

Ulnar Neuropathy

Theories regarding the cause of ulnar neuropathy of the elbow in throwers have been postulated [6]. Ulnar nerve changes can result from tensile forces, compressive forces, or nerve instability. A combination of any of these mechanisms may be responsible for ulnar nerve symptoms.

Valgus stress can lead to tensile injury of the ulnar nerve. This may be coupled with an external rotation-supination stress overload mechanism. The traction forces are magnified with medial instability of the elbow following an ulnar collateral ligament sprain.

Hypertrophy of the surrounding soft tissues or the presence of scar tissue may cause compression of the nerve, or the nerve may be entrapped between the two heads of the flexor carpi ulnaris.

Repetitive flexion and extension of the elbow with an unstable ulnar nerve can irritate or inflame the nerve. Up to 16.2% of patients may be found to have this problem [7]. The nerve may subluxate or rest on the medial epicondyle (type A), rendering it vulnerable to direct trauma. Complete dislocation of the nerve may occur anteriorly (type B) leading to friction neuritis.

There are three stages of ulnar neuropathy [1]. The first includes an acute onset of radicular symptoms. The second stage is manifested by a recurrence of symptoms as the athlete attempts to return to throwing. The third stage is associated with persistence of motor weakness and sensory changes. Once this stage is reached, a reversal of symptoms by intervention with conservative measures such as rehabilitation would be compromised.

Often, ulnar neuropathy is a secondary pathology and symptomatic of medial elbow joint laxity caused by the ulnar collateral ligament (UCL) insufficiency. Thus, careful examination to determine UCL integrity is critical. Most throwers we see clinically are in stage one and more frequently stage two of ulnar neuropathy.

Table 2. Nonoperative treatment for ulnar neuritis

I. Acute Phase
A. Goals
1. Diminish ulnar nerve inflammation
2. Restore normal motion
3. Maintain/improve muscular strength
B. Brace: (optional)
C. Range of motion: Restore full nonpainful ROM as soon as possible. Initiate stretching exercises for wrist, forearm and elbow musculature
D. Strengthening exercises: if elbow is extremely painful and/or inflamed, use isometrics for approximately 1 week
1. Initiate isotonic strengthening
2. Wrist flexion/extension
3. Forearm supination/pronation
4. Elbow flexion/extension
5. Shoulder program
E. Pain/inflammation control
1. Warm whirlpool
2. Cryotherapy
3. High voltage galvanic stimulation
II. Advanced strengthening phase (week 3–6)
A. Goals
1. Improve strength, power, and endurance
2. Enhance dynamic joint stability
3. Initiate high speed training
B. Exercise
1. Throwers' ten program
2. Eccentrics wrist/forearm muscles
3. Rhythmic stabilization drills for elbow joint
4. Isokinetics for elbow flex/extensor
5. Plyometric exercise drills
C. Continue stretching exercises
III. Return-to-Activity Phase (week 4–6)
A. Goals
1. Gradual return to functional activities
2. Enhanced muscular performance
B. Criteria to Begin Throwing
1. Full nonpainful ROM
2. Satisfactory clinical exam
3. Satisfactory muscular performance
C. Initiate interval sport program
D. Continue throwers' ten program
E. Continue all stretching exercise

The conservative treatment program is focused on diminishing ulnar nerve irritation to enhance dynamic medial joint stability and return the athlete gradually to throwing. The rehabilitation protocol can be found in Table 2.

Following the evaluation process and, once the diagnosis of ulnar neuritis has been made, the athlete is instructed to discontinue throwing for approximately 4 to 5 weeks. This depends greatly on the severity of

Table 3. Isokinetic assessment

Bilateral comparison		
Elbow flexor	180/s	300/s
Elbow extensor	110%–120%	105%–115%
	105%–115%	100%–110%
Flexion: extension ratio	70%–80%	63%–69%

45' Phase

Step 1
A. Warm-up Throwing
B. 45' (25 throws)
C. Rest 15 min
D. Warm-up throwing
E. 45' (25 throws)

Step 2
A. Warm-up throwing
B. 45' (25 throws)
C. Rest 10 min
D. Warm-up throwing
E. 45' (25 throws)
F. Rest 10 min
G. Warm-up throwing
H. 45' (25 throws)

60' Phase

Step 3
A. Warm-up throwing
B. 60' (25 throws)
C. Rest 15 min
D. Warm-up throwing
E. 60' (25 throws)

Step 4
A. Warm-up throwing
B. 60' (25 throws)
C. Rest 10 min
D. Warm-up throwing
E. 60' (25 throws)
F. Rest 10 min
G. Warm-up throwing
H. 60' (25 throws)

90' phase

Step 5
A. Warm-up throwing
B. 90' (25 throws)
C. Rest 15 min
D. Warm-up throwing
E. 90' (25 throws)

Step 6
A. Warm-up throwing
B. 90' (25 throws)
C. Rest 10 min
D. Warm-up throwing
E. 90' (25 throws)
F. Rest 10 min
G. Warm-up throwing
H. 90' (25 throws)

120' Phase

Step 7
A. Warm-up throwing
B. 120' (25 throws)
C. Rest 15 min
D. Warm-up throwing
E. 120' (25 throws)

Step 8
A. Warm-up throwing
B. 120' (25 throws)
C. Rest 10 min
D. Warm-up throwing
E. 120' (25 throws)
F. Rest 10 min
G. Warm-up throwing
H. 120' (25 throws)

150' phase

Step 9
A. Warm-up throwing
B. 150' (25 throws)
C. Rest 15 min
D. Warm-up throwing
E. 150' (25 throws)

Step 10
A. Warm-up throwing
B. 150' (25 throws)
C. Rest 10 min
D. Warm-up throwing
E. 150' (25 throws)
F. Rest 10 min
G. Warm-up throwing
H. 150' (25 throws)

180' phase

Step 11
A. Warm-up throwing
B. 180' (25 throws)
C. Rest 15 min
D. Warm-up throwing
E. 180' (25 throws)

Step 12
A. Warm-up throwing
B. 180' (25 throws)
C. Rest 10 min
D. Warm-up throwing
E. 180' (25 throws)
F. Rest 10 min
G. Warm-up throwing
H. 180' (25 throws)

Step 13
A. Warm-up throwing
B. 180' (25 throws)
C. Rest 10 min
D. Warm-up throwing
E. 180' (25 throws)
F. Rest 10 min
G. Warm-up throwing
H. 180' (25 throws

Step 14
Begin throwing off the mound or return to respective position

Table 4. Interval throwing program, phase I

symptoms. A strengthening program is begun consisting of isometric exercises for the wrist, forearm, and arm musculature as well as shoulder strengthening exercises. Flexibility exercises also are begun to prevent muscular tightness and restore normal motion. The initial acute phase usually lasts approximately 2 weeks.

The second phase is considered the advanced strengthening period. The goals of this phase are: (1) improve strength, power, and muscular endurance, (2) enhance dynamic elbow joint stability, and (3) initiate higher special muscular training drills such as plyometrics. During this phase, the athlete continues the isometric strengthening program, but a greater emphasis is placed on eccentrics. Additionally, dynamic stability drills are initiated for the elbow stabilizers. Plyometric exercise drills also are initiated to prepare the athlete for throwing. The numerous specific plyometric drills are discussed later. This phase usually takes 2–4 weeks to prepare the athlete for the return to activity.

Table 5. Interval throwing program starting off the mound, phase II

Stage one: fastball only
Step 1: Interval throwing
15 throws off mound 50%
Step 2: Interval throwing
30 throws off mound 50%
Step 3: Interval throwing
45 throws off mound 50%
Step 4: Interval throwing
60 throws off mound 50%
Step 5: Interval throwing
30 throws off mound 75%
Step 6: 30 throws off mound 75%
45 throws off mound 50%
Step 7: 45 throws off mound 75%
15 throws off mound 50%
Step 8: 60 throws off mound 75%
Stage two: fastball only
Step 9: 45 throws off mound 75%
15 throws in batting practice
Step 10: 45 throws off mound 75%
30 throws in batting practice
Step 11: 45 throws off mound 75%
45 throws in batting practice
Stage three
Step 11: 30 throws off mound 75% warm-up
15 throws off mound 50%, breaking balls
45–60 throws in batting practice (fastball only)
Step 12: 30 throws off mound 75%
30 breaking balls 75%
30 throws in batting practice
Step 13: 30 throws off mound 75%
60–90 throws in batting practice 25%, breaking balls
Step 14: Simulated game: progressing by 15 throws per work-out (use interval throwing to 120' phase as warm-up). All throwing off the mound should be done in the presence of your pitching coach to stress proper throwing mechanics. (Use speed gun to aid in effort control)

The criteria we use to allow an athlete to initiate a throwing program are (1) full nonpainful ROM, (2) satisfactory clinical exam (in this case no neurologic symptoms, with adequate medial stability), and (3) satisfactory muscular performance. The criteria we use for muscular performance are based on isokinetic assessment (Table 3).

Once the athlete fulfills those criteria, the throwing program can be initiated. We start all throwers on an interval long-toss program beginning with light tossing from 45 feet. The throwing program's progression is based on increasing the distance, intensity, and number of throws gradually over the next several weeks. Once the thrower successfully completes step eight of the interval throwing program (phase I), he can initiate phase II, which is throwing from the pitching mound (Tables 4, 5). During this return-to-activity phase, the thrower is placed on a continuation of the strengthening program referred to on the throwers' ten program (Table 5). Once he successfully completes the throwing program, he may return to gradual play.

Medial Epicondylitis and Flexor-Pronator Tendinitis

Medial epicondylitis (golfer's elbow) in adults occurs because of changes within the flexor-pronator mass. During adolescence, chronic elbow pain referred to as "little leaguer's elbow" includes the diagnosis of medial epicondylitis [8, 9]. Associated ulnar neuropathy has been reported in 25% to 60% of patients with medial epicondylitis [10–12]. The underlying pathology is a microscopic or macroscopic tear within the flexor carpi radialis or pronator teres near their origin on the medial epicondyle. Tenderness over this site along with pain and resisted flexion or pronation distinguishes this diagnosis from ulnar neuropathy or ulnar collateral ligament injury. Throwers who exhibit flexor-pronator tendinitis may have an associated UCL partial tear or sprain. The tendinitis may develop as a secondary phenomenon. Differential diagnosis often is difficult. Steroid injection into the involved area should be used with caution, not be used early in the disease process, and be limited in number. Care must be taken not to inject the UCL because that could weaken its integrity.

The nonoperative treatment approach for athletes exhibiting flexor-pronator tendinitis is focused on diminishing the tendinitis inflammatory response and gradually improving muscular strength. Initially, treatment may consist of warm whirlpool baths, ultrasound with hydrocortisone cream (phono phoresis), stretching exercises, transverse massage, light strengthening to maintain musculature, high voltage galvanic stimulation to promote tendon healing, and ice massage. Once the patient's symptoms are significantly diminished, an aggressive strengthening exercise that uses concentrics, eccentrics, and isometrics may be used.

Table 6. Interval tennis program*

	Monday	Wednesday	Friday
First week	12 FH	15 FH	15 FH
	8 BH	8 BH	10 BH
	10-min rest	10-min rest	10-min rest
	13 FH	15 FH	15 FH
	7 BH	7 BH	10 BH
Second week	25 FH	30 FH	30 FH
	15 BH	20 BH	25 BH
	10-min rest	10-min rest	10-min rest
	25 FH	30 FH	30 FH
	15 BH	20 BH	15 BH
	10 BH		
Third week	30 FH	30 FH	30 FH
	25 BH	25 BH	30 BH
	10 OH	15 OH	15 OH
	10-min rest	10-min rest	10-min rest
	30 FH	30 FH	30 FH
	25 BH	25 BH	15 OH
	10 OH	15 OH	10-min rest
			30 FH
			30 BH
			15 OH
Fourth week	30 FH	30 FH	30 FH
	30 BH	30 BH	30 BH
	10 OH	10 OH	10 OH
	10-min rest	10-min rest	10-min rest
	Play 3 games	Play set	Play 1 1/2 sets
	10 FH	10 FH	10 FH
	10 BH	10 BH	10 BH
	5 BH	5 OH	3 OH

OH, overhead shots; FH, forehand shots; BH, backhand shots.
*Ice after each day of play.

Table 7. Interval golf program*

	Monday	Wednesday	Friday
First week	10 putts	15 putts	20 putts
	10 chips	15 chips	20 chips
	5' rest	5' rest	5' rest
	15 chips	25 chipping	20 putts
			20 chips
			5' rest
			10 chips
			10 short irons
Second week	20 chips	20 chips	15 short irons
	10 short irons	15 short irons	10 medium irons
	5' rest	10' rest	10' rest
	10 short irons	15 short irons	20 short irons
	15 chips	15 chips putting	
Third week	15 short irons	15 short irons	15 short irons
	15 medium irons	10 medium irons	10 medium irons
	10' rest	10 long irons	10 long irons
	5 long irons	10' rest	10' rest
	15 short irons	10 short irons	10 short irons
	15 medium irons	10 medium irons	10 medium irons
	10' rest	5 long irons	10 long irons
	20 chips	5 wood	10 wood
Fourth week	15 short irons	Play 9 holes	Play 9 holes
	10 medium irons		
	10 long irons		
	10 drives		
	15' rest		
	Repeat		
Fifth week	Play 9 holes	Play 9 holes	Play 18 holes

*Use flexibility exercises before and ice after.
Key to strokes: chips, pitching wedge; short irons, 8, 9; medium irons, 5–7; long irons, 2–4; woods, 2, 5; drives, driver.

Once the patient's strength and endurance have reached suitable levels, an aggressive strengthening program using plyometrics and a gradual return to sports may be initiated. We utilize interval sport programs to progress the patient successfully back to unrestricted sports (Tables 6, 7). An analysis of the patient's overhead sport mechanics may be helpful in recognizing faulty motions that may be contributing to this condition. This is especially true with recreational tennis players.

Ulnar Collateral Ligament Strain/Tear

Pain in the medial aspect of the elbow is common in both throwing and racquet sports. This results from repetitive valgus forces applied across the elbow [13]. A number of structures can contribute to symptoms in this location, causing a potential diagnostic dilemma. These include the UCL and flexor-pronator mass in addition to the ulnar nerve. A detailed history of the patient and physical exam usually can lead to specific diagnosis, although ancillary testing is helpful to confirm it. This is especially true when distinguishing UCL sprains from tears.

Ulnar collateral ligament ruptures occur in throwing athletes, most commonly in pitchers but also in javelin throwers, arm wrestlers, and collegiate wrestlers. The anterior band of the UCL is the main stabilizing structure in the elbow and thus the main elbow structure involved with throwing [9, 14]. Treatment requires open repair or reconstruction using an autologous tendon graft, commonly the palmaris longus tendon [15, 17].

Conservative treatment is reserved for UCL sprains or partial tears. The nonoperative treatment program for throwers with strained or partially torn UCLs is somewhat controversial. There is doubt whether or not to use immobilization or immediate motion. Additionally, it has been questioned whether a nonoperative treatment approach can be successful in throwing athletes.

The program we use employs motion of the elbow restricted from 20° to 90° immediately following injury (Table 8). This is used to allow the torn tissue's inflammation to calm and proper collagen formation and

Table 8. Conservative treatment following ulnar collateral sprains of the elbow

I. Immediate motion phase (weeks 0–2)
A. Goals
1. Increase range of motion
2. Promote healing of ulnar collateral ligament
3. Retard muscular atrophy
4. Decrease pain and inflammation

B. ROM
1. Brace (optional) nonpainful ROM [20–90°]
2. AAROM, PROM elbow and wrist (nonpainful range)

C. Exercises
1. Isometrics – wrist and elbow musculature
2. Shoulder strengthening (no ext. rotation strengthening)

D. Ice and compression

II. Intermediate phase (weeks 3–6)
A. Goals
1. Increase range of motion
2. Improve strength/endurance
3. Decrease pain and inflammation
4. Promote stability

B. ROM
1. Gradually increase motion 0–135° (increase 10° per week)

C. Exercises
1. Initiate isotonic exercises
2. Wrist curls
3. Wrist extensions
4. Pronation/supination
5. Biceps/triceps
6. Dumbbells: external rotation, deltoid, supraspinatus, rhomboids, internal rotation

D. Ice and compression

III. Advanced phase (weeks 6 and 7 to 12 and 14)
A. Criteria to progress
1. Full ROM
2. No pain or tenderness
3. No increase in laxity
4. Strength 4/5 of elbow flexor/extensor

B. Goals
1. Increase strength, power, and endurance
2. Improve neuromuscular control
3. Initiate high speed exercise drills

C. Exercises:
1. Initiate exercise tubing, shoulder program
2. Throwers' ten program
3. Biceps/triceps program
4. Supination/pronation
5. Wrist extension/flexion
6. Plyometric throwing drills

IV. Return-to-activity phase (weeks 12–14)
A. Criteria to progress to return to throwing
1. Full nonpainful ROM
2. No increase in laxity
3. Isokinetic test fulfills criteria
4. Satisfactory clinical exam

B. Exercises
1 Initiate interval throwing
2. Continue throwers' ten program
3. Continue plyometrics

alignment. The elbow most commonly is placed in a ROM brace to prevent a valgus condition to the joint. Isometric strengthening exercises are performed to the wrist and elbow joint musculature. We instruct the injured athletes to ice their elbows four to six times per day to control inflammation and pain.

The primary goals of the second phase are to restore full motion and gradually improve strength and endurance. During this phase, motion is increased by 5° to 10° per week for both flexion and extension. Therefore, by 6 weeks the patient should exhibit full motion. Additionally during this second phase, isometric muscle strengthening drills are initiated for the entire upper extremity. Rhythmic stabilization drills also are performed in this phase. The goals of these drills are to enhance neuromuscular control of the surrounding elbow musculature to improve dynamic joint stability.

The advanced strengthening phase usually is initiated at approximately 6–7 weeks after injury, and its primary goals are to enhance muscular strength, power, and endurance and gradually initiate higher speed drills in the position of throwing. During this time frame, the athlete performs an isotonic strengthening program referred to as the thrower's ten program (thrower's ten-exercise program) (Table 9). This program should be modified based on each patient's weakness and/or deficiencies. In addition, a plyometric program is initiated in this phase to prepare the athlete for throwing. Most frequently, we use several specific plyometric drills, including the two-hand overhead soccer, two-hand chest pass, two-hand side-to-side, and two-hand overhead side throws and the one-hand baseball throw.

An interval throwing program is initiated once the patient exhibits the criteria listed in Table 3. The long-toss program in Table 4 can be initiated as soon as the patient exhibits the criteria listed. Then the thrower is progressed to an off-the-mound throwing program (Table 5). However, our experience has indicated that throwers who exhibit a UCL sprain usually take 3–4 months for a return to play. Once the throwing program is completed, the athlete may return to competition. If symptoms persist, then reassessment is indicated and may lead to possible surgical reconstruction of the UCL.

Table 9. Throwers' ten program

Diagonal pattern D2 flexion and extension
External/internal rotation strengthening
Shoulder abduction
Empty can
Prone horizontal abduction
Press ups
Prone rolling
Push-ups
Elbow flexion/extension
Wrist flexion/extension
Forearm supinator/pronator

Table 10. Epicondylitis rehabilitation protocol

I. Phase I, Acute Phase
A. Goals
   1. Decrease inflammation
   2. Promote tissue healing
   3. Retard muscular atrophy

B. Cryotherapy

C. Whirlpool

D. Stretching to increase flexibility
   1. Wrist extension/flexion
   2. Elbow extension/flexion
   3. Forearm supination/pronation

E. Isometrics
   1. Wrist extension/flexion
   2. Elbow extension/flexion
   3. Forearm supination/pronation

F. HVGS

G. Phonophoresis

H. Friction massage

I. Iontophoresis (with anti-inflammatory agents, i.e., dexamethasone)

J. Avoid painful movements (i.e., gripping, etc)

II. Phase II, subacute phase
A. Goals
   1. Improve flexibility
   2. Increase muscular strength/endurance
   3. Increase functional activities/return to function

B. Exercises
   1. Emphasize concentric/eccentric strengthening
   2. Concentration on involved muscle group
   3. Wrist extension/flexion
   4. Forearm pronation/supination
   5. Elbow flexion/extension
   6. Initiate shoulder strengthening (if deficiencies are noted)
   7. Continue flexibility exercises
   8. May use counterforce brace
   9. Continue use of cryotherapy after exercise/function
   10. Gradual return to stressful activities
   11. Gradually reinitiate once-painful movements

III. Phase III, chronic phase
A. Goals
   1. Improve muscular strength and endurance
   2. Maintain/enhance flexibility
   3. Gradual return to sport/high level activities

B. Exercises
   1. Continue strengthening exercises (emphasize eccentric/concentric)
   2. Continue to emphasize deficiencies in shoulder and elbow strength
   3. Continue flexibility exercises
   4. Gradually decrease use of counterforce brace
   5. Use of cryotherapy as needed
   6. Gradual return to sport activity
   7. Equipment modification (grip size, string tension, playing surface)
   8. Emphasize maintenance program

Lateral Pathology

Lateral Epicondylitis

Lateral epicondylitis was first described by Major in 1883 [18]. It is also known as "tennis elbow," although it is estimated that approximately 5% of all cases actually result from playing tennis [19, 20]. However, it has been estimated that up to 50% of all people who play tennis will experience this pathology at least once [21, 22]. It occurs most frequently in the fourth to sixth decades and the incidence is equal between men and women except with tennis players, among whom it is more prevalent in men [19, 20, 23]. Treatment is directed toward conservative management and surgical intervention is reserved for refractory cases. The use of strapping has been shown to stimulate skin receptors with facilitation of muscle contraction [24]. As discussed with treatment of medial epicondylitis, steroid injections should be minimized.

The rehabilitation program for epicondylitis progresses through three sequential stages (Table 10). In the first or acute phase, the primary goals are to diminish inflammation and pain of the involved tissues and to minimize activities that aggravate the condition. Modalities such as cryotherapy, high voltage galvanic stimulation, ultrasound, iontophoresis, and whirlpool can be effective in reducing acute inflammation and pain. Gentle stretching exercises are performed to normalize motion. Submaximal strengthening exercises can be performed during this phase to prevent muscular atrophy. Frequently, isometrics can be initiated first, then isotonic exercises. It is important that painful movements and aggravating activities be avoided or minimized in an attempt to reduce inflammation and repetitive microtraumatic stresses.

During the subacute phase, the emphasis of the program is on restoring flexibility and the gradual progression of muscular strength. In this phase, strengthening exercises are progressed to use concentric and eccentric muscle loading. The emphasis is on eccentric muscular training. The patient is encouraged to use caution with excessive gripping activities.

The final phase is marked by the return of the patient to the sport activities that were aggravating in the past. The patient is encouraged to continue the strengthening, flexibility, and endurance exercises. Often they are encouraged to alter body mechanics or sports movements to prevent the recurrence of symptoms. The recreational tennis player or golfer is often instructed to seek the analysis of a teaching pro to ensure proper mechanics.

Osteochondritis Dissecans

Osteochondritis dissecans of the elbow was first described by Panner [25]. He reported this lesion in the capitellum, which is its most common location in the elbow. The etiology is unclear. Theories include vascular compromise and repetitive trauma [26, 27]. There also have been reports of familial tendencies [28, 29]. A majority of these cases have been reported in baseball players and gymnasts because of excessive loading to the lateral side of the elbow [30, 33]. In throwers, repetitive forceful extension and pronation of the elbow result in compressive forces that are transmitted from the radius to the capitellum. In addition, the capitellum receives end arteries terminating in the subchondral plate that are vulnerable to disruption. The capitellum usually appears in males at about 2 years of age and fuses at around 14 to 15 years. Thus, skeletal maturity is near completion when this condition occurs in adolescence.

Treatment options depend on the clinical and radiographic findings. Three stages have been identified for purposes of classification and treatment [36]. Stage 1 lesions include those without radiographic evidence of subchondral displacement or fracture. Stage 2 lesions are those showing evidence of subchondral detachment or articular cartilage fracture. Stage 3 lesions involve chondral or osteochondral fragments that have become detached and resulted in an intra-articular loose body or bodies. If there are no findings consistent with detachment of subchondral bone or articular cartilage or loose body, conservative treatment is indicated. This should consist of initial rest and immobilization of the elbow until irritability has resolved and is followed by institution of a rehabilitation program.

The nonoperative treatment program begins with 3 to 6 weeks of immobilization with the elbow flexed at 90°. The patient is instructed to perform ROM exercise three to four times per day. Once the symptoms are resolved, a gentle strengthening program can be initiated. The authors prefer to initiate isometric strengthening exercises for approximately 1 week, then progress to isotonic strengthening. The patient also performs stretching exercises for the entire upper extremity during this phase, with emphasis on the wrist and flexion musculature. Plyometric strengthening drills, eccentric muscle strengthening, and aggressive strengthening exercises can be initiated. Once these are successfully completed, an interval sport program can be started and progressed to a return to unrestricted sports.

If conservative treatment fails or there is evidence of an impending or documented loose body, surgery is indicated. This consists of arthroscopic abrading and drilling of the lesion with fixation or removal of the loose body [35]. Long-term follow-up has not supported a favorable effect on symptoms or radiographic changes from drilling or reattaching the lesions [36, 37]. Prevention and early detection appear to be the best form of treatment.

Posterior Pathology

Valgus Extension Overload

Valgus extension overload was first described in professional baseball pitchers by Bennett in 1941 [38]. This syndrome occurs during the acceleration and deceleration phases of throwing [39]. During these phases, excessive valgus forces coupled with medial elbow stresses cause a wedging of the olecranon into the medial wall of the olecranon fossa [40]. Repetitive extension stresses from triceps contraction also contribute to this condition. This eventually leads to posterior osteophyte development on the olecranon process that is responsible for the pain elicited posteriorly. Valgus instability of the elbow may further enhance osteophyte formation. Repetitive impact of the spur within the olecranon fossa may cause fragmentation and eventually loose body formation within the joint. These changes are mainly seen in baseball pitchers but also occur in javelin throwers who use the overhead throwing style.

A nonoperative rehabilitation program frequently is used before any surgical intervention is considered. The program initially is focused on diminishing any pain, soreness, and/or inflammation the patient exhibits in the posterior elbow flexors. By enhancing the eccentric strength efficiency or the biceps, brachioradialis, and brachialis muscles, we attempt to control the rapid elbow extension during the deceleration phase of throwing. This may be helpful in reducing the magnitude of the compressive load posteriorly. Occasionally, a young thrower who develops valgus extension overload may undergo a biomechanical pitching analysis to determine if faulty or undesirable pitching mechanics are present. Alterations in the throwing mechanics can then be detected by the player's pitching coach or biomechanist. A patient diagnosed with valgus extension overload is placed on a rehabilitation program similar to the one in Table 11. The standard program in Table 9 is altered to the individual's pathology, characteristics, and desired goals.

If conservative treatment fails, surgical excision of the posterior and posteromedial olecranon tip is indicated. This can be accomplished arthroscopically or through an open approach. We prefer the arthroscopic technique as it minimizes soft tissue involvement and allows for more aggressive rehabilitation.

Stress Fracture

Stress fracture of the olecranon has been reported in throwers and can occur at any part of the olecranon, especially the midarticular area [41]. This is likely caused by repetitive stresses from triceps extension during the acceleration, deceleration, and follow-through phases. It typically presents as an insidious onset of pain in the posterolateral elbow while throwing and afterwards.

Table 11. Nonoperative rehabilitation program for elbow injuries

I. Acute phase (week 1)
A. Goals
1. Improve motion
2. Diminish pain and inflammation
3. Retard muscle atrophy

B. Exercises
1. Stretching for wrist and elbow joint, stretches for shoulder joint
2. Strengthening exercises isometrics for wrist, elbow, and shoulder musculature
3. Pain and inflammation control cryotherapy, HVGS, ultrasound, and whirlpool

II. Subacute phase (weeks 2–4)
A. Goals
1. Normalize motion
2. Improve muscular strength, power, and endurance

B. Week 2
1. Initiate isotonic strengthening for wrist and elbow muscles
2. Initiate exercise tubing exercises for shoulder
3. Continue use of cryotherapy, etc

C. Week 3
1. Initiate rhythmic stabilization drills for elbow and shoulder joint
2. Progress isotonic strengthening for entire upper extremity
3. Initiate isokinetic strengthening exercises for elbow flexion/extension

D. Week 4
1. Initiate throwers' ten program
2. Emphasize eccentric biceps work, concentric triceps and wrist flexor work
3. Program endurance training
4. Initiate light plyometric drills
5. Initiate swinging drills

III. Advanced strengthening phase (weeks 4–8)
A. Goals
1. Preparation of athlete for return to functional activities

B. Criteria to progress to advanced phase
1. Full nonpainful ROM
2. No pain or tenderness
3. Satisfactory isokinetic test
4. Satisfactory clinical exam

C. Weeks 4–5
1. Continue strengthening exercises, endurance drills, and flexibility exercises daily
2. Throwers' ten program
3. Progress plyometric drills
4. Emphasize maintenance program based on pathology
5. Progress swinging drills (i.e., hitting)

D. Weeks 6–8
1. Initiate interval sport program once determined by physician
2. Phase I program

IV. Return-to-activity phase (weeks 6–9)
A. Weeks 6–9 – when you return to play depends on your condition and progress. Your physician will determine when it is safe
1. Continue strengthening program throwers' ten program
2. Continue flexibility program
3. Progress functional drills to unrestricted play

Symptoms are similar to triceps tendinitis; however, there is usually tenderness over the involved site of the olecranon. Bone scan or magnetic resonance imaging may be required to confirm the diagnosis if plain radiography is normal.

Conservative treatment consists of initial activity restriction for 6 to 8 weeks from aggressive strengthening exercises (such as heavy lifting), participation in sports, and any activities that aggravate elbow symptoms. During this time, the patient is instructed on stretching and ROM exercises to maintain motion. Additionally, isometrics and light isotonic strengthening exercises are initiated for the entire upper extremity musculature. If any exercise causes pain near the stress fracture site, the patient is instructed to discontinue that exercise and contact the therapist or physician. Usually by 6 to 8 weeks, the authors allow patients to begin a program to promote upper extremity strength and endurance. No aggressive strengthening exercises such as one-hand heavy weight lifting, plyometrics, or sports-related drills are allowed until bony healing can be shown by clinical and radiographic evaluation. This may require 8–12 weeks after the onset of symptoms. At this time, a light throwing program may be initiated. The throwing program consists of a long toss program (Table 5) progressing to a throwing program from the pitching mound (Table 6). Complete recovery may require 3–6 months.

If conservative treatment fails, surgery is indicated for internal fixation of the stress fracture with or without bone graft. Bony union can be expected in approximately 95% of cases with this treatment.

Shoulder Program

Any elbow rehabilitation program is not complete without inclusion of a shoulder program. These exercises should be initiated no later than the final stages of the elbow program and most appropriately in the second or subacute phase. Emphasis is placed on rotator cuff strengthening, with specific focus on the abductors and external rotators.

The concept of total arm strength is included in this program. This involves the development or maintenance of proximal stability and distal mobility to ensure adequate strength and neuromuscular performance. Thus, the rehabilitation program should include scapular muscle training and glenohumeral muscle exercise programs to help accomplish this (Table 9) [42–44]. These exercises are intended to focus on specific muscle groups active in the throwing motion.

Rehabilitation Following Elbow Surgery

Rehabilitation plays a vital role in restoring full unrestricted function following elbow surgery. Due to the excessive forces that are applied to the elbow joint, this joint appears susceptible to specific elbow injuries. Often these injuries require surgery to restore full pain-free function. The unique orientation of the elbow joint complex and particularly the high degree of joint congruency may account for much of the difficulty experienced by therapists in obtaining full motion and preinjury function. Therefore, postoperative complications such as loss of motion, persistent elbow pain, and muscular weakness may be due in part to the postsurgical rehabilitation program. The purpose of this section is to discuss these challenges and suggest treatment options that may lead to successful rehabilitation outcomes in the postsurgical elbow [45].

Rehabilitation following elbow surgery progresses through a multiphase approach that is sequential and progressive. The ultimate goal of this process is to return the athlete to his sport as quickly and as safely as possible. To enable a return to throwing, the elbow should exhibit the following criteria: full nonpainful ROM, no pain or tenderness, satisfactory muscular strength, and satisfactory clinical examination. Once these criteria have been met, the athlete may gradually return to sport-specific training and a progressive interval throwing program.

Elbow Arthroscopy

Elbow arthroscopy performed for diagnostic purposes or procedures such as debridement, loose body removal, or synovial resection generally causes minimal postoperative pain and stiffness. The postsurgical rehabilitation program can be somewhat aggressive in situations such as these [44] (Table 12).

In phase 1 of the rehabilitation process, the immediate motion phase, the goals are (1) to reestablish full nonpainful ROM, (2) diminish pain and inflammation, and (3) retard muscular atrophy. The exercises used during this phase are designed to restore motion, preventing the formation of adverse collagen tissue while respecting the healing constraints of the tissue involved.

Early motion exercises are performed to assist in collagen synthesis and alignment to assist in nourishing the articular cartilage [46–49]. Active assisted and passive motion exercises are performed for the humeroulnar joint to restore flexion/extension as well as supination/pronation exercises for the humeroradial and radioulnar joints. A major advantage of arthroscopic elbow surgery appears to be minimizing tissue morbidity; thus, aggressive immediate motion exercises can be performed following most arthroscopic elbow procedures. Reestablishing full elbow extension is a primary and critical goal during this initial phase of the rehabilitation program. A common side effect when this goal is not successfully accomplished is an el-

Table 12. Postoperative rehabilitative protocol for elbow arthroscopy

I. Initial Phase (week 1)
A. Goal: full wrist and elbow ROM, decrease swelling, decrease pain, retardation or muscle atrophy

B. Day of surgery: begin gently moving elbow in bulky dressing

C. Postop days 1 and 2
  1. Remove bulky dressing and replace with elastic bandages
  2. Immediate postop hand, wrist, and elbow exercises
  a. Putty/grip strengthening
  b. Wrist flexor stretching
  c. Wrist extensor stretching
  d. Wrist curls
  e. Reverse wrist curls
  f. Neutral wrist curls
  g. Pronation/supination
  h. A/AAROM elbow ext/flex

D. Postop days 3–7
  1. PROM elbow ext/flex (motion to tolerance)
  2. Begin PRE exercises with 1 lb weight
  a. Wrist curls
  b. Reverse wrist curls
  c. Neutral wrist curls
  d. Pronation/supination
  e. Broomstick roll-up

II. Intermediate phase (weeks 2–4)
A. Goal: Improve muscular strength and endurance; normalize joint arthrokinematics

B. Week 2 ROM exercises (overpressure into extension)
  1. Addition of biceps curl and triceps extension
  2. Continue to progress PRE weight and repetitions as tolerable

C. Week 3
  1. Initiate biceps and triceps eccentric exercise program
  2. Initiate rotator cuff exercises program
  a. External rotators
  b. Internal rotators
  c. Deltoid
  d. Supraspinatus
  e. Scapulothoracic strengthening

III. Advanced phase (weeks 4–8)
A. Goal: preparation of athlete for return to functional activities

B. Criteria to progress to advanced phase
  1. Full nonpainful ROM
  2. No pain or tenderness
  3. Isokinetic test that fulfills criteria to throw
  4. Satisfactory clinical exam

B. Weeks 3–6
  1. Continue maintenance program, emphasizing muscular strength, endurance, and flexibility
  2. Initiate interval throwing program phase I

bow flexion contracture [50, 51]. This can be a deleterious side effect in the overhead athlete. Flexion contractures can place abnormal stresses on various elbow structures, and this repetitive pattern may lead to further microtraumatic and/or macrotraumatic injuries.

Numerous factors may contribute and predispose patients to developing elbow flexion contracture, including (1) the intimate congruency of the elbow complex, especially of the humeroulnar joint, (2) the tightness of the elbow joint capsule, and (3) the tendency of the anterior capsule to scar and become adhesive. The anterior capsule is relatively thin and is very sensitive to injury. This may lead to many alterations in its anatomy that adversely affect normal elbow motion. The medial and lateral ligamentous structures are subject to contracture and occasionally calcification that can also severely compromise normal joint motion. Post-traumatic thickening of the lateral ligamentous structure can often cause impingement and snapping during active elbow movements [51]. Timmerman and Andrews [52] reported significant scar formation within the anterior, posterior, and lateral capsules of the elbow joint capsule in post-traumatic dislocated elbows with exhibited loss of motion. In addition, the anterior anatomy of the elbow is unique in that the brachialis muscle inserts directly into the anterior capsule, crossing as a muscle and not as a tendinous unit. Injury to the elbow may lead to formation of excessive scar tissue by the brachialis muscle and also cause functional splinting of the elbow because of pain. Once motion is limited or lost, changes can occur to the sarcomere of the muscle which may lead to additional motion restriction [53, 54].

To counteract the potential capsular restrictions, immediate motion is performed and joint mobilization [55] can also be used. Joint mobilization should be performed to the humeroulnar and radioulnar joints as well to promote the restoration of full motion. Another extremely effective technique designed to regain motion is a low-load long-duration stretching technique. An example of this technique to improve elbow extension is illustrated in Fig. 2. This type of stretch is performed for 10–12 min. The low-load long-duration stretching principle has been reported in the literature to produce a plastic response within the collagen tissue that will result in permanent elongation [56–59]. This type of stretching has proven to be extremely beneficial and superior to other techniques in restoring elbow motion and can be successfully used at home.

A second goal in this phase is to decrease the patient's pain and inflammation. Gentle joint mobilization techniques, oscillations of the joint, and gentle motion can all be beneficial in neuromodulating pain by stimulating the type I and II articulate receptors of the joint [55]. Additional modalities that can be helpful in decreasing pain and inflammation include ice, high voltage pulsed galvanic stimulation, ultrasound, whirlpool, and transcutaneous neuromuscular stimulation.

Also during this phase, muscular strengthening exercises for the wrist and elbow are initiated to prevent muscular atrophy. Patients are instructed to perform submaximal pain-free isometric exercises for the elbow and wrist flexors/extensors, pronators, and supinators.

During this first phase of elbow rehabilitation, the primary goal is motion, particularly in restoring full elbow extension. By attaining this goal, the most common postsurgical complication, elbow flexor contracture, is prevented. Stretching should be performed with caution to ensure that healing tissues are not overstressed and that the patient's pain complaints are not exacerbated.

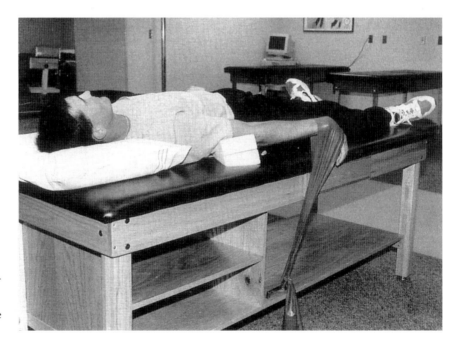

Fig. 2. A low-load long-duration (LLLD) stretch performed to enhance elbow extension. A low-resistance theraband is secured at one end and wrapped around the pateint's distal forearm

Phase 2, the intermediate phase, emphasizes the advancement of elbow mobility and improvement of strength, endurance, and neuromuscular control of the elbow complex. The criteria to progress to this phase include (1) full ROM, (2) minimal pain and tenderness, and (3) at least a good (4/5) manual muscle test grade for elbow flexors and extensors. If the patient has not fulfilled these criteria for progression, then we would continue with phase 1 activities until all of them are met.

In this phase, stretching exercises are continued to maintain full elbow and wrist ROM. Elbow extension and forearm pronation are important components to the thrower's elbow, making their flexibility paramount. In addition, wrist and shoulder flexibility stretching are also performed.

Muscular strengthening exercises are advanced using isotonic contractions (concentrics/eccentrics). Dumbbell isotonic progressive resistive exercises and/or elastic exercise tubing exercises are performed for the entire arm musculature. The muscles of the shoulder complex are also placed on a strengthening program during this phase, with a special focus on the rotator cuff musculature, abductors, and adductors. The concept of total arm strength is encouraged using proximal stability and enabling distal mobility to ensure adequate muscular performance and dynamic joint stability. In addition, neuromuscular control exercises are performed to enhance dynamic stability and proprioceptive skill. These exercise drills include proprioceptive neuromuscular facilitation exercises such as rhythmic stabilizations and slow reversal holds which can progress as tolerated to rapid diagonal movements (Figs. 3, 4).

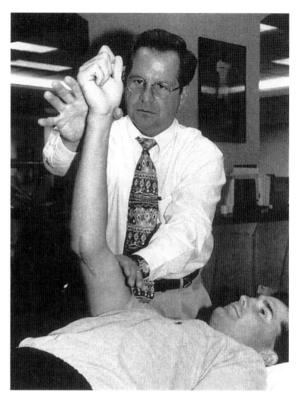

Fig. 4. Manual resistance proprioceptive neuromuscular facilitation drills to strengthen the entire upper extremity

The advanced strengthening phase, phase 3, is focused on progressively increasing activities to prepare the athlete for a return to sport. The specific goals of this phase are to increase total arm strength, power, en-

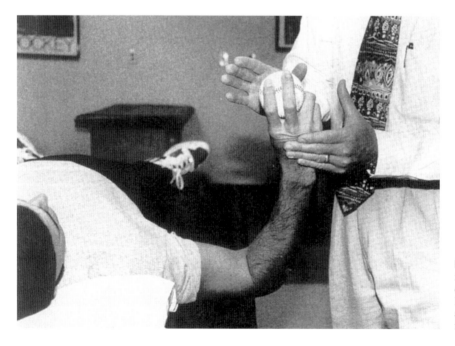

Fig. 3. Proprioceptive neuromuscular facilitation exercises for arm and forearm. Rhythmic stabilization drills are performed in a specific functional position

durance, and neuromuscular control. Meeting these goals will allow the patient a gradual return to sports-related activities such as throwing, tennis, or golf.

The criteria that must be fulfilled before entering this phase are (1) full nonpainful ROM, (2) no pain or tenderness, and (3) strength that is 70% of that on the contralateral side. These criteria should be fulfilled before initiating the specific exercises in this phase because of the explosive and aggressive movements required to perform these exercises.

Advanced strengthening exercises specific for the patient's activity are emphasized during this phase. These generally include high-demand modalities such as plyometrics and high-speed high-energy strengthening in addition to concentric and eccentric muscle loading [60].

Specifically, muscular training for the elbow extensors and wrist and eccentrics for the elbow flexors are all incorporated. The elbow extensors act concentrically to accelerate the arm rapidly during the overhead motion in many sports, whereas the elbow flexors act eccentrically to decelerate the elbow and prevent elbow hyperextension or the potentially pathologic abutting of the olecranon into its fossa during deceleration and follow-through phases. Thus, exercises are specifically designed to stimulate these specific muscle functions.

Plyometric muscle training is a form of exercise that is extremely beneficial in rehabilitating the overhead athlete [60, 61]. The basic principle of plyometric exercise is to use an eccentric muscle contraction to prestretch the muscle before a concentric muscular contraction. This stretch stimulates the muscle spindle that facilitates a greater or enhanced concentric contraction

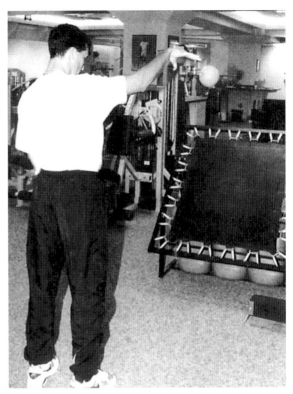

Fig. 5. Plyometric exercise drills replicating the throwing motion

during the exercise. Thus, plyometric neuromuscular training encompasses three phases: a stretch phase (eccentric loading), an amortization phase, and finally the response phase or concentric contraction. The throw-

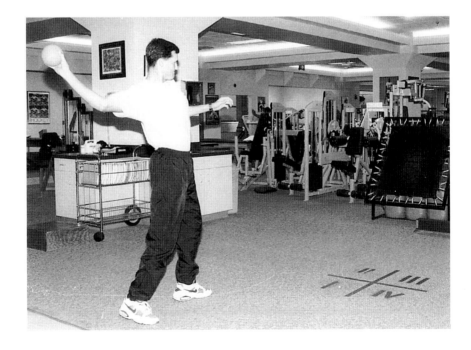

Fig. 6. Plyometric exercise drill, one hand baseball throw

ing motion is an example of a plyometric movement where cocking the arm produces a stretch on the anterior muscles to stimulate the acceleration (concentric) phase of the throw. Almost all sport movements use a plyometric form of muscular contraction.

Additionally, plyometric exercise drills are performed for the entire upper extremity and body using plyoballs and a plyoback (Functionally Integrated Technology, Dublan, Cal., USA). These drills can be used to replicate the throwing motion (Figs. 5, 6), improve flexibility (Figs. 7, 8), and/or teach weight trans-ferring and use of the legs to accelerate the arm (Figs. 9, 10). These drills can also be performed using a plyoball and a rebound wall. For a more complete description, a wide variety of upper extremity plyometric activities can be found in an article by Wilk et al. [60].

The shoulder complex musculature, especially the rotator cuff and scapular muscles, are also placed on an aggressive exercise program. Several years ago we established a thorough exercise program specifically designed for the overhead athlete called the "thrower's ten" exercise program [61]. These exercises are based

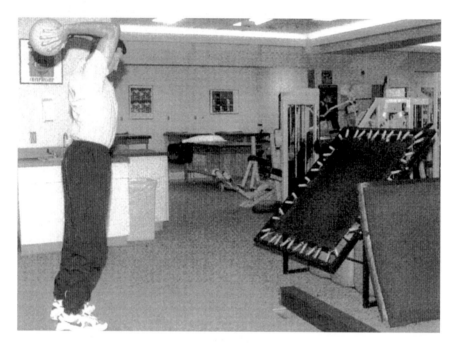

Fig. 7. Plyometric exercise drill, a two-hand soccer throw

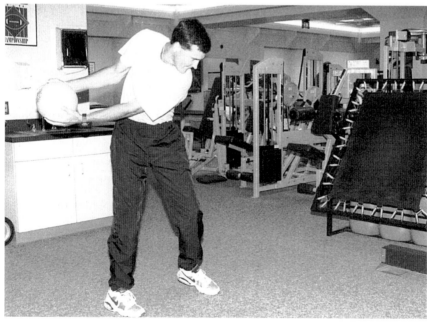

Fig. 8. Plyometric exercise drill, a two-hand side throw with rotation

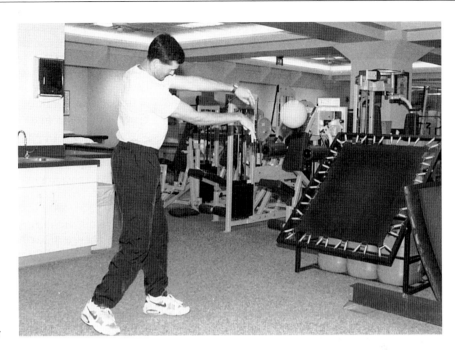

Fig. 9. A plyometric drill, two-hand side-to-side throw

on the collective works of numerous investigators and numerous electromyographic studies of the shoulder and arm musculature during exercise [62–66] (Table 9).

The last rehabilitation phase for the athlete's elbow is the return to activity phase. Its goal is to ensure that adequate motion, strength, and functional drills are performed to prepare throwers to return to their specific sports and positions. An interval throwing program is used to ensure gradual progression to unrestricted throwing activities (Tables 4, 5) or an interval

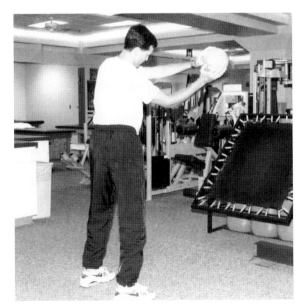

Fig. 10. A plyometric drill, two-hand side throw

tennis (Table 6) or golf program (Table 7). The principle of the interval throwing program is to increase demands on the shoulder, elbow, and arm progressively by controlling the intensity, duration, distance, type, and the number of throws performed.

Before an athlete is allowed to return to competitive throwing, specific criteria must be met. These are (1) full ROM, (2) no pain or tenderness, (3) an isokinetic test that fulfills set criteria, and (4) a satisfactory clinical examination.

The specific criteria of the isokinetic test are part of an ongoing study we are currently conducting. Routinely, the throwing elbow is tested at 180°/s and 300°/s in the seated position. The bilateral comparison at 180°/s indicates the throwing arm's elbow flexors to be 10–20% stronger and the dominant extensors 5–15% stronger than the nonthrowing arm. These data may be useful in providing objective muscular performance data regarding the thrower.

Following elbow arthroscopy, the immediate and primary goals are to reestablish full elbow ROM as quickly as possible. Immediately after surgery, the emphasis is placed on full elbow extension to prevent the formation of scar and elbow flexion contracture. Rehabilitation following elbow arthroscopy is intended to reinstate full motion as quickly and safely as possible; in most cases, this is accomplished 10–12 days after surgery. The advanced strengthening phase normally extends from week 3 or 4 post surgery until week 7 or 8. In addition, usually between weeks 3 and 6 after surgery (depending on the severity of the pathology), the athlete may initiate an interval throwing program.

Rehabilitation Following Ulnar Collateral Ligament Reconstruction

The rehabilitation programs following UCL reconstruction vary significantly based on the type of surgery performed, method of transposition of the ulnar nerve, and extent of injury within the elbow joint. There is a limited number of articles written describing rehabilitation programs following UCL reconstruction [67, 68].

Our rehabilitation program is based on the surgical technique described by Andrews et al. [17, 68]. Following UCL reconstruction, the patient is placed in a postoperative posterior splint and the elbow immobilized at 90° flexion for 1 week (Fig. 11). This is performed to allow initial healing of the UCL graft and soft tissue healing of the fascial slings for the transferred ulnar nerve. The wrist is free to move, and submaximal isometric muscle contractions are initiated for the wrist

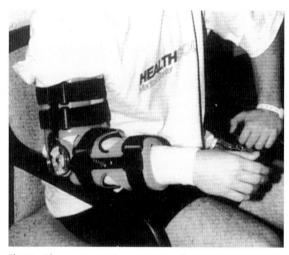

Fig. 11. The postoperative posterior elbow splint is used to maintain the elbow at 90° flexion

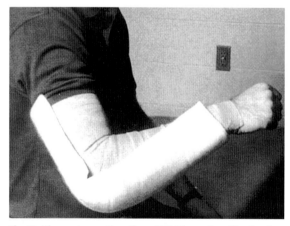

Fig. 12. The postoperative elbow ROM brace is utilized to improve elbow flexion and extension gradually. (Don Joy Brace, Smith and Nephew, Carlsbad, Cal., USA)

and elbow musculature. The patient also performs gripping exercises and cryotherapy with a bulky compression dressing to control inflammation and pain. At the end of the second week, the patient is placed in a ROM brace adjusted to allow motion from 30° to 100° of flexion (Fig. 12). During the third week, the brace is opened to allow 15° to 110° of motion. Every week thereafter, motion is increased by 5° of extension and 10° of flexion; therefore, by the end of the sixth week the patient should exhibit full ROM of the elbow joint (0°–145°). The complete rehabilitation program following UCL reconstruction can be found in Table 13.

Immediately after surgery and for the next several weeks, the physician and/or therapist must assess the status of the transferred ulnar nerve. Jobe et al. [69] and later Conway et al. [16] noted a 31% and 22% incidence, respectively, of ulnar neuropathy following UCL surgery with ulnar nerve transposition. Sensory changes of the little finger and ulnar half of the ring finger and/or the inability to adduct the thumb, weakness of the finger abductor/adductors, and abduction of the little finger and/or the flexor carpi ulnaris may suggest possible ulnar nerve injury. Often the patient conveys a slight sensory change along the ulnar side of the hand, but this is usually transient and should be resolved within 7 days. Often, immediately following surgery, the compression dressing may be too tight and simply loosening the wrap may alleviate the symptoms.

Strengthening exercises for the elbow, forearm, and wrist musculature are initiated immediately after surgery in the form of pain-free submaximal isometrics to prevent muscular atrophy. At 4 weeks, light-resistance isotonic strengthening exercises are initiated for the wrist and elbow musculature. By week 6, the patient is performing concentric/eccentric strengthening exercises for the entire upper quadrant. At approximately 8 to 9 weeks, the emphasis of the strengthening program is placed on sport-specific muscle training. The exercise program is designed to emphasize the muscle training and specificity of muscle contraction required by the muscle during the throwing motion.

During the intermediate and advanced strengthening phases, specific muscles are emphasized based on their roles during the overhead throwing motion. We have already discussed the important role played by the flexor carpi radialis, flexor digitorum superficialis, flexor carpi ulnaris, triceps brachii, and pronator teres muscles during the acceleration phase of throwing; these muscles should be exercised concentrically. The elbow flexors should feature an eccentric training program. In an anatomic study, Davidson et al. [70] noted that the flexor carpi ulnaris and flexor digitorum superficialis muscles directly overlay the anterior band of the ulnar collateral ligament and may provide synergistic support to the ligament. Because of this anatomic feature, we perform rhythmic stabilization exercises

Table 13. Postoperative rehabilitation following chronic ulnar collateral ligament reconstruction using autogenous graft

I. Phase I, immediate postoperative phase (0–3 weeks)

A. Goals
1. Protect healing tissue
2. Decrease pain/inflammation
3. Retard muscular atrophy

B. Postoperative week 1
1. Posterior splint at 90° elbow flexion
2. Wrist AROM ext/flexion
3. Elbow compression dressing (2–3 days)
4. Exercises such as gripping exercises, wrist ROM, shoulder isometrics (except shoulder ER), biceps isometrics
5. Cryotherapy

C. Postoperative week 2
1. Application of functional brace 30–100°
2. Initiate wrist isometrics
3. Initiate elbow flex/ext isometrics
4. Continue all exercises listed above

D. Postoperative week 3: advance brace 15–110° (gradually increase ROM; 5° extension/10° flexion per week)

II. Phase II, intermediate phase (weeks 4–8)

A. Goals
1. Gradual increase in range of motion
2. Promote healing of repaired tissue
3. Regain and improve muscular strength

B. Week 4
1. Functional brace set (10–120°)
2. Begin light resistance exercises for arm (1 lb) wrist curls, extensions pronation/supination elbow ext/flexion
3. Progress shoulder program emphasize rotator cuff strengthening (avoid ER until 6th week)

C. Week 6
1. Functional brace set (0–130°); AROM 0–145° (without brace)
2. Progress elbow strengthening exercises
3. Initiate shoulder external rotation strengthening
4. Progress shoulder program

III. Phase III, advanced strengthening phase (weeks 9–13)

A. Goals
1. Increase strength, power, endurance
2. Maintain full elbow ROM
3. Gradually initiate sporting activities

B. Week 9
1. Initiate eccentric elbow flexion/extension
2. Continue isotonic program; forearm, wrist
3. Continue shoulder program – throwers' ten program
4. Manual resistance diagonal patterns
5. Initiate plyometric exercise program

C. Week 11
1. Continue all exercises listed above
2. May begin light sport activities (i.e., golf, swimming)

IV. Phase IV, return-to-activity phase (weeks 14–26)

A. Goals
1. Continue to increase strength, power, and endurance of upper extremity musculature
2. Gradual return to sport activities

B. Week 14
1. Initiate interval throwing program (phase I)
2. Continue strengthening program
3. Emphasis on elbow and wrist strengthening and flexibility exercises

C. Weeks 22–26: return to competitive throwing

for the elbow to train these muscles and others near them to provide dynamic support to the joint and perhaps dynamically reduce the UCL load. We also focus on posterior shoulder girdle and scapular strengthening exercises to assist in decelerating the entire arm and diminish some of the compressive, valgus, and extension torques that could injure the elbow.

During the intermediate phase (weeks 4–8), the therapist and physician must continuously assess the patient's motion progression for contractures and/or joint stiffness, particularly the development of elbow flexion contracture. This can develop readily following any operative elbow procedure and is also common in overhead pitchers. Thus, prevention of elbow flexion contracture ensues through early intervention and progressive motion and stretching exercises. However, occasionally a patient's elbow may become stiff. To negate joint stiffness, particularly flexion contracture, we have found the following program to be extremely beneficial in rectifying the motion restriction. The patient may be placed in a splint to wear during the day and at night. A static splint can be used to hold the joint in a constant position or a dynamic splint can also be used. The latter uses a spring to exert a force to create progressive stretch. The patient is encouraged to remove the brace and perform motion and strengthening exercises two to three times daily and elbow stretching at least five to six times per day for approximately 10–15 min. Three vital components of the stretch are emphasized, namely duration (10–15 min), intensity (low to moderate), and frequency (five to six times per day). The advanced strengthening phase (weeks 9–14) is initiated only when the patient fulfills specific criteria. During this phase, an aggressive strengthening program is instituted consisting of plyometrics, eccentrics, concentric muscular contractions, and neuromuscular control drills. An interval sport program (Tables 4–7) can be initiated approximately 4 months after surgery. In most cases, throwing from the mound can be performed approximately 6 weeks later and a return to competitive sports at approximately 6 to 7 months following surgery.

Returning competitive throwers to preinjury levels is a significant challenge for the physician, therapist, athletic trainer, and athlete. Jobe et al. [69], reporting on surgically corrected UCL, noted that 63% returned to previous levels of throwing. Later, Conway et al. [16], reporting on 68 patients (average follow-up 6.3 years) found that 14 UCLs were repaired and 54 were reconstructed. Thirty-eight of the 54 reported reconstructions (72%) returned to throwing at previous levels, whereas only seven of the 14 in the UCL-repaired group were able to return to their previous athletic levels. Azar et al. [17] reported on 78 UCL reconstructions in athletes. The authors noted that 79% returned to their previous levels of competition or higher. In overhead throwers, the length of recovery (until return to competitive sport) was approximately 1 year.

In summary, appropriate rehabilitation is vital to the successful outcome following UCL surgery. Early motion should be used to prevent complications from loss of motion. An advanced strengthening program should be initiated before beginning a throwing program and include strengthening exercises to enhance joint stability, arm speed, power, and endurance. Because the flexor carpi ulnaris and flexor digitorum superficialis muscles are located directly over the anterior band of the UCL, these muscles are emphasized to provide dynamic support to the UCL. In addition, the biceps brachii are emphasized to control elbow extension and the shoulder arm scapular muscles (especially the posterior rotator cuff) are stressed to provide proximal stability.

Rehabilitation Following Posterior Olecranon Osteophyte Excision

A somewhat common pathology seen in the overhead thrower and other overhead athletes is the valgus extension overload syndrome [39, 40, 71, 72]. Because of the enormous stresses imparted onto the elbow joint during the acceleration and deceleration phases of the throw, the olecranon compresses against the olecranon fossa. Coupled with medial elbow stress during extension, the valgus stress causes impingement of the olecranon process against the medial wall of the olecranon fossa [72, 73]. This eventually leads to posterior osteophyte development on the olecranon process. Valgus instability of the elbow may accentuate this osteophyte formation. Surgical excision of the posterior and posteromedial olecranon tip is indicated in instances of pain and throwing disability. This can be accomplished arthroscopically or through an open posterolateral approach. We will discuss rehabilitation following arthroscopic technique, the procedure most frequently performed at our center.

The rehabilitation program following arthroscopic elbow arthroplasty is similar to that following elbow arthroscopy; however, the program is slightly more conservative. Elbow extension is often slightly slower to normalize, usually secondary to postoperative pain.

Range of motion is progressed as expeditiously as pain and patient tolerance allow. Usually by 10 days after surgery, the ROM is at least 15° to 100° and by 14 days it is 5° – 10° to 115°. In most cases, full ROM (0° – 145°) is accomplished by 20 to 25 days after surgery. Motion progression is often retarded because of osseous structure pain and synovial joint inflammation. If full motion is restored before 21 days, it is not a concern.

The strengthening program is similar to those in the previously discussed programs, with isometric strengthening during the first 10 – 14 days and isotonic strengthening during weeks 3 – 6. In the overhead athlete, a shoulder strengthening program should be instituted by week 6. In most cases, an athlete can begin an interval sport program 10 – 12 weeks after surgery. Again, the rate of progression should be advanced individually and closely monitored by the physician and therapist.

In throwers diagnosed with valgus extension overload, the nonoperative and postoperative rehabilitation programs should attempt to train the patient to control the rapid elbow extension during the acceleration and deceleration phases of throwing and also to stabilize the elbow dynamically against the valgus strain during arm acceleration. We have previously discussed the important role of the wrist flexor-pronator muscles in dynamic elbow joint stability with valgus stress. Additionally, the elbow flexors, particularly the biceps brachii, brachioradialis, and brachialis contract eccentrically to control the rapid rate of elbow extension and the abutting of the olecranon within the medial aspect of fossa. Therefore, this type of muscle control must be emphasized in the rehabilitation program. Andrews and Timmerman [74], reporting on 72 professional baseball players, noted that 47 (65%) exhibited a posterior olecranon osteophyte. Additionally, they noted that 25% of the individuals who had an isolated olecranon resection later required UCL reconstruction [74]. This may suggest that, in some throwers, subtle medial laxity may accelerate osteophyte formation on the olecranon.

Rehabilitation Following Ulnar Nerve Transposition

The rehabilitation process following an isolated subcutaneous ulnar nerve transposition is outlined in Table 14. This therapy uses fascial slings to stabilize the relocated ulnar nerve. Thus, rehabilitation must initially be fairly conservative to allow soft tissue healing to occur [67]. We use a posterior splint to immobilize the elbow at 90° flexion to prevent elbow extension and thus tension on the ulnar nerve. During the second week, the patient removes the splint and performs ROM exercises. By 3 to 4 weeks, full ROM is normally restored. Vigorous strengthening exercises are restricted until the fourth week. An isotonic program for the entire arm can then be initiated until the eighth postoperative week. Between weeks 7 and 8, an aggressive strengthening program can safely be used. An interval sport program may be initiated at 8 to 9 weeks if all the previously outlined criteria have been met. A return to competitive sports (i.e., throwing, tennis, etc.) can usually take place between 12 and 16 weeks after surgery [67].

Table 14. Postoperative rehabilitation following ulnar nerve transposition

I. Phase I, immediate postoperative phase (week 0–1)
A. Goals
  1. Allow soft tissue healing of relocated nerve
  2. Decrease pain and inflammation
  3. Retard muscular atrophy

B. Week 1
  1. Posterior splint at 90° elbow flexion with wrist free for motion (sling for comfort)
  2. Compression dressing
  3. Exercises such as gripping exercises, wrist ROM, shoulder isometrics

C. Week 2
  1. Remove posterior splint for exercise and bathing
  2. Progress elbow ROM (PROM 15–120°)
  3. Initiate elbow and wrist isometrics
  4. Continue shoulder isometrics

II. Phase II, intermediate phase (weeks 3–7)
A. Goals
  1. Restore full pain free range of motion
  2. Improve strength, power, and endurance of upper extremity musculature
  3. Gradually increase functional demands

B. Week 3
  1. Discontinue posterior splint
  2. Progress elbow ROM, emphasize full extension
  3. Initiate flexibility exercise for wrist extension/flexion, forearm supination/pronation, and elbow extension/flexion
  4. Initiate strengthening exercises for wrist extension/flexion, forearm supination/pronation, elbow extensors/flexors, and a shoulder program

C. Week 6
  1. Continue all exercises listed above
  2. Initiate light sport activities

III. Phase III, advanced strengthening phase (weeks 8–12)
A. Goals
  1. Increase strength, power, endurance
  2. Gradually initiate sporting activities

B. Week 8
  1. Initiate eccentric exercise program
  2. Initiate plyometric exercise drills
  3. Continue shoulder and elbow strengthening and flexibility exercises
  4. Initiate interval throwing program

IV. Phase IV, return-to-activity phase (weeks 12–16)
A. Goal: gradually return to sporting activities

B. A. Week 12
  1. Return to competitive throwing
  2. Continue throwers' ten exercise program

Rehabilitation After Arthroscopic Arthrolysis

The elbow is one of the body joints that most commonly develop loss of motion [75]. The elbow may be subjected to significant trauma such as a fracture or dislocation, although these are relatively uncommon in baseball. This type of trauma may cause both intra- and extra-articular injury. Periarticular soft tissue may be injured and become edematous and hemorrhagic and the elbow flexes in response to pain and the ensuing hemarthrosis. As a result, the particular soft tissue and joint capsule became shortened and fibrotic, and loss of motion develops [76–78]. Once this clinical sequela develops, a nonoperative treatment is used. If this conservative treatment fails, then arthroscopic arthrolysis may be necessary in selected cases [75].

The rehabilitation program following arthroscopic arthrolysis of the elbow capsule is aggressive in reestablishing full elbow motion (Table 13). During the first week after surgery, the patient is instructed to perform hourly ROM exercises, with special attention to restoring full elbow motion. We want to obtain full motion quickly but at the same time are cautious not to inflame the joint capsule, which may lead to further pain and reflex splinting. It is imperative to control joint swelling and effusion. During the second week, usually by 10 to 14 days, full passive ROM is restored. The use of the low-load long-duration stretching technique (previously discussed) is extremely beneficial in restoring motion. Isometric strengthening exercises are used during the first 2 weeks, with progression to isotonic dumbbell exercises during the third and fourth weeks. Once the patient accomplishes full ROM, a motion maintenance program should be used. Stretching exercises should be performed several times a day, especially before and after sports activities, for 2 to 3 months from the time of surgery to ensure that full motion is maintained.

Summary

In summary, immediate motion exercises that respect the healing constraints of the surgical procedure performed are imperative to ensure successful rehabilitative outcome in overhead athletes. Paramount to activities is the restoration of full elbow motion, which is essential to symptom-free elbow function. As the postoperative rehabilitation progresses, strengthening exercises must also be advanced to ensure the athlete has appropriate total arm strength, power, and endurance to return to symptom-free throwing. It should be remembered that there is more to strengthening than just dumbbells or exercise tubing. Rehabilitation programs should incorporate plyometric training, manual resistance techniques, and neuromuscular control drills, which are paramount to reaching power and endurance levels necessary for proper sport movements. In addition, by improving the muscular strength of the elbow, the extreme forces generated at the elbow joint may be dissipated. Finally, a systematic, progressive, and functional sports program including interval sport is also necessary for successful gradual increase in demands on the arm. It is not any one of these elements

but their coordinated and timely combination that allow the throwing athlete to return to free unrestricted
throwing after an operative elbow procedure.

References

1. Alley RM, Pappas AM (1995) Acute and performance-related injuries of the elbow. In: Pappas AM (ed) Upper extremity injuries in the athlete. Churchill Livingstone, New York, pp 339–364
2. Werner SL, Fleisig GS, Dillman CJ et al. (1993) Biomechanics of the elbow during baseball pitching. J Orthop Sports Phys Ther 17:274–278
3. Fleisig GS, Escamilla RF (1996) Biomechanics of the elbow in the throwing athlete. Op Tech Sports Med 4(2):62–68
4. Wilson FD, Andrews JR, Blackburn TA et al. (1983) Valgus extension overload in pitching elbow. Am J Sports Med 11:83–88
5. Andrews JR, Craven WM (1991) Lesions of the posterior compartment of the elbow. Clin Sports Med 10:637–652
6. Glousman RE (1990) Ulnar nerve problems in the athlete's elbow. Clin Sports Med 9:365–377
7. Regan WD (1994) Acute traumatic sports injuries of the elbow in the athlete. In: Griffin LY (ed) Sports medicine orthopaedic knowledge update. American Academy of Orthopedic Surgeons, Rosemont USA, 191–203
8. Deaven KE, Evarts CM (1972) Throwing injuries of the elbow in athletes. Orthop Clin North Am 4:801–808
9. Schwab GH, Bennett JB, Woods GW (1980) Biomechanics of elbow instability. Clin Orthop 146:42–52
10. Gabel GT, Morrey BF (1994) Medial epicondylitis: Surgical management, influence of ulnar neuropathy. J Shoulder Elbow Surg 3:511–516
11. Nirschel RP (1983) Medial tennis elbow, surgical treatment. Orthop Trans 7:298
12. Vangsness T, Jobe F (1988) The surgical treatment of medial epicondylitis. Orthop Trans 12:733
13. Bennett GE (1936) Elbow and shoulder lesions of baseball players. Am J Surg 18:921–940
14. Morrey BF, An KN (1984) Stability of the elbow joint: A biomechanical assessment. Am J Sports Med 12:315–319
15. Jobe FW, Stark H, Lombardo SJ (1986) Reconstruction of the ulnar collateral ligament in athletes. J Bone Joint Surg 28:1158–1163
16. Conway JE, Jobe FW, Glousman RE et al. (1992) Medial instability of the elbow in throwing athletes. Treatment by repair or reconstruction of the ulnar collateral ligament. J Bone Joint Surg 74:67–83
17. Azar FM, Andrews JR, Wilk KE, Groh D (2000) Operative treatment of ulnar collateral ligament injuries of the elbow in athletes. Am J Sports Med 28(1):16–23
18. Major HP (1883) Lawn-tennis elbow. B Med Joint Surg 2:557
19. Coonrad RW (1986) Tennis elbow. Instr Course Lect 35:94–101
20. Werner CO (1979) Lateral elbow pain and posterior interosseous nerve entrapment. Acta Orthop Scand Suppl 174:1–62
21. Nirschl RP, Pettrone FA (1979) Tennis elbow: The surgical treatment of lateral epicondylitis. J Bone Joint Surg 61:832–839
22. Nirschl RP (1988) Prevention and treatment of elbow and shoulder injuries in the tennis player. Clin Sports Med 7:289–308
23. Nirschl RP (1973) Tennis elbow. Orthop Clin North Am 4:787–800
24. McLean DA (1989) Use of adhesive strapping in sport. Br J Spots Med 23:147–149
25. Panner HJ (1929) A peculiar affection of the capitellum humeri resembling Calve-Perthes disease of the hip. Acta Radiol 10:234–242
26. Haraldsson S (1959) On osteochondritis deformans juveniles capitula humeri including investigation of intra-osseous vasculature on distal humerus. Acta Orthop Scand 38[Suppl]:1–232
27. Kvidera A, Madera D, Pedegano AL (1983) Stress fracture of the olecranon: A report of two cases and a review of the literature. Orthop Rev 12:113–116
28. Gardiner JB (1955) Osteochondritis dissecans in three members of one family. J Bone Joint Surg Br 37:139–142
29. Sougaard J (1964) Familial occurrence of osteochondritis dissecans. J Bone Joint Surg Br 46:542–543
30. Jackson DW, Silvino N, Reiman P (1989) Osteochondritis on the female gymnast's elbow. Arthroscopy 5:129–136
31. Naguro S (1960) The so-called osteochondritis desiccans of Konig. Clin Orthop 18:100–122
32. Smith MGH (1964) Osteochondritis of the humeral capitellum. J Bone Joint Surg Br 46:50–54
33. Pappas AM (1981) Osteochondritis dissecans. Clin Orthop 158:57–69
34. Morrey BF (1994) Osteochondritis dissecans. In: DeLee JC, Drez D (eds) Orthopaedic Sports Medicine. Saunders, Philadelphia, pp 908–912
35. Roberts W, Hughes R (1950) Osteochondritis dissecans of the elbow joint: A clinical study. J Bone Joint Surg Br 32:348–360
36. Baur M, Jonsson K, Josefsson PO et al. (1992) Osteochondritis dissecans of the elbow; a long-term follow-up study. Clin Orthop 284:156–160
37. Woodward AH, Bianco AJ Jr (1975) Osteochondritis dissecans of the elbow. Clin Orthop 110:35–41
38. Bennett GE (1941) Shoulder and elbow lesions of the professional baseball pitcher. J AMA 117:510–514
39. Indelicato PA, Jobe FA, Kerlin RK et al. (1979) Correctable elbow lesions in professional baseball players. Am J Sports Med 7:72–75
40. Andrews JR, McCluskey GM, McLeod WD (1976) Musculotendinous injuries of the shoulder and elbow in athletes, Schering symposium. Athletic Training 11:68–71
41. Nuber GW, Diment MT (1992) Olecranon stress fractures in throwers: A report of two cases and a review of the literature. Clin Orthop 278:58–61
42. Wilk KE, Arrigo CA (1993) Current concepts in the rehabilitation of the athletic shoulder. J Orthop Sports Phy Ther 18:365–378
43. Wilk KE (1994) Current concepts in the rehabilitation of athletic shoulder injuries. In: Andrews JR, Wilk KE (eds) The Athlete's Shoulder. Churchill Livingstone, New York, pp 335–354
44. Wilk KE, Andrews JR, Arrigo CA et al. (1997) Preventive and rehabilitative exercises for the shoulder and elbow. American Sports Medicine Institute, Birmingham USA
45. Wilk KE (1994) Rehabilitation of the elbow following arthroscopic surgery. In: Andrews JR, Soffer SR (eds) Elbow arthroscopy. Mosby, St. Louis, USA, pp 109–116
46. Coutts R, Rothe C, Kaita J (1981) The role of continuous passive motion in the rehabilitation of the total knee patient. Clin Orthop 159:126–132
47. Dehne E, Tory R (1971) Treatment of joint injuries by immediate mobilization based upon the spiral adaption concept. Clin Orthop 77:218–232, 1971
48. Noyes FR, Mangine RE, Barber SE (1987) Early knee motion after open and arthroscopic anterior cruciate ligament reconstruction. Am J Sports Med 15:149–160
49. Akeson WH, Amiel D, Woo SLY (1980) Immobilization effects on synovial joints. The pathomechanics of joint contracture. Biorheology 17:95–107

50. Green DP, McCoy H (1979) Turnbuckle orthotic correction of elbow flexion contractures. J Bone Joint Surg Am 61A:1092

51. Nirschl RP, Morrey BF (1985) Rehabilitation. In: Morrey BF (ed) The elbow and its disorders. Saunders, Philadelphia, pp 147–152

52. Timmerman L, Andrews JR (1994) Arthroscopic treatment of post-traumatic elbow pain and stiffness. Am J Sports Med 22:230–235

53. Gossman MR, Sahrmann SA, Rose SJ (1982) Review of length associated changes in muscles: Experimental evidence and clinical implications. Phys Ther 62:1799–1807

54. Tabary JC, Tabary C, Tardiev C (1972) Physiological and structural changes in the cat's soleus muscle due to immobilization at different lengths by plaster casts. J Physiol (Lond) 224:231–244

55. Kaltenborn KM (1980) Mobilization of extremity joints. Examination and basic treatment techniques. Olaf Norlis Bokhard, Oslo, pp 86–91

56. Kottke FJ, Pauley DL, Ptak RA (1966): The rationale for prolonged stretching for correction of shortening of connective tissue. Arch Phys Med Rehabil 47:345–352

57. Sapega AA, Quedenfeld TC, Moyer RA et al. (1976) Biophysical factors in range of motion exercise. Arch Phys Med Rehabil 57:122–126

58. Warren CG, Lehmann JF, Koblanski JN (1976) Heat and stretch procedures: An evaluation using rat tail tendon. Arch Phys Med Rehabil 57:122–126

59. Warren CB, Lehmann JF, Koblanski JN (1971) Elongation of rat tail tendon: Effect of load and temperature. Arch Phys Med Rehabil 52:465–474

60. Wilk KE, Voight M, Keirns MJ et al. (1993) Plyometrics for the upper extremities: Theory and clinical application. J Orthop Sports Phys Ther 17:225–239

61. Wilk KE, Arrigo CA, Courson RE et al. (1991) Preventive and rehabilitation exercises for the shoulder and elbow (edn 3). American Sports Medicine Institute, Birmingham, USA

62. Moseley JS, Jobe FW, Pink M et al. (1991) Electromyographic analysis of the glenohumeral muscles during a baseball rehabilitation program. Am J Sports Med 19:264–269

63. Townsend H, Jobe FW, Pink M et al. (1991) Electromyographic analysis of the glenohumeral muscles during a baseball rehabilitation program. Am J Sports Med 19:264–269

64. Blackburn TA, McLeod WD, White B (1990) EMG analysis of posterior rotator cuff exercises. Athl Training 25:40–45

65. Jobe FW, Moynes DW (1985) Delineation of diagnostic criteria and a rehabilitation program for rotator cuff injuries. Am J Sports Med 10:336–340

66. Pappas AM, Zawacki RM: (1985) Rehabilitation of the pitching shoulder. Am J Sports Med 13:223–226

67. Wilk KE, Arrigo CA, Andrews JR (1993) Rehabilitation of the elbow in the throwing athlete. J Orthop Sports Phys Ther 17:305–317

68. Andrews JR, Joyce M, Jelsma R et al. (1996) Open surgical procedures for injuries to the elbow in throwers. Op Tech Sports Med 4:109–113

69. Jobe FW, Stark H, Lombardo SJ (1986) Reconstruction of the ulnar collateral ligament in athletes. J Bone Joint Surg 68:1158–1163

70. Davidson PA, Pink M, Perry J et al. (1995) Functional anatomy of the flexor pronator muscle in group relation to the medial collateral ligament of the elbow. Am J Sports Med 23:245–250

71. Bennett GE (1941) Shoulder and elbow lesions of the professional baseball pitcher. J Am Med Assoc 117:510–514

72. Andrews JR, Frank W (1985) Valgus extension overload in the pitching elbow. In: Andrews JR, Zarins B, Carson WB (eds) Injuries to the throwing arm. Saunders, Philadelphia, pp 250–257

73. Wilson FD, Andrews JR, Blackburn TA et al. (1983) Valgus extension overload in the pitching elbow. Am J Sports Med 11:83–87

74. Andrews JR, Timmerman L (1995) Outcome of elbow surgery in professional baseball players. Am J Sports Med 23:407–413

75. Soffer SR, Andrews JR (1994) Arthroscopic surgical procedure of the elbow: Common cases. In: Andrews JR, Soffer SR (eds) Elbow arthroscopy. Mosby, St. Louis, USA, pp 74–78

76. Green DP, McCoy H (1979) Turnbuckle orthotic correction of elbow flexion contractures after acute injuries. J Bone Joint Surg Am 61A:1092–1096

77. Buxton JD (1985) Ossification in the ligaments of the elbow. Contemp Orthop 11:21–26

78. Morrey BF (1985) The elbow and its disorders. W.B. Saunders, Philadelphia

8 Rehabilitation of Hand and Wrist Injuries

Antonio Castagnaro

Introduction

Sport has become a widespread social phenomenon at both professional and amateur levels. The number of participants is also increasing, but very often these athletes lack necessary physical training and in many cases expect their bodies to perform beyond capacity. As a consequence, sports injuries to the hand and wrist are on the increase. If we consider the overall view, hand and wrist injuries have an important place in general sport pathology inasmuch as they represent 5% to 31% of all sport traumatisms (Table 1).

Table 1. Incidence rate of hand traumas compared with general muscle-skeletal traumas in sports activities

Sport	Percentage
Boxing	31
Handball	30
Volleyball	23
Basketball	19
Gymnastics	17
Ski	16
Judo	10
Ice hockey	5

Very often, these injuries are only examined and treated subsequently, and this accentuates the therapeutic and rehabilitation problems. The sportsman as such is not the ideal patient, because he tends to minimise the seriousness of injuries. He does not want to interrupt his sporting activity (perhaps also for economic reasons) or he wants to resume too soon to avoid losing his place in the team, which obviously complicates rehabilitation treatment.

In this chapter the main sports injuries to the hand and wrist are listed, along with their relative treatments.

Hand

Metacarpal Fractures

The majority of metacarpal fractures are stable and treated with a brace or set in plaster. The time before resumption of sporting activity is clearly correlated to the type of sport practised. Usually it takes at least 15 days before training can be resumed and at least 25 before competitive activity may begin. For unstable fractures, open reduction is necessary and metal fixation must be used (screws or wire). In this case, the time needed for a return to the sport is shortened (12 days before starting training and 20 days before competitive activity).

Fractures at the base of the metacarpals or the proximal metaphysis are not treated surgically and modelled braces are applied which leave the fingers free. To avoid rotation, the metacarpal in question is normally fixed to an adjacent finger by means of a Velcro strip (in a figure of eight), and the athlete is encouraged to mobilise his fingers to decrease the edema. Furthermore, the limb is elevated, and an ice pack is applied and wrapped in coban.

Flexion movement of the interphalanges (IP) while the metacarpal phalanges (MCP) are held flexed not only aids the pump action and therefore lessens the hand's swelling, but the mobilisation of the fingers aids the compressive forces on the fracture, stimulating healing without provoking its dislocation [9]. Furthermore, early mobilisation prevents tendon adherence and diminishes ligament stiffness. Finger movement begins only when the fracture is stable (in the first weeks). Fractures treated surgically are also mobilised right from the first weeks, but only passively.

Cutaneous lesions are also very often associated with some fractures, and therefore scar adhesions tend to form between the tendons and the cutaneous layer. Such a problem can be resolved with early passive mobilisation, massages on the scar (which must be carried out along the scar in the opposite direction to the action of the tendon) [2], and electrical muscle stimulation (EMS).

In order to aid precocious passive mobilisation and avoid scar adherence or stiffness of the joints, continuous passive motion (CPM) is used for the hand (Fig. 1), which allows the patient to mobilise his hand repeatedly during the course of the day (4–6 times) for about 15–20 min at a time.

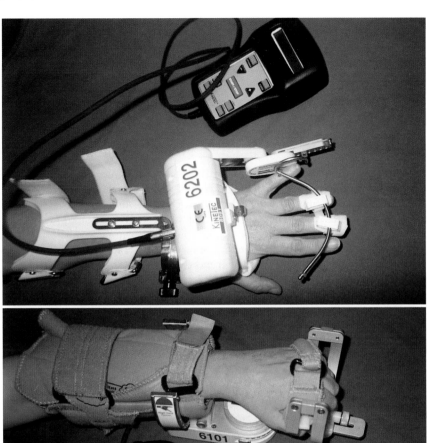

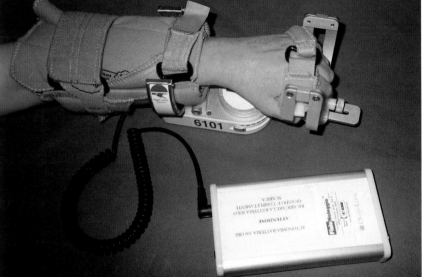

Fig. 1. CPM for hand and wrist

Fracture of the Proximal Phalanx

If stable, fractures of the first phalanx of the fingers (P1), excluding thumb, are usually treated with a valve brace and fastened with a plaster glove or plastic static splint. Unstable fractures must be treated with a closed reduction and plaster (and K-wires) or with an open reduction and internal fixation (microscrews). In this case, the patient is also advised to mobilise the fingers as soon as possible in order to facilitate tendon motion and reduce the risk of scar adherence. To improve movement of the interphalangeal joints, an analytic exercise is advised which consists of keeping the MCP fixed in extension and actively bending the PIP; therefore the PIP is fixed in extension while the DIP is actively bent.

In order to differentiate the movement of the flexor digitorum superficialis (FDS) and the flexor digitorum profundus (FDP), the patient is invited to carry out the so-called four fists exercise: starting with the hand in an open position, the hook position is performed (bending the PIP and DIP with MCP extended); then the MCP and the PIP (at 90°) are bent while the DIP is extended; then the hand is made into a fist with overall bending of the three joints.

Intra-articular fractures of the DIP which are slightly dislocated are treated with a brace for 3–4 weeks. The active movements are carried out after 15 days and only after an x-ray. Unstable intra-articular fractures need to be treated surgically (open reduction and internal fixation with microscrews or K-wires). Actively assisted exercises start right from the first week. A splint is kept on for at least 6 weeks.

Such injuries often provoke rigidity of the joints and contractures. For this reason, it is indispensable to start passive mobilisation as soon as possible, especially if the fixation obtained is very stable.

Fractures of the Second and Third Phalanges of the Fingers

Fractures of the middle phalanx (P2) often occur due to a direct trauma; they are not dislocated and heal with the application of a finger brace held in an extended position. Sports activity can be resumed at a very early stage wearing the brace. Fractures of the third phalanx (P3) are also treated by applying a simple brace, and the athlete can resume sport activities after 10 days (always wearing the Stax splint) (Fig. 2).

The so-called mallet finger needs special treatment, especially when the fracture at the base of the distal phalanx (Segond lesions) (Fig. 3) concerns the portion where the extensor tendon is inserted. The traction of the extensor tendon determines a diastasis of the fracture. Such lesions are dealt with in the chapter regarding lesions of the extensor tendon.

Collateral Ligament Lesions of the PIP and MCP

Collateral ligament lesions of the PIP (grade I) are treated with a Velcro splint (figure of eight) joining the injured finger to the proximal one (Fig. 4). The athlete is invited to move his finger gently by flexion and extension and can resume sporting activity very soon, depending on the type of sport practised. The brace should be worn for about a month.

With grades II and III lesions, a plaster cast brace is applied with 30° flexion of the PIP, which allows the ligaments to cicatrise more easily. Grade III lesions with complete joint instability need to be treated surgically. With both types of treatment, mobilisation of the finger starts with limited range of motion (ROM) after 12 days and continues until the 21st day. The resumption of competitive activity (with a splint) is allowed toward the 35th day.

Collateral ligament lesions of the MCP occur following a stress in the radial or ulnar direction with the joint in a flexed position. The treatment consists of immobilising the involved finger with an adjacent one using a soft brace (for grade I) (Fig. 5) or by applying a rigid splint which blocks two contiguous fingers in a semiflexed position at an angle of 60° for 2 or 3 weeks

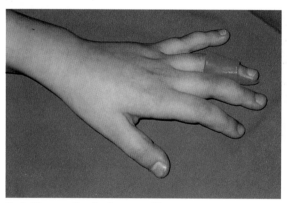

Fig. 2. Finger splint for fracture of P3

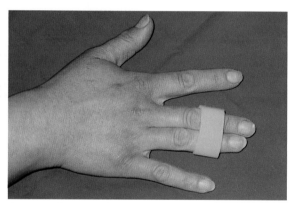

Fig. 4. Two-finger splint for PIP collateral legament tears

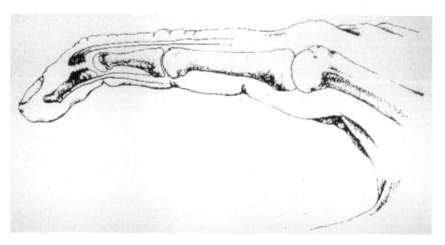

Fig. 3. Segond's fracture

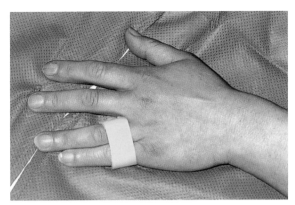

Fig. 5. Two-finger splint for MCP collateral ligament tears

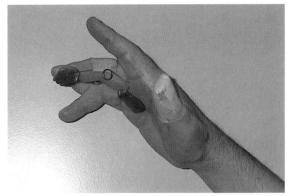

Fig. 6. Capener splint

(for grades II and III). The athlete can resume his sport using the brace, and cautious passive mobilisation can start from the 6th to 21st day after the injury (depending on degree of the lesion). After the initial splint is placed, a soft brace must be applied for a significant period, at least until the joint is stable for stress tests and any pain has ceased.

A particular injury is that to the radial collateral ligament of the second finger MCP. This type of injury is very painful, especially when performing the thumb-index finger pincer movement. It requires surgical treatment in the ligaments that are completely damaged or else in the interarticular fractures [26] of the base of the first phalanx. A brace is applied after the operation and kept on for 2 weeks with the MCP flexed at an angle of 60°. A rehabilitation programme can start after 3 weeks in order to recover complete movement and strength of the hand.

Distortions of the PIP

Many dislocations of the PIP are called coach's finger (or jammed finger) because they are treated at the time of trauma by the trainer or coach. This type of dislocation can involve more than one direction, but most frequent is the dorsal one due to trauma in hyperextension with a lesion in the volar plate. If stable, it is treated with a palmar splint flexed at an angle of 30°, which allows the volar plate to heal. Passive exercises do not start until 15 days after the trauma.

The dislocations that accompany detachment of the joint affecting more than 50% of the joint surface require surgical treatment (open reduction and fixation with wires or screws). Postoperative treatment consists of immobilisation for 2 weeks, after which active flexion can begin with a brace which impedes extension of the finger and is worn for 3 – 4 weeks. The therapeutic programme in these cases is similar to that for intra-articular fractures, and by using a dynamic brace (Capener splint) (Fig. 6) it is possible to recover complete ex-

tension. Resumption of sporting activity is not allowed before 6 – 8 weeks.

Ulnar Collateral Ligament Lesions of the Thumb

Lesions of the thumb MCP are particularly common sports injuries. The thumb's MCP joint is condyloid and principally allows two types of movement, flexion and extension. There are two ligaments in both the radial and ulnar parts: the principal ligament (metacarpal phalanx) and an accessory ligament (metacarpal glenoidal). The glenoidal fibrous cartilage or volar plate insures stability in the anterior-posterior direction. From a biomechanical point of view, the principal ligament is contracted when flexed and not contracted when extended.

In the radial side, the same ligaments are present, the only difference being that the ulnar collateral ligament is damaged in 86% of cases while only 14% in cases of radial collateral ligament lesion [19]. Such lesions usually occur from falls while skiing with the ski poles in hand (ski pole lesion) and with the thumb in forced abduction and slightly flexed (Fig. 7). These lesions are normally classified as:

1. Mild strains, characterised by a simple pain of the ligament without any instability. In such cases, elastic strapping is sufficient. This support allows active mobilisation while allowing continuation of the sporting activity without further lesions to the ligaments.
2. Grade 1 and 2 strains. Grade 1 is treated with a resin brace which blocks the thumb in slight opposition with 40° abduction and flexed at 20° (Fig. 8) for 2 – 3 weeks. During this period, the patient must mobilise his thumb with the brace in place to insure complete movement. The athlete is able to return to sport activity (training) with a padded brace after 15 days of immobilisation (Fig. 9), while competitive sport will be allowed only when the pain has

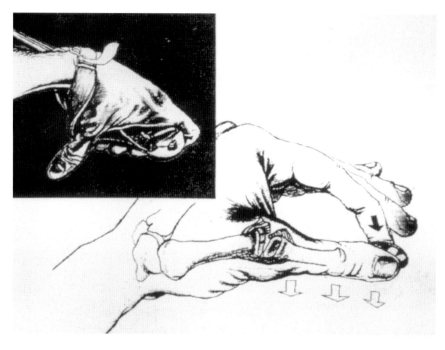

Fig. 7. Sky thumb tear

completely ceased. After 2–3 weeks with the splint, active movements of the thumb joints can begin. After 4 weeks, the counter-resistance pincer movement of the thumb and forefinger can begin. Grade 2 distortion, in which the ligament has undergone a partial lesion, is treated in the same way, but the brace is worn for 5–6 weeks before starting active movement. Depending on the stability of the joints and the sporting requirements, a plaster glove (including the thumb) can substitute the brace. A small plastic brace can be worn under the ski glove to prevent further lesions of the IP during a fall. Athletes with types 1 and 2 lesions can continue skiing with their splints inserted under the ski glove.

3. Grade 3 strains: A laxity of more than 25%–30% compared with the contralateral thumb signals a serious lesion and the need for systematic surgical treatment. The thumb must be tested when it is slightly flexed (which will indicate a lesion of the principal ligament). Rotary instability must be systematically searched for, as well as anterior subluxation of the proximal phalanx, a sign of overall lesion of the extensor apparatus. The need for surgical treatment in serious dislocations is due to the so-called Stener effect [28] (Fig. 10). In fact, the damaged ligament passes above the abductor's expansion and the thumb's long extensor, and it is definitely separated from the distal stump. Only surgical treatment can return it to the anatomical side. The ligament often ends behind a bone fragment, which tends to rotate and separate. Also in these cases, only surgical treatment can reposition the fragment in its anatomical side. This is not always carried out in the time scale established and the athlete is often examined when the lesion is stabilised and the ligament can no longer be sutured.

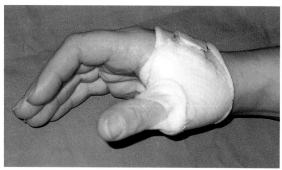

Fig. 8. Plastic brace for MCP ulnar collateral ligament tear

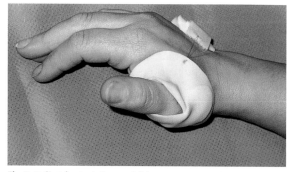

Fig. 9. Splint for training activities

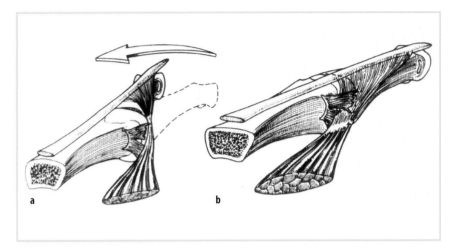

Fig. 10. Stener effect

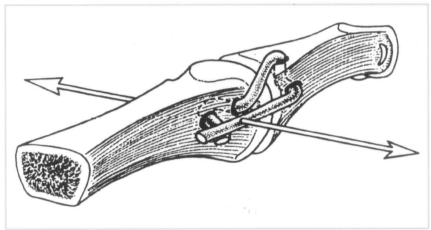

Fig. 11. Ligament reconstruction according Verdan-Simonetta

In these *inveterate strains*, the surgical treatment advised Gore-Tex synthetic ligament reconstruction (or palmaris longus graft) passing through the bone tunnels several times. The synthetic material gives stability and holding strength that persist over time. From a technical standpoint, we prefer the Verdan-Simonetta [29] (Fig. 11) or Littler methods: in the postoperative stage, a splint is applied which blocks the MCP, leaving the IF and wrist free. This brace is worn for 6 weeks, following which rehabilitation begins. With application of the brace, sporting activity can continue (both training and competition); in fact, this type of splint can easily be worn inside the ski glove.

Mallet Finger

The mallet finger is an injury which occurs when there is a break of the distal portion of the extensor tendon in the insertion of the bone (Fig. 12). The tendon can also break with a small portion of bone (Segond's fracture). The treatment of mallet finger is carried out with a finger brace with the DIP fixed in hyperextension to pro-

mote healing of the tendinous lesion (Fig. 13). This splint blocks the DIP while leaving the PIP free to flex. It is worn continuously for 35 days and then removed during the day (allowing the flexion-extension movement of P3) and applied only at night for another 40 days. There are various splint types on the market which are, however, all based on the same principle. The patient can remove the brace from time to time to wash his finger, but the DIP must be held extended. In cases that are examined 10–30 days after the lesion, the splint is kept on uninterruptedly for 8 weeks and at night for another 6. Patients are examined weekly in order to evaluate their skin condition and to see if the P3 tends to yield while flexed. After 6–8 weeks, when the splint is removed, the patient is advised to carry out active and passive flexion-extension exercises four to five times a day for the first week, then six to eight times a day during the second week. If the finger tends to reposition itself during flexion, the patient is advised to wear the extension splint. Athletes can train with the splint and even take part in competitive sport (always wearing the brace). This obviously depends on the type

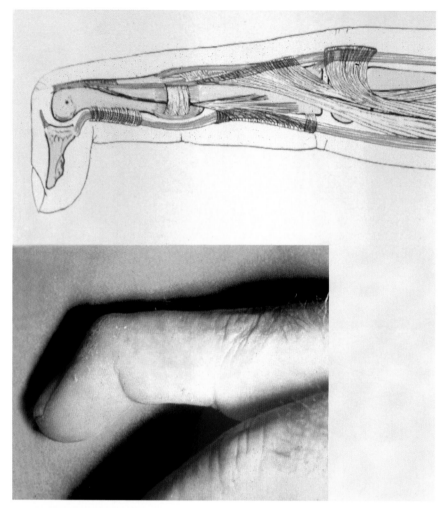

Fig. 12. Mallet finger

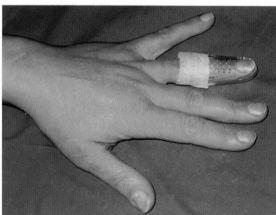

Fig. 13. Stax splint for mallet finger

of sport practiced. The rehabilitation treatment is the same as for Segond's fractures, which require surgical treatment only when the articular fragment is large (more than half of the P3 base) or when it is clear after the splint application and lateral x-ray that the desired reduction has not been obtained. In these cases, it must be operated on and repositioned in the appropriate position.

Boutonnière Deformity

The break of the central position of the extensor apparatus (at the P2 base) provokes what is called boutonnière deformity (Fig. 14). This can arise following isolated trauma or volar dislocation of the PIP. It is treated at first using an extension splint on the PIP, leaving the DIP free to move for 6 weeks. The DIP is moved repeatedly during the day both passively and actively. The athlete can resume sporting activity wearing this splint. After 6 weeks, active exercises begin and are carried out five to six times a day. The splint is kept on at night for another 8 weeks. Following this, a dynamic splint can be applied to treat the flexion. If the lesion is treated secondarily, normally a flexion contracture develops that has to be resolved using a dynamic or progressive static splint or a series of plaster braces. The

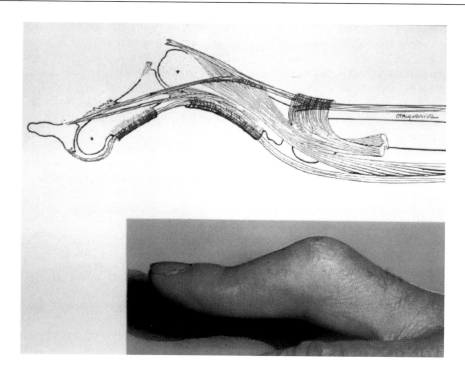

Fig. 14. Boutonniere lesion

plaster braces must be modified every 5 to 7 days. During this period, it is important to mobilise the DIP. Once total extension of the PIP is achieved, a boutonnière splint is applied. It is called *pseudoboutonnière*, a deformity that provokes flexion contracture of the PIP, which also affects the DIP. The damaging mechanism is usually hyperextension with lesion of the proximal insertion of the volar plate (Fig. 15). An oblique retraction of the ligament (ORL) is verified in such a lesion where the ligament is held in the scar callus of the initial lesion. When healed, the scar tissue creates a flexion contracture of the PIP. Various plasters in progressive extension are used to regain passive extension. In case there is no response to the rehabilitation treatment, surgical treatment is advised, with lysis of the volar plate.

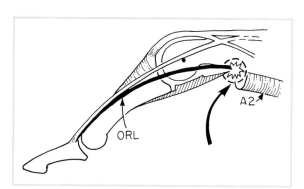

Fig. 15. Pseudo-boutonnière

Rupture of the Flexor Digitorum Profundus

This usually happens when an athlete grabbing an opponent's shirt undergoes forced extension of the DIP while it is flexed [18]. For this reason, it is called "grasping jersey finger" or "rugby finger". The ring finger is involved more often. Sometimes the FDP disconnects from the base of P3, taking with it a small corticocancellous or bone fragment. This fragment can be seen in lateral x-ray of the finger, especially if enlarged, and can aid diagnosis. In other cases, the bone avulsion of flexor insertion is very large, so the P3 undergoes traction of the extensor and tends to subluxate dorsally. The level of the retraction, the presence of a detached bone fragment, and age of the lesion allow the physician to suggest a classification of this type of lesion:

1. Type 1. The distal portion of the FPD withdraws until the crossing of the FDS and is sometimes blocked in this seat by a small bone fragment in front of the P1. The vincula longa is intact. In this most frequent type of lesion, especially if recent, the vascularization is retained and allows the tendon to be reinserted with a good chance of success.
2. Type 2. The FDP is retracted (usually found in the palm). The vincula longa are broken and the whole extremity is devascularized. These forms are frequently seen in older lesions.
3. Type 3. There is a large epiphysial fragment of the P3 that is blocked at the entrance of the digital canal. The DIP is destabilised in subluxations.

In recent type 1 lesions, treatment consists of distal reinsertion of the FDP and a Kleinert type of postoperative treatment, that is, with precocious passive mobilisation by means of an elastic band fastened to the brace (with the wrist slightly flexed) allowing active extension and passive flexion. In type 3 lesions, good results are guaranteed only by reinsertion of the large bone fragment in the distal seat and by stabilisation of the DIP. From a prognostic point of view, results are the same as those for joint fractures and directly related to the quality of the setting. In type 2 lesions with the devascularized tendon in the distal portion, it is necessary to avoid reinsertion of the tendon at all costs, because this type of treatment is bound to fail. In these cases, resection of FDP to the palm is more efficient and a tenodesis with a DIP flexed (therefore allowing the PIP to be mobile and the DIP to be stable). When presented with avulsion which is not recent, the surgical method must be well evaluated, taking into account the functional loss of passive mobility of the IP and also the patient's expectations. It is absolutely impossible to reinsert a DPF in inveterate lesions, because the risk of rigidity is very high. Palmaris longis pro-DPF grafting is reserved for exceptional cases with consenting patients wishing greater mobility and full strength and who have soft interphalanges. Precocious passive mobilisation is carried out postoperatively with Kinetec in both recent and older lesions to allow rapid functional recovery.

Digital Pulley Lesions

Since the 1970s, a new type of sport has become popular: "bare hands" climbing. With this free-climbing technique commonly called rock climbing, the upper limb is not only a safety anchor but becomes a means of climbing. In certain positions, all the body weight is sustained by one or two fingers. In these cases, rupture of the digital pulleys can occur, which is particularly frequent for the A2 and A4 [2, 4, 6] (Fig. 16). Usually such lesions are examined only tardily (after at least a month). The sportsman recounts that while climbing he felt a strong whiplash pain that made him release his hold, accompanied by a sensation of internal breaking. When examined, the fingers in question are usually the middle and ring fingers, which are swollen at the P2 level in semiflexed position and show pain when completely extended. The A2 pulley on the P1 is the one usually affected by the lesions, while the A4 on the P2 and sometimes both the A2 and the A4 are rarely damaged. Such lesions are explained by the particular way in which the athletes attach themselves to the rock they are climbing. In fact, the fingers are in a position with the PIP hyperflexed and the DIP hyperextended such that the pulleys are under extreme stress, even to the point of breaking. Magnetic resonance imaging (MRI) currently allows us to verify these lesions clearly. The treatment is a conservative type used in isolated lesions of the A2 and A4 and in partial lesions. It consists in abstention from the sport for 45 days, combined with a syndactylism of the adjacent fingers to avoid rigidity in PIP semiflexion and anti-inflammatory active and passive kinesis for total recovery of the joints. After 45 days, the athlete can gradually resume training and after another 3 weeks he can resume sport activity. When two pulleys are damaged, the flexor tendons lose strength because of the so-called bowstring phenomenon, and therefore surgery is necessary, which consists in reconstruction of the two pulleys (especially when

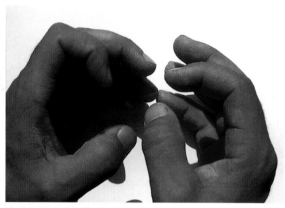

Fig. 16. Digital pulley lesions

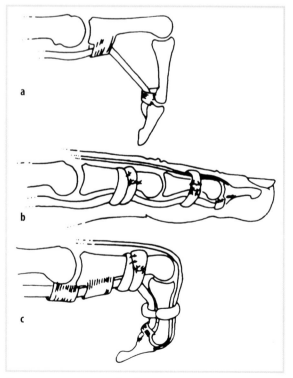

Fig. 17. Reconstruction of pulleys according to Littler

the lesion is very old) with a strip of tendon of the long palm passed twice around the P1 and the P2 respectively below and above the extensor tendon (Fig. 17). Rehabilitation consists of passive mobilisation in flexion and active mobilisation in extension.

Compression of the Digital Collateral Nerves

Ten-pin bowling players hold the ball using three fingers. The thumb is usually placed in a hole on the ball and the hold is carried out with the internal margin, so the ulnar collateral nerve of the first finger can have microtraumatisms which provoke the formation of pseudoneuromas (Fig. 18). Patients complain of paresthesia on the apex of the thumb with Tinel's sign in the compression zone. In this area, there is a painful nerve tumefaction that can simulate a cyst. Treatment consists of holding the ball using a brace [10] or otherwise modifying the thumb grip. Only in inveterate cases and when there is no improvement with these procedures, surgical treatment can be undertaken (neurolysis and possible transposition of the collateral nerve behind the thumb's abductor).

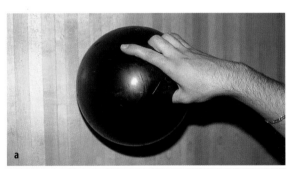

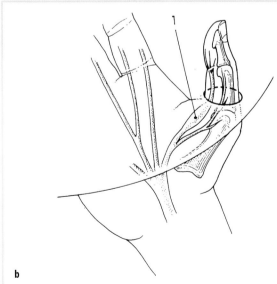

Fig. 18. Neuromas of thumb in a bowler

Wrist

Wrist Tendinopathies

De Quervain's Tendinopathies

De Quervain's tenosinovity appears at the level of the first extensor compartment occupied by the short extensor (ECP) and long abductor of the thumb (APL). It is provoked by angled lateral movements of the thumb and is a very common injury in skiing, fencing, volleyball, tennis, and gymnastics. There is a specific manoeuvre described by Finkelstein [11] which aggravates the pain when tensing the tendons and confirms the diagnosis. Tenosinovitis is often combined with a sensitive neuritis of the radial nerve called Wartenberg's disease [30]. This neuritis can be found with a Tinel's sign 9 cm from the radial styloid. Foucher claims to have found this association (tenovaginalitis neuritis) in 15% of De Quervain's tendinitis. From the rehabilitative point of view, patients are treated with braces for 2 weeks, laser therapy, ultrasound therapy, and local steroid injections. In case of failure of conservative therapy, surgical treatment can be carried out which, even if it appears simple, is not without complications [15, 16, 32]. In fact, this type of surgery is simple only when the local anatomy is well known, and only then is it possible to avoid obvious errors: the absence of complete freedom, neuroma of the sensitive ramifications of the radial nerve, painful subluxation of the long abductor, tendon adherence, and cheloid scars. For these reasons, we prefer to open the first compartment using a zed of the pulley that allows us to resuture it, thereby enlarging the first compartment.

Extensor Muscle Tendinopathies

This condition is much rarer, even if characterised by two typical signs: crepitation in the dorsal part of the forearm and pain at the intersection of the two distal tendons. It is frequent in some sports (canoeing, skiing, volleyball) and treated with a resting brace with the wrist extended at an angle of 20°, radial inclination, abduction, and retropulsion of the thumb. In case of failure, surgical treatment must remove the bursitis described by Wood [33].

Tendinopathy of Ulnar Extensor Carpis

Where the ulnar extensor carpis (EUC) passes above the wrist, the tendon is fastened to the ulnar head by means of a tendon sheath. In forced supination movements, ulnar deviation, and wrist flexion (which frequently happens playing tennis), this sheath can break and the EUC starts to subdislocate with ulnar deviation movements and the wrist in supination. When the tendon is subdislocated, the athlete feels a painful 'snapping' sensation. Acute lesions are treated with a Muenster splint, with the wrist in slight radial deviation and dorsiflexion and the forearm kept prone for 4–6 weeks. Chronic lesions do not respond very well to conservative treatment and require surgical treatment with reconstruction of the sheath. A Muenster splint is therefore applied for 4 weeks. The strengthening exercises are carried out after 8 weeks and progressively increased. Complete return to sport activity with wrist bandage normally occurs after the third or fourth month.

Nerve Lesions to the Wrist

Ulnar Nerve Lesions to the Wrist

First described in 1861 by Felix Guyon [13], these lesions cause pain of the ulnar nerve at the wrist level. Guyon's tunnel is characterised by a dorsal portion made up of the annular ligament of the carpus, pisouncinate, and pisometacarpal ligaments, a volar portion made up of the short palm and medial portion (transversal ligament of the carpus), and lateral portions (pisiform and FUC, Flexor Ulnaris Carpi). Inside the plaster cast, the ulnar nerve divides into two branches, one sensitive and one motor.

The tunnel is characterised by two fibrous arches, one at the entrance and one at the exit that can act as a scythe and compress the nerve. This pathology is frequent in cyclists and players of racquet sports (racquet player's pisiform). Especially with cyclists, compression of the nerve can happen both when the hand is kept for long periods in hyperextension and ulnar inclination and for microtraumatisms on the nerve between the ulnar portion of the wrist and the handlebar [14]. Therefore, the aetiology can be postural, microtraumatic, or both. Only the motor branch of the nerve can be affected, the sensitive branch as well as the nerve in its entirety. The paralysis can manifest itself in acute form (rapid occurrence of a typical ulnar 'griffe') and also in progressive form (paresthesia starting in the fourth and fifth fingers, reduction of the thumb-index finger pincer, then atrophy of the first interosseous space, etc.). Treatment consists in the absolute prohibition of riding a bicycle and the prognosis is usually benign, with complete healing. It is rarely necessary to intervene surgically. At the resumption of sport activity, it is important to advise the patient of necessary precautions to avoid the return of ulnar pain: changing hand position often, wearing gloves padded with foam rubber in the ulnar seat, only riding short distances, applying the ulnar splint, etc.

Fracture of the Carpal Bone

Unciform Apophysis Fracture of the Hamate Bone

Unciform apophysis fracture of the hamate bone is very rare in traumatology and occurs following a fall on the ulnar border of the hand. In sport traumatology, it is more frequent in golf, tennis, baseball, squash, and hockey and due to microtraumas provoked by repetition of the action and therefore by the impact of the sport equipment against the unciform apophysis or rubbing of the sport equipment on the hypothenar prominence. Unfortunately, it is rarely diagnosed at the time of the trauma and is falsely classified as tendinitis or dislocation. In fact, with standard x-rays the pathology is easily recognised. Exact diagnosis, therefore, very often happens at a later stage when only a possible complication (a break of the flexor of the fourth and fifth fingers) leads to the discovery of this fracture. Clinically, the patient complaints of violent pain corresponding to the pisiform which is accentuated by playing the sport and decreases with rest. There is swelling in the ulnar seat and the pain is accentuated by pressing the pisiform and with palm ulnar flexion of the wrist. To arrive at a correct diagnosis, it is important to carry out not only standard x-rays but also targeted projections for the carpal tunnel which allow the lesion to be clearly seen. Computed tomography scan and MRI allow this. Treatment of acute and chronic forms must be differentiated. Those cases diagnosed precociously must be divided into forms without shifting (in which the treatment consists of a brace or plaster immobilising the forearm up to the IP of the fourth and fifth fingers) and detached forms (in which the fragment must be surgically removed). In forms examined at a later stage, surgical treatment with exeresis of the fragment is the only possibility.

Scaphoid Fracture

To underline the importance and frequency of scaphoid fractures, we quote the aphorism of Watson-Jones, who observes: "Every dislocation of the wrist is a scaphoid fracture, at least until an x-ray proves the contrary." In fact, such fractures are very common in football, basketball, rugby, and American football. They are the result of indirect trauma due to a fall on the wrist in a hyperextended position and with the radial inclined.

Some 70% of fractures to the scaphoid concern the 1/3 medium and are stable. They are treated in plaster up to the forearm-thumb and heal in about 3 months. To avoid absenting an athlete from competitive activity for such a long time or in the case of detached fractures, an arthroscopy to the wrist treatment and synthesis with a Herbert screw have been proposed [31]. For detached fractures, another type of treatment is possible:

open reduction and internal fixation. A brace or plaster is applied postoperatively for 4 weeks and then rehabilitation treatment for another 3 weeks. In this way, the athlete can resume training with a brace 7–8 weeks after the trauma. In cases treated with a plaster brace, the patient is requested to move his fingers actively and passively during the period of immobilisation. The hand is held elevated. Once the fracture is healed, the plaster is removed during the day to allow recovery and less often during the night. Active and passive ROM exercises for the thumb, wrist, and forearm are carried out six to eight times an hour. Then the thumb-index finger pincer exercises and strengthening exercises of the wrist and thumb can start. Dynamic splints can also be applied, which helps to recover the passive movements.

Various types of dynamic splints are utilised (made by hand therapists or various companies). The dynamic splint is worn for about 20 min more during the day and used to recover flexion/extension.

When carrying out the rehabilitation programme (exercises with weights), it is important to apply a plastic brace that protects the wrist from hypertension. Such splints are kept on until the fracture is completely healed.

Triangular Fibrocartilage Complex Lesions

The triangular fibrocartilage complex (TFCC) [22] is a structure distally placed between radius and ulna and is part of a complex fibrous system beginning at the carpal edge of the sigmoidal incisure of the radius and attached to the volar base of the ulnar styloid. The TFCC provides a flowing surface between the radius and ulna in wrist movements and is a flexible mechanism for rotary movements of the radius-carpical(s) around the ulnar axis. In fact, it connects the ulnar edge to the carpus and cushions the forces through the ulna-carpal axis.

Palmer [21] introduced a classification that divides TFCC lesions into traumatic and degenerative types. The former are verified by an axial compression mechanism (a fall on the palm of the hand and/or rotation of the external distal of the ulna). The degenerative lesions result from prolonged and repetitive overload of the distal radius-ulnar, e.g., in repeated movements of prone supination. Furthermore, Palmer [22] demonstrated how the concentration of load forces of the distal radio-ulnar vary in relation to its length. In fact, the longer the ulna (ulna-plus), the greater the burden on the ulnar column; and this predisposes to the onset of degenerative lesions. For this reason, it is easy to associate such lesions with sport activities or the repetitive movements typical in many sports. Patients with traumatic lesions of the TFCC often explain that their wrist trauma symptomatology began with brusque torsion movements. The pain is localised at the ulnar edge of the wrist, exacerbated by prone-supination movements, and can be accompanied by a snapping sensation. A big step in the diagnosis and treatment of TFCC lesions was introduced by wrist arthroscopy, which is more accurate and specific than artrography, giving positive diagnosis in 95% of cases [20]. Pederzini et al. [24] compared artrography RMN and arthroscopy in the diagnosis of some TFCC lesions. The arthroscopy not only proved as reliable as RMN but goes further, as it allows therapeutic resolution of the pathologies identified.

The most common type of TFCC lesion is that to the articular disc. As the central portion of the disc is avascular, it does not tend to heal with conservative treatment. The peripheral lesions, especially if they are not detached, have a greater possibility of healing by rest (with a brace), while those that are dislocated need surgical treatment followed by a long period of immobilisation with a brace for 6 weeks. If the lesion is stable and there are no associated fractures, a slightly flexed wrist brace with ulnar deviation worn for 4 weeks will lead to healing (Fig. 19). Palmer furthermore observed that, when treated conservatively, some central lesions become asymptomatic. For symptomatic ones, however, the only possible treatment is surgical and consists in arthroscopic debridement.

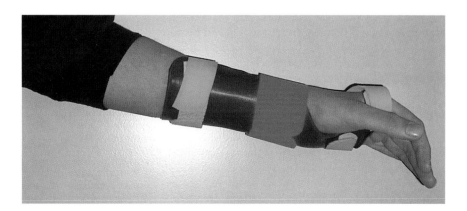

Fig. 19. Wrist splint

One day after arthroscopy, the patient can begin the rehabilitation programme with movement of the wrist and forearm and with examination of the edema. A wrist brace is applied during the night for a few weeks. If pain and swelling have ceased, the muscle strengthening programme can begin 7 days after operation (EMS and isometric exercises). Resumption of sporting activity takes place around the sixth week.

A degenerative lesion often provokes lesion of the central portion of the articular disc with associated chondromalacia of the ulna and semilunar. In such cases, debridement of the TFCC and chondromalacia are necessary. It can also be important to shorten the ulna to decrease load forces on the wrist. In case the TFCC is stable but there is a positive ulna-plus measuring less than 2–3 mm, a wafer procedure is carried out to remove 2 mm of thickness from the ulna. However, if the ulna-plus is greater than 3 mm, the ulna is shortened using the open technique and application of a plate and screws so as to stabilise the lunopyramidal ligament and DRUJ (Distal Radio-Ulnar Joint) with an increase in tension of the ulnacarpal ligaments.

Rehabilitation after debridement of the TFCC or a wafer procedure begins 1–2 days after the operation. When a shortening of the ulna is carried out, it is necessary to wait at least 1 week. Immediately after the operation, active and cautiously passive ROM exercises can begin, and cryotherapy is used to control edema and pain. Once the wound is healed, home exercises and massage of the scar can begin. In the case of a wafer procedure, hand strengthening exercises are carried out after a week. However, with shortening of the ulna, it is necessary to wait at least 6 weeks.

Ganglion of the Wrist

A cystic formation can appear on the wrist following a stress. Such a condition is typical in young gymnasts who repeatedly carry out exercises with the wrist extended. Even if the wrist is stable, after a short time a cystic formation appears in these athletes above the scapholunate ligament. These cysts are quite painful, but the pain is accentuated with flexion-extension and after competition. Conservative treatment can be attempted and usually consists in wearing a wrist brace for 2–3 weeks. As soon as the pain disappears, strengthening exercises can begin. Splints are worn when the athletes train and soft splints when they resume competitive activity.

A surgical procedure of the ganglion is necessary when the pain does not diminish. A week after the operation, the movements can begin. After 14 days, massages on the scar can begin. The brace is usually worn for 3 weeks. Passive flexion exercises are carried out to avoid the rigidity which is common after such operations. After 3 weeks, strengthening exercises can start which are continued until the return to competitive sport.

Recommended Reading

1. Aulicino PL (1990) Neurovascular injuries in the hands of athletes. Hand Clin 6:455–459
2. Bollen SR (1990) Injures to the A2 pulley in rock climbers J Hand Surg 15B(2):268–270
3. Bowers WH (1987) The interphalangeal joints. Churchill Livingstone, New York
4. Bowers WH, Kusma GR, Bynum DK (1994) Closed traumatic rupture finger flexor pulleys. J Hand Surg 19A(5):782–787
5. Carroll RE, Match RM (1970) Avulsion of the prufundus tendon insertion. J Traum 10:1109–1112
6. Cartier JL, Toussaint B et al (1985) Approche d'une nouvelle pathologie de la main, liée à la pratique de l'escalade. A propos d'une revue de 51 grimpeurs professionels. J Traumat Sportiv 2:35–39
7. Chang WH, Thoms OJ, White WL (1972) Avulsion injury of the long flexor tendons. Plast Reconstr Surg 19:35–39
8. Chery A, De Carlo M (1998) Rehabilitation and use of protective devices in hand and wrist injuries. Clin Sports Med 17(3):635–654
9. Colditz JC (1995) Functional fracture bracing. In: Hunter JM et al (eds) Rehabilitation of the hand. Surgery and Therapy. Vol 1. Mosby, St Louis USA, p 395
10. Dobins JH, O'Brien ET, Linscheid RL, Farrow GM (1972) Bowler thumb: Diagnosis and treatment. Journal of Bone and Joint Surgery 54A:751–756
11. Filkenstein H (1930) Stenosing tendovaginalitis at the radial stiloid process. Journal of Bone and Joint Surgery 12A:509–515
12. Folmar RC, Nelson CL, Phalen CS (1972) Rupture of the flexor tendons in hand of nonrheumatoid patients. Journal of Bone and Joint Surgery 54A:579–584
13. Guyon F (1861) Note sur une disposition anatomique propre a la face anterieure de poignet et non encore déscrite. Bull Soc Anat Paris 2:184–186
14. Halova JP (1995) La compression du nerve ulnaire chez les coureures cyclistes. In: Allieu Y (ed) La main du sportif. GEM, Paris, pp 96–99
15. Lapidus PW, Fenton R (1952) Stenosing tenovaginalitis at the wrist and finger: Report of 423 cases in 369 patients with 354 operations. Arch Surg 64:475–479
16. Lipscomb PR (1994) Chronic nonspecific tenosinovitis and peritendinitis. Surg Clin North Am 24:780–789
17. Maneaud M, Littler W (1978) La reconstruction du ligament lateral interne de la mètacarpo-phalangienne du pouce. Ann Chir 32(9):605–607
18. Mansat M, Bonnevialle P (1995) L'avulsion traumatique du flechisseur commun profond des doigts chez le sportif. In: Allieu Y (ed) La main du sportif. GEM, Paris, pp 118–121
19. Moutet F, Guinard D, Massart P et al (1995) Entorses de la métacarpo-phalangienne du pouce en pratique sportive. In: Allieu Y (ed) La main du sportif. GEM, Paris, pp 27–34
20. Ostermann L, Mikulics M (1988) Scaphoid manunion. Hand Clin 4:437–455
21. Palmer AK (1989) Triangular fibrocartilage complex lesions: A classification. J Hand Surg 14A:594–596
22. Palmer AK, Werner FW (1984) Biomechanics of the distal radioulnar joint. Clin Orthop 187:26–35
23. Pederzini L (1999) Artroscopia di polso. Ortopedia e Chirurgia mininvasiva. Springer-Verlag, Milan
24. Pederzini L, Luchetti R et al (1992) Evaluation of the trian-

gular fibrocartilage complex tears by arthroscopy, arthrography, and magnetic resonance imaging. Arthroscopy 8:191–197

25. Rettig AC (1991a) Current concepts in management of football injuries of the hand and wrist. J Hand Ther 3:4–42

26. Rettig AC (1991b) Hand injuries in football players. Phys Sports Med 19:97

27. Rettig AC, Patel DV (1992) Wrist and hand injuries in athletes. Physician's Handbook. American College of Sports Medicine, Indianapolis USA

28. Stener B (1981) Displacement of the ruptured ulnar collateral ligament of the metacarpal-phalangeal joint. The Hand 13(3):257–266

29. Verdan C (1971) Traitement chirurgical des séquelles des entorses métacarpo-phalangienne du pouce. In: Vilain R (ed) Traumatismes osteo-articolaires de la main. GEM, Paris, pp 115–121

30. Wartenberg R (1932) Cheiralgia parestetica (isolierte Neuritis des Ramus superficialis nervi radialis). Ger Neurolog Psychiatr 141:145–155

31. Wipple TL (1992) The wrist. Arthroscopic Surgery. J.B. Lippincott, Philadelphia

32. Wood MB, Dobins JH (1986) Sports-related extraarticular wrist syndromes. Clin Orthop 202:93–102

33. Woods THE (1964) De Quervain's disease: A plea for early operation. A report on 40 cases. Brit J Surg 51:358–359

9 Rehabilitation of Low Back Pain

Pierre A. d'Hemecourt, Lyle J. Micheli, Carl Gustafson

Introduction

Back injuries are a common phenomenon in sports, estimated to occur in 10% – 15% of all participants [23, 36]. However, the rate of injury varies between sports and often the position played. Back injuries have been reported in 11% of gymnasts and up to 50% of American football linemen [43]. As athletes are increasingly required to perform repetitive training skills, overuse injuries appear to be increasing. Of concern to sports physicians is the recurrence of these debilitating problems in 26% of males and 33% of females [66].

Early intervention and appropriate rehabilitation often reduce the chronicity and progression of injury. Rehabilitation is directed by the diagnosis, which in turn is derived from an understanding of lumbar spine anatomy, biomechanics, and the injury patterns of different sports.

Anatomy

Spinal injuries are especially prevalent in adolescence and young adulthood. During this maturation period, the spine is subject to both structural and flexibility changes. Structural changes are derived from the growth tissues in the vertebral bodies and neural arch. During growth, these are often the weakest link in force transfer [58].

The vertebrae are divided into anterior and posterior columns. The former consists of the vertebral body, intervertebral disc, and the attached anterior and posterior longitudinal ligaments. The posterior column is the neural arch, including the facet joints, spinous process, and pars interarticularis.

In the anterior column, the vertebral body ends at the superior and inferior margins with the epiphyseal growth plate and its contiguous ring apophysis. The vertebral end plate develops from the cartilaginous portion of the growth epiphysis and functions to nourish the disc through hydrostatic motion (Fig. 1). Injury to the end plate hinders disc metabolism. Herniation through the end plate can result in a Schmorl's node, usually seen in the thoracolumbar region. The anulus fibrosus is attached to the ring apophysis and inner end

plate [3]. The apophysis represents the weak link and fails first with distraction and compression forces. This may result in either disc herniation into the vertebral body at the apophysis (limbus vertebrae) or avulsion of the apophysis with the attached anulus.

Additionally, the disc itself is subject to changes with age. This includes dehydration of the nucleus pulposus. The loss of water content begins in childhood and adolescence [5]. The intervertebral disc loses elastin and gains collagen. The anulus becomes fibrillated. The resulting disc is less mobile and less able to recover from creep deformation [5]. Except for the outer anular fibers, the disc is avascular and requires motion to provide hydrostatic forces through the end plate to deliver nutrition.

In the posterior column, a single ossification center is present in each pedicle. Ossification proceeds in a posterior direction and may be incomplete on the superior aspect of the pars interarticularis, predisposing to stress fracture from the abutting inferior articular facet above [56]. Incomplete lysis of the superior aspect of the pars has been demonstrated in cadaver studies [36]. The posterior arch also has growth cartilage on the facet joints and spinous process apophysis, which are subject to traction by the dorsolumbar fascia and impingement with excessive lordosis [38].

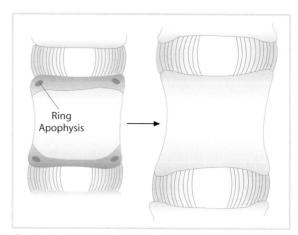

Ring Apophysis

Fig. 1. Development of the end plate

The facet joints and vertebral bodies form a segmental triple joint complex at each level. In standing posture, the facet joints assume up to a third of the weight-bearing force.

The sacroiliac (SI) joint is a complex joint of the lower spine and pelvic ring. Forces are transferred and dissipated across the SI joint between the lower extremities and trunk. The motion of the ipsilateral ileum during hip flexion is a posterior rotation with increased SI compression. With hip extension, the ileum rotates anteriorly with SI distraction. Often the lower extremities move in opposite directions, utilizing the symphysis pubis as the pivot point [5]. The SI joint is flat until after puberty. Corrugations develop in late adolescence and early adulthood, ultimately ankylosing later in life [2]. The inferior portion is synovial, while only 25% are superiorly synovial [12].

The muscle and fascial attachments of the lumbar spine and pelvis are important to the rehabilitation of low back pain. Lumbar flexors include the rectus abdominus and psoas. Lumbar extension is accomplished with the intrinsic polysegmental multifidus and the long polysegmental erector spinae group. The multifidus is the largest group in diameter and functions to extend the lumbar spine as well as control rotation with its oblique orientation [11]. The extrinsic group of lumbar extensors includes the latissimus dorsi and gluteus maximus. They perform with attachments to the thoracolumbar fascia.

The thoracolumbar fascia serves multiple functions with attachments to the transverse processes, transversus abdominis, and internal obliques. Activation provides lumbar stability in lifting and forward bending. Another role is to provide the link for abdominal and lumbar extensor coactivation, which increases intra-abdominal hydrostatic pressure for load attenuation across the spine [33].

Biomechanics

In sports, the lumbar spine is subject to motion and reactive forces, specifically kinematics and kinetics. Kinematic describes body motion. Kinetics relate force to a mass and its motion [47].

The kinematics of lumbar flexion and extension involve a constantly changing instantaneous axis of rotation. In flexion, the pivot point centers near the nucleus pulposus with compression of the anterior disc and distraction of the facet joints. Extension transfers compression to the posterior disc and facet joints, while tensile forces move from the facets to the anterior disc [30, 45]. Consequently, injury patterns are often seen in anterior and posterior columns simultaneously [24]. Flexion and extension occur predominantly at the L4–L5 and L5–S1 discs. The motion is part of a concerted lumbopelvic rhythm.

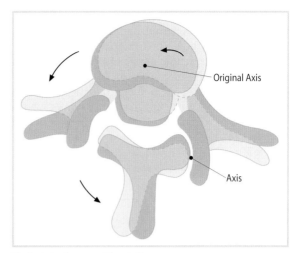

Fig. 2. Axis change with rotation

Axial rotation is also a complex motion with the initial axis of rotation in the posterior aspect of the disc until the facet contralateral to rotation is engaged, transferring the axis to this zygoapophyseal joint [5]. At this point, the disc is subject to shear forces along with the original torsion forces [16] (Fig. 2). The maximal stress is at the posterolateral disc.

The kinetics of lumbar spine motion in sports include both intrinsic (individual musculotendinous and anatomic variants) as well as extrinsic (collision and ground reactive) forces applied to the spine. Appropriate spinal motion relies on coordinated trunk muscle activation and pelvic flexibility. Increased lumbar lordosis places stress on the posterior elements while excess flexion places compression on the disc. Intrinsic biomechanical risk factors include iliopsoas inflexibility, femoral anteversion, thoracolumbar fascia tightness, abdominal weakness, genu recurvatum, and thoracic kyphosis.

Iliopsoas tightness increases lordosis as well as anterior compression forces to the disc [69]. Lumbar lordosis is also increased with thoracolumbar tightness, lower abdominal weakness, thoracic kyphosis, and genu recurvatum. In dancers, a unique cause of lordosis is attempting hip turnout with femoral anteversion. The increased lordosis releases the ileoinguinal ligament allowing greater aesthetic turnout.

Trunk muscle weakness is a risk to spinal stability. Injury to the lumbar spine has been shown to cause dysfunction of the lumbar stabilizers [54]. Lumbar stability is best understood using the concept of global and local muscles of the lower trunk [2]. The global (extrinsic) muscles refer to the large groups that link the pelvis to the thoracic wall and serve to provide motion and general stabilization against external forces. The local (intrinsic) muscles, predominantly the multifidi, transversus abdominus, and internal obliques, control local motion and segmental stability. These act functionally in a coactivated manner and provide joint stiffness during force application [54]. An analogy would be the interaction between large-muscle shoulder movers and fine motor control of the rotator cuff.

Finally, volume of training and nutrition are additional risk factors for injury. Training in excess of 15 h per week in gymnastics increases the risk of injury from 13% to 57% [21]. Poor caloric intake in the female athlete is manifested with diminished bone mineralization and stress fractures [7, 14, 31].

Injury Patterns

Gymnastics involves repetitive flexion and extension of the lumbar spine. Disc degeneration has been strongly associated with this sport (11% in pre-elite, 43% in elite, and 63% in Olympic level athletes) [21]. Weight lifting, crew, collision sports, and bowling involve lumbar flexion, axial compression, and rotation. These are associated with herniation of the nucleus pulposus [37, 43, 64]. Hyperextension in dancers, figure skaters, and interior linemen is associated with posterior element overuse and spondylolysis [18, 19]

Appropriate rehabilitation and avoidance of reinjury requires an understanding of injury patterns and their classification. Sports injuries to the lumbar spine are classified in several ways. First, they are separated as macrotraumatic (acute) or microtraumatic (overuse) injuries. Macrotraumatic injuries include fractures of the vertebrae, apophyseal avulsions from the spinous process or iliac crest, and acute herniation of the nucleus pulposus as well as sprains and contusions.

Table 1. Flexion- and extension-based injuries

Flexion-based	Extension-based
Disc herniation	Spondylolysis
Disc degeneration	Spondylolisthesis
Disc derangement	Transitional vertebrae
Atypical Scheuerman	Lordotic low back pain

Overuse injuries to the spine occur in both the anterior and posterior columns. Anterior injuries occur with lumbar flexion and are often coupled with rotation [16]. With rotation, the posterolateral disc is subject to shear as the pivot transfers from the posterior third of the disc to the zygoapophyseal joint. If the posterior disc lamella is preloaded in flexion, this force is magnified [52].

Posterior injuries occur with an extension mechanism. However, rotation may be an additional mechanical factor, because a secondary axis of rotation occurs at the facet joint with distraction forces at the contralateral facet capable of inducing capsular avulsions and fractures of the facet or pars interarticularis [16].

These injuries may be separated according to whether they are flexion-based or extension-based (Table 1).

Evaluation

Description of the pain is helpful in classifying the injury. Axial pain (including buttock and thigh) is distinguished from radicular pain. Aggravating factors are considered. Pain that worsens with sitting is often discogenic, while pain with standing often represents a

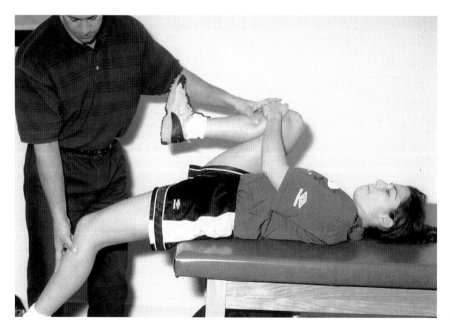

Fig. 3. Thomas angle testing for hip flexion contracture

posterior element injury. However, crossover of symptoms is quite frequent. Posterior element injury with spasm may be stretched in the sitting posture. Pain with transitional motion often represents inflammation. Nocturnal pain and urinary and gastrointestinal complaints should elicit immediate investigation for the underlying cause.

The examination confirms the history. Pain elicited in flexion may indicate an anterior element injury. The forward flexion test also allows assessment for scoliosis and structural abnormalities such as kyphosis or "flat back." Posterior element pain is aggravated in exten-sion. The sensitivity for a spondylolytic stress fracture is enhanced with a single-leg lumbar extension test.

Pelvic flexibility is assessed. Hip flexor tightness is a risk factor for anterior and posterior element injury. Thomas angle testing detects psoas tightness, while Ely's test is specific for rectus femoris tightness (Figs. 3, 4). Hamstring tightness is assessed measuring the popliteal angle. This angle is formed between the femur and the tibia as the extending knee reaches passive resistance (Fig. 5).

Tests for sacroiliac inflammation are variable in their clinical reproducibility. The Patrick's ("fabere"

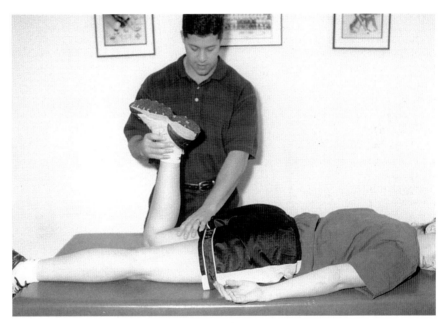

Fig. 4. Ely testing

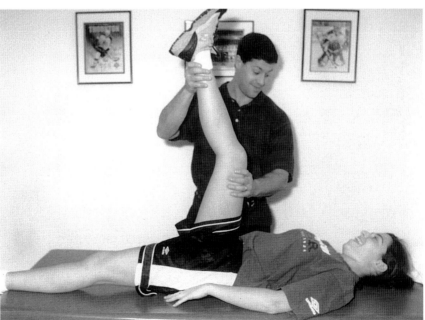

Fig. 5. Popliteal angle between the vertical axis of the femur and the tibia

sign) and Gaenslen's tests are common. Patrick's test is performed with an ipsilateral force to the abducted and externally rotated lower extremity ("figure of four" position) with an opposing force to the contralateral pelvis. The Gaenslen's test applies a saggital shear force across the pelvis with the patient supine and passively extending one hip while flexing the other. Piriformis impingement is reproduced with hip extension and internal rotation.

Lower trunk muscle strength testing is performed on the lumbar extensors and abdominals (Figs. 6, 7). The Biering-Sorensen test is predictive of lumbar extensor endurance strength [4]. This is performed with the upper torso prone and suspended with the pelvis resting on a pad. The time maintaining a neutral posture is measured. A full neurologic exam is also essential.

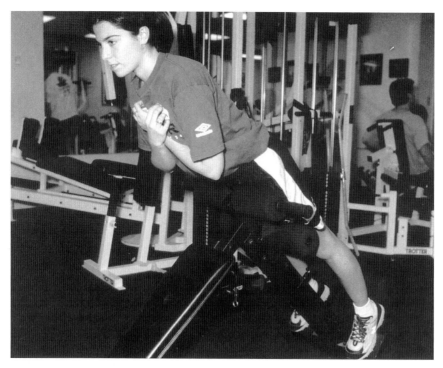

Fig. 6. Lumbar extension strength

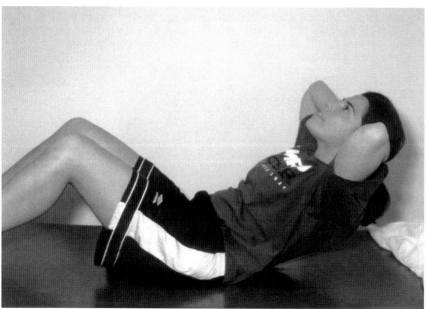

Fig. 7. Abdominal strength

Methods of Rehabilitation

Rehabilitation of the athlete should follow an orderly progression based on specific diagnosis. Initially, pain and inflammation are controlled. While allowing the tissues to heal, the athlete maintains general conditioning and motion within a protected zone. Biomechanical deficits are addressed. Truncal musculature strengthening is advanced in stepwise fashion with the goal of restoring normal functional lumbar stability.

Rehabilitation advances along the kinetic chain with attention to hip stabilizers such as the often weak abductors. Ground reactive forces are transmitted through the lower extremities to the pelvis and spine. Therefore, the entire lower extremity is addressed for flexibility and strength and incorporated into the sport-specific training. The muscular support system is trained for recruitment in a programmed manner specific to the sport. For example, preactivation of the quadriceps is necessary in preparation for landing from a jump [54].

A number of treatment programs have been described for spinal rehabilitation, including McKenzie, Williams' flexion, and spine stabilization exercises. This text describes an approach combining elements of each.

The McKenzie approach separates patient problems into postural, dysfunctional, and derangement types. The postural patients have pain from prolonged end-range positioning with static loads. Dysfunctional patients develop pain once the connective tissue shortens with scar and then is stretched with motion. The derangement patients represent an advanced stage with disc derangement manifesting pain with motion and static loading. Exercises and posture are determined which centralize the symptoms. These are often extension-based. However, a posterolateral or central disc protrusion may be exceptions where extension increases symptoms [44].

The Williams' flexion exercises were developed with the concept that flexion diminishes stress on the posterior aspect of the disc and widens the neuroforamen. This reduces radicular symptoms. However, flexion increases intradiscal pressure and radicular symptoms may actually increase. Patients with central canal stenosis and posterior element pain may benefit from this approach.

The spine stabilization approach defines the neutral position that places the least stress on the spine [55]. This is individual-specific for spine and pelvis position. Exercises are advanced as long as the patient is able to maintain the neutral posture. This approach may not be feasible for athletes who require increased spinal motion in their sport.

Acute Phase

The early phase of treatment may be subdivided into acute and subacute phases. Acutely, relative rest is utilized, not bed rest. Pain and inflammation are minimized with medication and modalities, primarily cryotherapy. Patient education for movement and positioning for comfort are important. Patients with discogenic pain will often benefit from extension-based exercise, while posterior element pain benefits from flexion-based exercises.

Subacute care is begun as the patient gains some pain control. The injured tissue remains at relative rest while mobilization is progressed in the alternate directions. Joint mobilization techniques apply forces to restore mobility [32]. The early joint motion in a protected range provides for cartilage nutrition and diminished capsule stiffness. Myofascial release techniques apply shear forces across fascial planes. This breaks adhesions limiting the normal fascial glide mechanisms.

Flexibility and some cardiovascular training are initiated early. The choice of cardiovascular exercise posture is determined by the injury. An athlete with a flexion-based injury is started on extension movements such as walking, treadmill, and breaststroke swimming. Extension-based injuries are started on the stationary bike and freestyle or backstroke swimming. Isometric strengthening is begun to avoid the muscular atrophy that accompanies immobilization.

The use of modalities is also helpful in the subacute phase. Cryotherapy is used to control pain, edema, and bleeding in the early stages of injury and inflammation. In the later stages of rehabilitation, ice helps regulate pain and spasm for mobilization [13]. Heat therapy may be initiated after 48 h to help control spasm and pain and to increase circulation. Moist heat delivers superficial heat with a reflexive increase in circulation. Ultrasound delivers deep heat for circulation and mobilization. Massage may be useful for mobilization in the early phases.

Medication is used to control pain. Acetaminophen and nonsteroidal anti-inflammatory drugs (NSAID) are effective in reducing acute pain. Inflammation causes pain and swelling. This can be limited with NSAID and corticosteroids. However, the utilization of corticosteroids is probably not warranted in the acute setting. The exception may be severe sciatica. Newer NSAID with cyclooxenase-2 specificity minimize the risk of gastrointestinal disturbances.

Recovery Phase

As pain and spasm subside, the level of exercise increases for strength and conditioning. This is the longest period of rehabilitation. Range of motion is increased. Aerobic conditioning is maintained. The biomechanical inflexibilities are aggressively addressed in this phase.

The strengthening progresses from isometric and floor exercises to dynamic progressive resistive exercises (Fig. 8). Isolated strengthening of muscle groups minimizes compensation from surrounding groups. This is specific for the lower abdominal, rotary torso, and lumbar extensor groups. Once full strength of isolated groups has been achieved, coactivation is emphasized with a Swiss ball program. This also enhances balance and proprioception. The kinetic chain is addressed with lower extremity and pelvic strengthening including the hip abductors, gluteus maximus, quadriceps, hamstrings, and gastrosoleus muscles. Impact training may be avoided with water therapy or pilates. Pilates is a series of recumbent exercises using spring resistance initially developed for ballet dancers but now used for many types of rehabilitation. It is particularly suited for back injuries, as gravitational forces are neutralized and peripelvic stabilization is emphasized.

Injured tissues continue healing in this phase. If there is concern about specific injuries such as a spondylolytic stress fracture, bracing is continued. Bracing allows healing while mobilization and strengthening are pursued. A lumbosacral orthosis can be positioned in antilordosis (unloading the posterior elements) or lordosis (unloading the anterior elements).

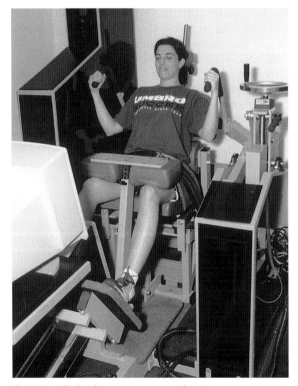

Fig. 8. Specific lumbar extensor strengthening

Modalities play a lesser role in this stage. However, ice and heat assist in mobilization. Electrical stimulation may have benefit. Transcutaneous electrical nerve stimulators (TENS) provide low voltage in varying frequencies to stimulate sensory nerve endings. Their efficacy is debated and they are not recommended as isolated therapy.

If uncertainty exists about the diagnosis and the athlete is experiencing problems advancing his program, selective analgesic/corticosteroid injections are helpful. Fluoroscopically guided nerve root injections will assist the strengthening process and return to sports. For undifferentiated axial low back pain, serial epidural, facet, and sacroiliac injections may be helpful diagnostically and therapeutically. Again, they are used to assist in the stabilization.

Functional Phase

At this point the athlete is back to nearly full strength and endurance. However, prior to returning to sports, functional and sport-specific training are engaged. These include plyometrics, particularly with jumping sports.

An important concern at this stage is to address the sport-specific ergonomics. A crew athlete is at risk with loaded flexion and rotation. Training emphasizes motion through the hips. Lumbar posture is maintained in the pull phase with exhalation and coactivation of the abdominal and lumbar extensor groups [33]. This increased intra-abdominal pressure buffers the forces across the spine. The ballet dancer focuses on pelvic posture and lower abdominal eccentric strength with extension in arabesque.

Athletes in a brace are weaned. If recurrent stress fracture is a concern, a semirigid transitional brace may be used.

Specific Clinical Applications

All spinal problems follow the guidelines delineated above. However, each diagnosis has specific considerations.

Lumbar Disc Herniation

Acute herniation of the nucleus pulposus occurs with a complete tear of the anulus fibrosus. The protruding nucleus is both inflammatory and cytotoxic to the dorsal root ganglion [51, 71]. Acutely, rest may be assisted with a lumbosacral orthosis in a lordotic posture. Oral corticosteroids may be a consideration for acute inflammation. Correction of trunk shifts and inflexibilities are addressed.

Extension-based stabilization is usually performed to centralize the pain. However, a large central or far lateral disc may respond to relatively more flexion. Lower trunk strengthening is advanced as tolerated. Epidural corticosteroids are useful for pain that persists for more than a month. The period before a return to sports may be as long as 6 months. Indications for surgical intervention include cauda equina syndrome, progressive motor loss, and unresponsiveness to at least 8 weeks of a well-directed physical therapy program, with continued incapacitating pain.

Atypical Scheuermann's Disease and Disc Degeneration

Atypical Scheuermann's disease represents thoracolumbar changes of apophyseal ring compressions with wedging, vertebral end plate fractures, and Schmorl's nodes. It is usually encountered in athletes with a "flat back," where there is structurally decreased thoracic kyphosis and decreased lumbar lordosis Disc degeneration is a desiccation of the disc. Rehabilitation starts with correction of inflexibilities. Attention is given to a tight thoracolumbar fascia. Extension-biased and kinetic chain stabilization exercises are employed. A lordotic brace may be useful for relative rest by unloading the disc and for the initial return to sports.

Spondylolysis and Spondylolisthesis

Spondylolysis is a stress fracture of the pars interarticularis. Spondylolisthesis is a secondary forward slippage of the superior vertebral body over its inferior vertebrae. This is best detected with SPECT bone scanning and defined with limited CT scanning. A treatment goal of a symptomatic stress fracture including a minimal spondylolisthesis is to achieve a stable bony or fibrous union. This is accomplished for a lumbosacral orthosis in 4–6 months with associated antilordotic exercises.

However, the rehabilitation may include a return to sports in 4–6 weeks. Athletes aggressively address hip flexor and peripelvic inflexibilities and strengthen antilordotic muscles. Once the athlete is asymptomatic and adjusted to the brace, he is allowed athletic competition as long as he is in the brace and remains symptom-free. Limited lumbar extensor strengthening is initiated at this time. The length of treatment is judged by symptoms and repeat limited CT scanning at 4 to 6 months to evaluate healing.

Lordotic Low Back Pain

This diagnosis is a diagnosis of several other posterior element overuse strains including facet inflammation and degeneration along with spinous process impingement and spinous process apophyseal avulsion injuries. These entities often respond to aggressive attention to hip flexor and thoracolumbar inflexibilities as well as strengthening of trunk and lower extremities. Facet arthropathy may be assisted in rehabilitation with corticosteroid injections.

Transitional Vertebrae

Incomplete segmentation of the lower lumbar and upper sacrum may result in a transitional bony extension to the sacral ala or ileum with a secondary pseudarthrosis. Hyperextension sports may result in inflammation of this pseudarthrosis. The bony extension also alters lumbar motion, increasing stress to the disc space above the transitional vertebrae. Pain may be generated in this disc space. The pain generator may be delineated with bone scan uptake in the pseudarthrosis or MRI changes in the disc.

Rehabilitation is assisted with corticosteroid injections of the inflamed pseudarthrosis or disc. Temporary bracing is also helpful as an anti-inflammatory measure. Flexibility and strength issues are addressed as previously described.

Sacroiliac Inflammation

Inflammation of the sacroiliac joint (SI) is often secondary to biomechanical deficits such as limb length discrepancy or laxity from the hormonal influence of relaxin in the pregnant female. Inherent inflammatory arthropathies are also considered. Rehabilitation progresses in a similar manner. Sacroiliac mobilization techniques are quite adjunctive to the flexibility and strengthening process. The standing bike ergometer is an excellent form of aerobic conditioning. Rotary torso strengthening advances SI stabilization. Correction of limb length greater than 1/2 inch and use of a compression belt limit abnormal SI motion. Corticosteroid injections are also ancillary to the rehabilitation program. These are best performed with fluoroscopically guided technique.

Summary

Rehabilitation of athletic low back pain should follow a logical and orderly pattern. Specific diagnosis assists in the direction of rehabilitation. Attention to age-specific factors is important. Tissue healing is allowed with relative rest. Biomechanical deficits should be addressed. Flexibility and strength along the kinetic chain are aggressively pursued as the inflammation subsides. Ancillary modalities are used only with the intent of enhancing the stabilization process. Sport-specific retraining is crucial step in injury prevention.

References

1. Bellah RD, Summerville DA, Treves ST, Micheli LJ (1991) Low back pain in adolescent athletes: Detection of stress injury to the pars intra-articularis with SPECT. Radiol 180:509–512
2. Bergmark A (1989) Stability of the lumbar spine. A study in mechanical engineering. Acta Orthop Scandinav Suppl 230(60):20–24
3. Bick EM, Copel JW (1950) Longitudinal growth of the human vertebrae. J Bone Joint Surg (Am) 32:803–814
4. Biering-Sorensen F (1984) Physical measurements as risk indicators for low back trouble over a one year period. Spine 9:106–119
5. Bogduk N (1997) Clinical anatomy of the lumbar spine and sacrum, third edn. Churchill Livingston, London
6. Brown T, Micheli L (1998) Where artistry meets injury. Biomechanics 5(9):12–22
7. Cann CE, Martin MC, Genant HK (1984) Decreased spinal mineral content in amenorrheic women. JAMA 251:626–629
8. Congeni J, McCulloch J, Swanson K (1997) Lumbar spondylolysis. A study of natural progression in athletes. Am J Sports Med 25(2):248–253
9. Derby R, Bogduk N, Schwarzer A (1993) Precision percutaneous blocking procedures for localizing pain. Part I: The posterior compartment. Pain Digest 3:89–100
10. Derby R, Howard M, Grant J et al. (1999) The ability of pressure-controlled discography to predict surgical and nonsurgical outcomes. Spine 24(4):364–372
11. Donisch W, Basmajian V (1972) Electromyography of deep back muscles in man. Am J Anat 133:25–36
12. Dreyfuss P, Cole A, Pauza K (1995) Sacroiliac joint injection techniques. Phys Med Rehab Clin North Am 6(4):112–140
13. Drez D (1989) Therapeutic modalities for sports injuries. Year Book Publishers, Chicago
14. Drinkwater BL et al. (1990) Menstrual history as a detriment to current bone density in the young athlete. JAMA 263:545–548
15. Elster AD (1989) Bertolotti's syndrome revisited. Transitional vertebrae of the lumbar spine. Spine 14(12):1373–1377
16. Farfan F, Cossette W, Robertson H et al. (1970) The effects of torsion on the intervertebral joints: The role of torsion in the production of disc degeneration. J Bone Joint Surg 52A:468–497
17. Fellander-Tsai L, Micheli LJ (1998) Treatment of spondylolysis with external electrical stimulation and bracing in adolescent athletes: A report of two cases. Clin J Sport Med 8(3):232–234
18. Ferguson RJ, McMaster JH, Staniski CZ (1974) Low back pain in college football lineman. J Sports Med 2:63
19. Garrick JG, Requa RK (1980) Epidemiology of women gymnast injuries. Am J Sports Med 8:261
20. Gerbino PG, Micheli LJ (1995) Back injuries in the young athlete. Clin Sports Med 14(3):571–589
21. Goldstein JD, Berger PE, Windler GE (1991) Spine injury in gymnasts and swimmers. An epidemiologic investigation. Am J Sports Med 19:463–468
22. Green TP, Allvey JC, Adams MA (1994) Spondylolysis. Bending of the inferior articular processes of lumbar vertebrae during simulated spinal movements. Spine 19(23):2683–2691
23. Hubbard DD (1974) Injuries to the spine in children and adolescents. CIRN Orthopedics 100:156
24. Itaka T, Miyake R, Katoh S, Morita T, Murasa M (1996) Pathogenesis of sports-related spondylolisthesis in adolescents. Radiographic and magnetic resonance imaging study. Am J Sports Med 24(1):94–98
25. Itaka T, Morita T, Katoh S Tachibani K et al. (1995) Lesions of the posterior endplate in children and adolescents. J Bone Joint Surg 77B:951–958
26. Jackson D, Forman W, Benson B (1980) Patterns of injury in college athletes: A retrospect of study of injuries sustained in intercollegiate athletics in two colleges in a two-year period. Mt Sinai J Med 47:423
27. Kawakami M Tamaki T, Hashizume H et al. (1997) The role phospholipase A2 and nitric oxide in pain-related behavior produced by an allograft of intervertebral disc material to the sciatic nerve of the rat. Spine 22:1074–1079
28. Kim N, Suk K (1997) The role of transitional vertebrae in spondylolysis and spondylolytic spondylolisthesis. Bull Hosp Jt Dis 56(3):161–166
29. Lane W (1886) A remarkable example of the manner in which pressure changes in the skeleton may reveal the labour history of the individual. J Anat Physiol 12:385–406
30. Letts M, Smallman T, Afanasiev R (1986) Fracture of the pars interarticularis in adolescent athletes: A clinical biomechanical analysis. J Pediatr Orthop 6:40–46
31. Louks AB, Callister R (1993) Induction and prevention of low T-3 syndrome in exercising women. Am J Physical 264:924–930
32. Maitland G (1993) Vertebral manipulation, fifth edn. Butterworth, London
33. Manning T et al. (1998) Intra-abdominal pressure and rowing: The effect of entrainment. Presented at the American College of Sports Medicine, Orlando USA (unpublished)
34. Martinez-Lage J, Poza M, Arcas P (1998) Avulsed lumbar vertebral rim plate in an adolescent: Trauma or malformation? Childs Nerv Syst 14(3):131–134
35. McKenzie R (1979) Prophylaxis in recurrent low back pain. N Z Med J 89:22–29
36. Merbs C (1995) Incomplete spondylolysis and healing. Spine 20(21):2328–2334
37. Micheli LJ (1979) Low back pain in the adolescent: Differential diagnosis. Am J Sports Med 7(6):362–364
38. Micheli LJ (1983) Overuse injuries in children's sports: The Growth Factor. Orthop Clin North Am 17:337–359
39. Micheli LJ (1985a) Back injuries in gymnastics. Clin Sports Med 4(1):85–93
40. Micheli LJ (1985b) Sports following spinal surgery in the young athlete. Clin Orthop 198:152–157
41. Micheli L, Wood R (1995) Back pain in young athletes. Arch Pediatr Adolesc Med 149:15–18
42. Morita T, Ikata T, Katoh S et al. (1995) Lumbar spondylolysis in children and adolescents. J Bone Joint Surg 77B:620–625
43. Mundt DJ, Kelsey JL, Golden AL et al. (1993) Northeast Collaborative Group on Low Back Pain. An epidemiologic study of sports and weight lifting as possible risk factors for herniated lumbar and cervical discs. Am J Sports Med 21(6):854–860
44. Muschik M (1996) Competitive sports and the progression of spondylolisthesis. J Ped Orthop 16(3):364–369
45. Nachemson A (1996) The load on lumbar disks in different positions of the body. Clin Orthop Rel Res 45:107–122
46. Nerlich A, Schleider E, Boos N (1997) Immunohistologic markers for age-related changes of human lumbar intervertebral discs. Spine 22(24):2781–2795
47. Nigg BM (1994) Biomechanics as applied to sports. In: Harries M, Williams C, Stanish WD, Micheli LJ (eds): The Oxford textbook of sports medicine. Oxford Medical Publications, New York, pp 94–111
48. Noakes TD, Jakoet I, Baalbergen E (1999) An apparent reduction in the incidence and severity of spinal cord injuries in schoolboy rugby players in the western cape since 1990. S Afr Med J 89(5):540–545

49. O'Sullivan P, Manip Phyty G, Twomey T, Allison G (1997) Evaluation of specific stabilizing exercise in the treatment of chronic low back pain with radiologic diagnosis of spondylolisthesis. Spine 22(24):2959–2967

50. Ohmori K, Ishida Y, Takatsu T et al. (1995) Vertebral slip in spondylolysis and spondylolisthesis. J Bone Joint Surg (Br) 77B:771–773

51. Olmarker K (1989) Edema formation in spinal nerve roots induced by experimental graded compression. Spine 14:569–573

52. Pearcy J (1990) Inferred strains in the intervertebral discs during physiologic movements. J Man Med 5:68–71

53. Peh WC, Griffith JF, Yip JK, Leong JC (1998) Magnetic resonance imaging of the lumbar vertebral apophyseal ring fractures. Australas Radiol 42(1):34–37

54. Richardson CA, Jull GA (1995) Muscle control-pain control. What exercises would you prescribe? Manual Therapy 1:2–10

55. Saal J (1990) Dynamic muscular stabilization in the nnonoperative treatment of lumbar pain syndromes. Orthop Rev 19:691–699

56. Sagi H, James G, Jarvis M, Uhthoff H (1998) Histomorphic analysis of the pars interarticularis and its association with isthmic spondylolysis. Spine 23:1635–1640

57. Saifuddin A, White J, Tucker S, Taylor BA (1998) Orientation of lumbar pars defects: Implications for radiological and surgical management. J Bone Joint Surg (Br) 80(2):208–211

58. Salter RB, Harris WR (1963) Injuries involving the epiphyseal plate. J Bone Joint Surg (Am) 45:587–622

59. Sammarco G (1983) The dancer's hip. Clin Sports Med 2:485–498

60. Seitsalo S, Antila H, Karrinaho T (1997) Spondylolysis in ballet dancers. J Dance Med Sci 1:51–54

61. Stewart T (1953) The age and incidence of neural arch defects in Alaskan natives. J Bone Joint Surg (Amer) 35:937

62. Stinson J (1993) Spondylolysis and spondylolisthesis in the athlete. Clin Sport Med 3:517–528

63. Sturesson B, Selvic G, Uden A (1989) Movements of the sacroiliac joints in roentgen stereophotogrammetric analysis. Spine 14:162–165

64. Swaard L (1992) The thoracolumbar spine in young elite athletes. Current concepts on the effects of physical training. Sports Med 13:357–364

65. Swaard L, Hellstrom M, Jacobsonn B (1990) Acute injury to the vertebral ring apophysis and intervertebral disc in adolescent gymnasts. Spine 15:144–148

66. Taimela S, Kujala UM, Salminen JJ et al. (1997) The prevalence of low back pain among children and adolescents. A nationwide, cohort-based questionnaire survey in Finland. Spine 22(10):1132–1136

67. Takata K, Inoue SI, Takahashi K et al. (1988) Fracture of the posterior margin of a lumbar vertebral body. J Bone Joint Surg (Am) 70(4):589–594

68. Tertti M, Paajanen H, Kujula U et al. (1999) Disc degeneration in young gymnasts: A magnetic resonance imaging study. Am J Sports Med 18:206–208

69. Trepman E, Walaszek A, Micheli L (1990) Spinal problems in the dancer. In: Solomon R, Minton S, Solomon J (eds) Preventing dance injuries: An interdisciplinary perspective. American Alliance for Health, Physical Education, Recreation and Dance, Reston USA, pp 103–131

70. Twomey T, Taylor R (1985) Age changes in lumbar intervertebral discs. Acta Orthop Scandinav 56:496–499

71. Yabuki S, Kikuchi Solmarker K et al. (1998) Acute effects of nucleus pulposus on blood flow and endoneural fluid pressure in rat dorsal ganglia. Spine 23(23):2517–2523

72. Yancey RA, Micheli LJ (1994) Thoracolumbar spine injuries in pediatric sports. In: Stanitsky CL, DeLee JC, Drez D (eds) Pediatric and adolescent sports medicine. WB Saunders, Philadelphia, pp 162–174

10 Rehabilitation of the Knee After Anterior Cruciate Ligament Reconstruction

Paolo Aglietti, Fabrizio Ponteggia, Francesco Giron

Introduction

Rehabilitation of the knee after anterior cruciate ligament (ACL) reconstruction is as important today as surgical technique for good clinical and functional results. Rehabilitation was not considered very much until few years ago because it was believed that the only postoperative goal was protection of the "weak" graft by immobilization. Histological and biomechanical studies of ACL autografts performed on animals and humans lead to conflicting results, because human studies showed a faster recovery of the graft characteristics after implantation and higher ultimate load [73]. The graft is mature in humans, the end of the so-called ligamentization process, between 1 [30] and 3 years after ACL reconstruction and is viable as early as 3 weeks without necrosis [67]. Since the return to sport activities is usually between 4 and 9 months after surgery without a significant percentage of graft failure, we can state that other parameters like fixation, tunnel placement, pretensioning, and rehabilitation program are more important than the graft healing process itself for good clinical outcomes.

To avoid complications like extension loss and graft failure, proper tunnel placement is necessary to allow full range of motion (ROM) [16, 41, 46]. Fixation devices are more important if a semitendinosus and gracilis (STG) graft is employed because there is an increased incidence of graft slippage in comparison to bone-patellar tendon-bone (BPTB) grafts; today, however, several methods for strong and stiff proximal STG fixation have been developed.

During recent years, rehabilitation protocols have become more aggressive, permitting sooner and safer return of patients to their sport or work activities with a lower percentage of complications [41, 42, 57, 71, 72, 75]. The improvement in biomechanical knowledge of the knee ligaments [84] by means of in vivo human studies allows us to prescribe safer exercises.

There is a large consensus in the world about the goals of pre- and postoperative rehabilitation (ROM, stability, muscle strength, proprioception, and preinjury level of activity), but agreement does not exist about the speed of progression. In the era of evidence-based medicine, we think that every exercise and device must be tested and validated in a quantitative way; clinical and functional results should also always be statistically analyzed.

In this chapter, the rehabilitation protocol used in the First Orthopaedic Clinic of the University of Florence will be described; a brief review of the literature about ACL rehabilitation-related issues will also be presented.

Biomechanical Studies and Specific Related Issues

In Vivo Biomechanical Studies

We must always remind ourselves that every joint movement (during clinical examination and also activities of daily living) may be more or less dangerous for healing grafts. The best way to measure the effects of movement on the ACL is to measure the forces directly on the ligament in vivo to evaluate strain in the ligament itself, also considering the role of the proprioceptive system, muscles, ligaments, tendons, soft tissues, and all other joint structures (not completely considered during studies performed on cadaveric knee and biomechanical models) [53, 54]. Only the local anesthesia used to perform the investigations could slightly alter the results.

Henning and colleagues [38] were the first to study ACL strain (injured ligament) in vivo, but no statistical evaluation of the data was made due to the small number of patients investigated (only two). Five years later, the first [40] of a long series of studies [11–13, 15, 32–35] from the University of Vermont was published: in this experience, Hall effect strain transducers (HEST) inserted arthroscopically on the anteromedial band of the ACL in vivo in healthy subjects showed for the first time the real amount of ACL strain during knee joint movement.

Analysis of the data obtained performing rehabilitation exercises in vivo [13] showed that at 10° and 20° of flexion, ACL anteromedial band strain for active extension of the knee with a weight of 45 N applied on the lower leg was significantly greater than during active extension without the weight. Isometric quadriceps muscle contraction at 15° and 30° produced a significant increase in anterior cruciate ligament strain, while the same muscle contraction at 60° and 90° of knee flexion displayed no change in strain in comparison with relaxed muscle. Cocontraction of quadriceps and hamstring muscles at 15° provoked a significant increase in ligament strain over the relaxed state while at 30°, 60°, and 90°, no strain was recorded. No ACL strain was recorded during isometric contraction of the hamstring muscle at any angle of ROM. In accordance with these results, it is possible to state that the exercises producing the lowest ACL strain are isometric hamstring contractions at any angle of ROM, active knee movement between 35° and 90°, and isometric quadriceps contraction with the knee flexed at 60° or more. In contrast, it is interesting to note that high ACL strain has been measured during Lachman's test.

Another useful investigation on ACL performed with a transducer implanted in vivo [15] was about ligament strain caused by closed kinetic chain exercises (CKC) and open kinetic chain (OKC) exercises. We remind the reader that, speaking of the lower leg, an OKC exercise occurs when the foot is free while a CKC exercise involves the foot placed on a surface. Some OKC exercises are for example leg extension (for quadriceps) and leg curl (for hamstrings) while squats and leg presses are CKC exercises. Closed kinetic chain exercises are thought to be more protective against ACL strain than OKC exercises due to lower anterior tibial translation from more compressive joint forces and more hamstring-quadriceps cocontraction.

The maximum ACL strain recorded during squatting is not different from that obtained during active flexion-extension. Moreover, squatting performed with an elastic resistance does not add strain over the same exercise without loads. These results seem to show that CKC is not safer than OKC, in contrast to results stated by previous clinical studies.

In any case, a significant difference exists concerning resistance, which provokes more strain if applied during OKC exercises but does not change values if CKC exercises are used.

Bicycling is another exercise often prescribed in many rehabilitation programs after ACL reconstruction. An investigation to measure ACL strain in vivo during stationary bicycling was performed on eight patients before arthroscopic meniscectomy [34]. Biking was performed at three different power levels (75 W, 125 W, and 175 W to simulate downhill, level, and uphill riding conditions) and two cadences (60 rpm and 90 rpm). Therefore, six riding conditions were tested.

The higher ACL strain was recorded during the test with 125 W at 60 rpm, but all the strain values recorded during the six different riding conditions (obtained combining the three different power levels and the two cadences) do not significantly differ. On average, the ACL was strained in the crank angle range from 110° to 180° (with knee ROM from 50° to 37°), with peak ACL strain recorded at a mean crank angle of 148° with the knee at a mean flexion angle of 38°. Moreover, in comparison with the rehabilitation activities described in the previously cited papers, the peak strain values during bicycling were relatively low (Table 1). These results indicate that bicycling is a safe exercise during the rehabilitation period after ACL reconstruction.

Stair climbing is a common activity of daily living and can also be considered a CKC exercise. The ACL strain during stair climbing was recorded in vivo in a study [35] on five subjects with normal ACL before arthroscopic meniscectomy. Climbing cadences of 80 and 112 steps per minute were evaluated on a Stairmaster device. In accordance with results from previous similar studies, strain values increased as the knee moved from flexion to extension. No significant difference was recorded by changing the cadence. In comparison with other rehabilitation activities, the strain values provoked during stair climbing were highly variable between subjects.

Table 1 summarizes the peak strain values during common rehabilitation activities as measured by researchers at the University of Vermont, USA [13].

Table 1. Peak strain values measured during common rehabilitation activities by researchers at the University of Vermont, USA

Activity	Peak strain
Isometric quadriceps contraction at 15° of knee flexion (to 30 Nm extension torque)	4.4%
Squatting with sport cord	4.0%
Active knee flexion-extension with 45 N weight boot	3.8%
Lachman's test (150 N of anterior shear load at 30° flexion)	3.7%
Squatting	3.6%
Active knee flexion-extension without weight	2.8%
Simultaneous quadriceps and hamstring contractions at 15°	2.8%
Isometric quadriceps contraction at 30° (to 30 Nm extension torque)	2.7%
Stair climbing	2.7%
Anterior drawer (150 N anterior shear load at 90° flexion)	1.8%
Stationary bicycling	1.7%
Isometric hamstring contraction at 15° (to −10 Nm flexion torque)	0.6%
Simultaneous quadriceps and hamstring contractions at 30°	0.4%
Passive knee flexion-extension	0.1%
Isometric quadriceps contraction at 60° (to 30 Nm extension torque)	0.0%
Isometric quadriceps contraction at 90° (to 30 Nm extension torque)	0.0%
Simultaneous quadriceps and hamstring contractions at 60°	0.0%
Simultaneous quadriceps and hamstring contractions at 90°	0.0%
Isometric hamstring contraction at 30°, 60°, and 90° (to −10 Nm flexion torque)	0.0%

Open Versus Closed Kinetic Chain

The effectiveness and safeness of OKC versus CKC exercises are matters of debate. Differences between these two types of kinetic chain exercise (ligament strain, joint compression forces, muscle activity, clinical results after ACL reconstruction) have been studied by several authors [15, 50, 60, 80, 86].

Wilk et al. [83] compared three exercises: squat (CKC), leg press (CKC), and leg extension (OKC). During isotonic exercises performed by 10 healthy subjects, the author recorded tibiofemoral joint kinetics (compressive force, anteroposterior shear force, and extension torque) and the electromyographic activity of quadriceps, hamstrings, and gastrocnemius. The results showed that isotonic CKC exercises produced significantly greater compressive forces than the OKC extension; during CKC exercises, a posterior shear force (the resisting forces to anterior drawer; posterior cruciate ligament stress) was generated throughout the entire ROM, with maximal shear from 85° to 105° of flexion, while during OKC exercises there was an anterior shear force (the resisting forces to posterior drawer; ACL stress) from 38° to 0° and a posterior shear force from 40° to 101°. A greater posterior shear force was produced during CKC than OKC exercises. Not all CKC exercises produce cocontraction of the hamstrings and quadriceps (more cocontraction during squat). Furthermore, the level of cocontraction depended on trunk position relative to the knee joint and also the application of force and knee flexion angle. There were significant differences in joint forces and EMG activity during the ascending and descending phases of both OKC and CKC exercises. This study let us know that not all CKC exercises have the same effects on joint compressive forces and cocontraction: for example, the difference in trunk position means that leg presses "should" be less protective than squats. The joint compression forces must be considered, especially when there are combined chondral lesions in primary weight-bearing areas.

Open and closed kinetic chain exercises were also investigated by Lutz [50] in 5 healthy subjects and a biomechanical model to compare tibiofemoral joint forces. The results showed that during OKC extension exercise the maximum anterior shear forces occurred at 30° of knee flexion and maximum posterior shear forces occurred at 90°. The CKC produced significantly greater compression forces and increased muscle cocontractions at the same angles where OKC produced maximum shear forces.

Quantification of the anterior tibial displacement occurring in ACL-deficient knees during OKC (resisted knee extension) and CKC (parallel squat) exercises was performed by Yack et al. [86] in comparison with Lachman's tests.

The results showed a greater displacement during OKC extension than during squats from 64° to 10° of knee flexion. The displacement during the Lachman's test was lower than that during OKC but more than during CKC.

Bynum et al. [17] conducted a clinical study in 100 patients undergoing ACL reconstruction to compare OKC and CKC exercises after ACL reconstruction (mean follow-up 19 months): the results showed that the CKC group had lower anterior tibial translation (measured with KT1000), less patellofemoral pain, more subjective satisfaction, and faster return to activities of daily living (ADL) and sports. A recent clinical study [55] seems to prove that there are better results (same stability, faster return to sports activities, and higher muscle torque) using both OKC and CKC instead of CKC alone; in this study, OKC exercises consisted of isokinetic concentric and eccentric quadriceps exercises starting from the seventh postoperative week, initially in the ROM from 90° to 40° and then from 90° to 10°.

Observing the overall results of the reported biomechanical studies (in vivo, clinical, and mathematical), in our opinion it is possible to state that an ACL rehabilitation protocol must combine both OKC and CKC exercises. The exercises should be modified and modulated depending on the specific sport activities and the combined lesions or syndromes (chondral damage or tendinitis, for example) of each patient [31].

Continuous Passive Motion

We do not use continuous passive motion (CPM) devices after ACL reconstruction, preferring to stimulate the patient to perform ROM exercises actively. Continuous passive motion does not help patients regain ROM and diminish pain after ACL reconstruction. Rigon et al. [64] studied 40 patients with chronic ACL lesions divided in two groups after ligament reconstruction with BPTB. After surgery, a group of patients performed CPM for 1 h three times a day in the ROM between 0° and 60° at a speed of ten cycles every minute; every day 10° were added. In the other group, patients performed passive knee flexion-extension assisting with their hands during the first 2 postoperative days, and from the third day they began active motion as tolerated. The rehabilitation program was the same in both groups concerning weight-bearing and other exercises. After 2 months there were no significant differences between the two groups in ROM, pain, or thigh circumference. To be noted: there was faster reduction of swelling in the second and third postoperative weeks for patients performing CPM.

Another study [66] evaluated the potential advantages of combining active motion and CPM in comparison with CPM or active exercises alone. Seventy-five patients were divided into three groups (active motion, CPM, and combination of both) after ACL reconstruction with BPTB. Continuous passive motion was used 20 h/day during the hospital stay and a minimum of 6 h/day at home for 4 weeks in a ROM from 0° to 90°. Subjectively, the patients appreciated CPM very much. No significant differences were found between the groups at follow-up of 6 months regarding ROM, joint stability, usage of analgesics, or length of hospital stay.

The duration of using CPM devices seems unimportant for improving postoperative parameters. Richmond et al. [63] compared 4-day CPM vs. 2-week CPM after ACL reconstruction with BPTB in 20 patients. The CPM device was used at least 6 h/day. Joint laxity measured with KT1000 was better in the 14-day CPM group. This finding is useful to demonstrate the safeness of CPM. There were no significant differences at 6-week follow-up in joint swelling, muscle atrophy, and ROM. The absence of risk to joint stability after surgery depends above all on the type of CPM machine. The CPM devices that support the leg at the calf could provoke undesired strain of the healing graft (such as an anterior tibial translation caused by a 20-lb Lachman's test). If the leg is supported at the heel and the posterior thigh risk of, there is no translation [25]. Moreover, a study on 13 anatomic knee specimens demonstrated a direct correlation between isometricity of the ACL substitution (defined as equal to or less than 1 mm of graft length change through a knee ROM of 0°–110°) and changes in knee stability after CPM [59]. These basic scientific and clinical results are also important from a financial point of view for patients, who need not rent the machine after discharge, and for the hospital because it frees CPM devices for patients that really need them [20].

We can state that, using CPM after ACL reconstruction, there is no change in laxity but no improvement in ROM, even though there is an increase in subjective patient satisfaction. The doubt concerns the cost effectiveness of this device.

Electrical Muscle Stimulation

In our rehabilitation program, electrical muscle stimulation (EMS) of the quadriceps muscle is allowed starting from the beginning of the second postoperative week. We warn the patient and the physical therapist on the protocol delivered: the stimulation must be performed in "isometric fashion," i.e., without provoked joint motion (knee extension or flexion > 60°) to protect the joint and the graft. When we prescribed EMS of the quadriceps in knee flexion (no ACL strain at 60° according to Beynnon's studies), many patients said that during the stimulation there was sudden knee extension; so it is safer in our opinion to stimulate at the 0° position to avoid active involuntary knee extension and to assure safe isometric contraction (so the ACL strain is the same as with straight leg raises). The effectiveness of EMS alone or combined with active exercises has been evaluated by several authors, as reviewed by Selkowitz [69]. Moreover, other authors studied the biochemical effects of EMS [6, 27].

High intensity EMS (2500-Hz triangular alternating current at a burst rate of 75 bursts/s) seems to be more effective than low intensity portable EMS in the recovery of quadriceps strength (15 min four times a day 5 days a week, pulse duration 0.3 ms, frequency 55 Hz, on time 15 s, off time 50 s). The stimulation was performed in isometric fashion at 65° of flexion [77, 78]. The patients who received EMS had more normal gait and showed better values for cadence, walking velocity, stance time, and flexion excursion [76]. Females seem to react better than males to electrical stimulation of the quadriceps after ACL reconstruction, showing a lower degree of muscle atrophy [6]. There is no consensus about the effectiveness of EMS after ACL reconstruction. A recent randomized, double-blinded, controlled study from Austria [61] showed no significant difference in isometric and isokinetic torque in the knee extensor and flexor muscles comparing a rehabilitation program based on early exercises alone with early exercises combined plus EMS. The study groups were composed of 49 patients. The EMS was performed daily during the first 6 weeks after ACL reconstruction, starting from the third or fifth day. Follow-up evaluation was conducted after 6, 12, and 52 weeks. Electrical stimulation parameters and protocol were as follows: stimulation intensity was enough for strong muscle contraction; impulse rectangular monophasic length 0.2 ms; first set of stimulation: frequency 30 Hz, on time 5 s, ramp 1 s, off time 15 s, 12 repetitions; the second set after 6 min of rest: frequency 50 Hz, on time 10 s, ramp 2 s, off time 50 s, 12 repetitions.

Nowadays, many EMS devices are integrated in handy minicomputers that allow sequential programs of stimulation, varying parameters such as impulse and pause duration. In our opinion, these devices could be effective and helpful in recovering muscle strength together with an active exercise program, but more controlled prospective studies should be published about this topic in peer-reviewed journals. Moreover, due to the complexity of computerized stimulation protocols, it is difficult to know the relevance of any single parameter.

Braces

Knee braces can be used preoperatively (when the patient is ACL-deficient) to protect the joint from giving-way episodes that could provoke chondral damage or meniscus lesions, postoperatively (to avoid ACL graft strain during the early healing period), and later as functional braces at the return to sport-specific activities.

In our opinion, the use of a protective brace prior to surgery is useful only if there is joint instability during activities of daily living and it is impossible to perform an ACL reconstruction soon. We do not use postoperative orthosis unless there is a combined ligamentous lesion or a meniscal repair because avoiding a postoperative brace has been reported to have no adverse effects on joint stability, ROM, hamstring-quadriceps strength, subjective assessment, and functional outcomes using BPTB or DSTG as grafts [43, 45, 56]

Functional braces help to protect the graft [14], diminishing anterior tibial translation when the patient begins sport-specific activities (protective effect on ACL strain up to 140 N) but, due to their biomechanical role, also have an influence on muscle function [24, 65, 85]. The role in reducing anterior tibial translation verified in most braces seems to be effective only if there are low forces [65]. Moreover, during the stance phase of walking there should be a reduction of protection [24]. In our opinion, as stated above, functional braces are important during the preoperative phase if there is an associated MCL lesion. Explaining to the patient the limited protective effect of the brace is of fundamental importance.

Water Therapy

If the healing process of the surgical wounds is completed, we allow swimming exercises starting between the third and fourth postoperative weeks. The decreased stress on the knee joint underwater helps in the gait retraining phase and during weight-bearing exercises. The advantages of exercises in water are accommodating resistance (such as the force exerted by the patient) and variable resistance (according to normal movements of the patient and not at a fixed speed, as with isokinetic devices). These advantages are helpful in regaining functional knee skills because, in nature, most human motion is variable [62].

Exercises performed in water seem to be less effective than traditional exercises on land in recovery of muscle strength, especially in flexion, but they provoke less joint effusion. In a recent comparative study [81], 20 patients were divided into two groups after ACL reconstruction with BPTB to perform "traditional" or "water" rehabilitation programs. During the first postoperative week, both groups followed the same program with active knee flexion, passive extension, and calf and hamstring stretching. Weight bearing was done as tolerated with two crutches (no crutches from the tenth day) and a brace locked in extension (90° from the second week and 120° from the third to sixth postoperative weeks). From the second to the eighth postoperative weeks, both groups performed the same exercise program three times a week, one group on the land and the other in water. The programs consisted of stationary cycling, gait training without brace, stepups, hip muscle exercises, and knee flexion. The muscle

strengthening exercises were performed in the water using Hydrotone resistance boots. A pedaling device was used in the water as a stationary bicycle. Neither program induced more knee joint laxity (measured with KT1000 arthrometer) than the other. At 8-week follow-up, there were no differences in ROM between the groups. It is interesting to note that significantly higher Lysholm scores were recorded in patients with water rehabilitation due to a lower incidence of reported pain and swelling during activities of daily living. In contrast, hamstring isokinetic torque was significantly better in traditional group. These results show that part of the rehabilitation program should be performed in water to allow earlier weight bearing and reduce joint swelling and pain without stopping exercise. But even though the patient might prefer the swimming pool program, we must also prescribe traditional land exercise to enable better muscle strengthening.

Cryotherapy

There are different methods to perform cryotherapy: simple bags of crushed ice, cold packs, and cooling and compression devices. Some authors studied the effect of cryotherapy in the knee recording skin, subcutaneous, and intra-articular temperatures [22] and comparing the role of various icing times in decreasing bone metabolism and blood flow [39]. Although cryotherapy is probably the "oldest modality in the world" due to its analgesic, anti-inflammatory, and antiedemagen effects, there is no consensus about its duration and mode of employment.

The clinical and functional effectiveness of cryotherapy after ACL reconstruction has been studied by several authors evaluating some parameters like knee swelling, ROM, pain, length of hospital stay, and drug consumption. The results are not homogeneous: some authors [23, 26, 47] found no benefits in the treated groups while others [7, 21, 58, 74] observed less postoperative pain, shorter length of hospitalization, and a reduction in drug requirements.

Continuous-flow cold therapy plus compression seems to be more effective than traditional methods in diminishing pain and swelling, but we do not know exactly if the benefit is due more to compression or to the lower temperature. The effectiveness of cryotherapy in the early postoperative phase could be largely due to the placebo effect, because there is often no significant reduction of skin and intra-articular temperature from applying the cold devices on the dressing.

Cryotherapy is surely more effective in pain and swelling reduction during the rehabilitation phase (after removal of the dressing) at the end of any exercise session. We must always remember that cryotherapy may induce nerve injury [8], so it is necessary to pay attention to the thickness of the subcutaneous fat and the duration of tissue cooling, especially on the peroneal nerve.

Proprioceptive Rehabilitation

In our opinion, rehabilitation of the proprioceptive system is as important as the restoration of ROM and the recovery of muscle strength after ACL reconstruction, especially in athletes. Proprioceptive training is a valid method of preventing ACL injuries and reducing new injuries after ACL reconstruction. A prospective study in two groups of 300 Italian soccer players each showed that the inclusion of balance exercises in the traditional training program significantly reduces the incidence of ACL injuries [18].

A functional sports agility program started in the first 4 weeks after ACL reconstruction to enhance proprioception is safe and does not provoke reductions in joint stability [70].

Another study demonstrates that a proprioceptive exercise program in ACL-deficient patients can be more useful than traditional rehabilitation for the improvement of knee function and reflex hamstring contraction latency [10]. Unfortunately, a good method of quantifying the function of a proprioceptive system does not exist. We can only measure some components such as proprioception (reproduction of joint position), kinesthesia (threshold to detect joint motion), static or dynamic balance (force platform, unstable board), and reflex hamstring contraction latency (via EMG). The basis of the proprioceptive system and its role in the prevention of joint lesion are treated in another chapter of this book.

Clinical Experience

We reported the rehabilitation methods and clinical results of three authors who published studies on "accelerated" (also called "aggressive") rehabilitation programs after ACL reconstruction, from the historical paper published by Noyes [57] to the more recent studies of Shelbourne (BPTB grafts) [70–72, 75] and Howell (STG grafts) [42–44]. In comparison with those from Shelbourne and Howell, our rehabilitation program in Florence is slower, especially for a return to sport-specific activities, but nearly the same for the first 2 weeks (except for the use of CPM).

Noyes

In our opinion, the prospective randomized study [57] published in 1987 by Noyes is a historic milestone for rehabilitation: in this paper, he reported the results of a comparison between early knee motion and delayed motion after ACL reconstruction, demonstrating the safety of the former treatment. The patients were divided in a randomized way into two groups, "motion" (brace limitation 0°–90°, 10 h/day continuous passive motion starting from second postoperative day until discharge, then intermittent passive motion) and "delayed motion" (soft hinged knee brace locked at 10° of flexion for 6 days after reconstruction, intermittent passive motion 0°–90°, 90°–30° active assisted motion, and 30°–0° passive motion from the seventh day). Both groups performed EMS (20 min three times a week), cryotherapy, straight leg raises (supine and prone without weight), and isometric exercises (quadriceps and hamstrings ten times holding the contraction for 10 s hourly). Weight bearing was not allowed for the first 6 days while, from the seventh day, all the patients began partial (25%) weight bearing. Patellar mobilization started from the second postoperative week for 5 min/h. The patients were discharged from the hospital when they were able to perform straight leg raises and quadriceps isometrics and could ambulate satisfactorily.

At home, both groups performed intermittent passive motion (0°–90°using the uninvolved leg to assist the involved limb for 5 min/h to 10 min/h. Partial weight bearing (50%) and stationary bicycling (20 min two times daily) started at the end of the fourth postoperative week. The results showed that early knee motion did not increase joint effusion (absent in all the patients at the end of the second week), hemarthrosis, and soft tissue swelling; moreover, no statistically significant differences were found in pain medication used, length of hospital stay, and ROM (however, a tendency to more knee extension and flexion at the end of the second and third postoperative weeks was observed in the early motion group). In both groups, a marked decrease in thigh circumference was recorded, so early motion did not seem to be effective in preventing the muscle atrophy due to joint injury and inactivity observed by several authors [28, 37]. Stability testing performed with a KT1000 arthrometer at 12-month follow-up showed no deleterious effect of early knee motion on stretching the ligament reconstruction. According to his results, Noyes recommends in conclusion an early motion program to reduce morbidity (for example, minimize scar tissue formation) of major intra-articular ligamentous procedures.

Shelbourne

The "accelerated" rehabilitation program [70–72, 75] prescribed by Shelbourne to his patients begins prior to surgery with a preoperative phase: the goals are restoration of full ROM, including hyperextension at the level of the uninjured knee, reduced swelling, and recovery of a normal gait. The exercises suggested to achieve these goals are prone hangs, heel prop extensions, wall slides, active assisted flexion, gait training, bicycling, use of the Stairmaster, leg presses, and squats. Continuous passive motion is started a few hours after the ACL reconstruction using patellar tendon as graft, with the knee moved from 0° to 30° of flexion and continuing full time for 1 week. The CPM together with cold compression device and bed rest is important to minimize the development of postoperative hemarthrosis, which is dangerous because it inhibits the quadriceps muscle and ROM. Once an hour for 10 min, the patient places his heel on the end of the bed frame to obtain hyperextension of the knee. Three times a day, he sits on the side of the bed (usually while eating) to reach 90° of knee flexion and perform straight leg raises and short-arc quadriceps exercises. Weight bearing is allowed immediately from the first day as tolerated, with two crutches during the first postoperative week only to go to the bathroom. The patient is discharged from the hospital if knee flexion is at least 90° and there is good leg control and full hyperextension. He must maintain full hyperextension, decrease swelling, maintain active quadriceps control, increase knee flexion to more than 90°, and allow wound healing. During the second week after surgery, the patient can return to work or school, limiting all other activities. At the end of second postoperative week, knee flexion must reach 110°, and if all other goals of the first 2 weeks are maintained and the wound is completely healed, the patient begins knee bends, step-ups, leg presses, squats, and stationary bicycling. In this period (from the second to fifth postoperative weeks), he can increase the activities and also perform functional agility exercises to improve muscle reaction time. After 5 weeks, an isokinetic test is performed: if quadriceps muscle strength is at least 65% of the contralateral leg's, the patient begins sport-specific activities requiring hand-eye coordination and foot agility to regain proprioception and confidence in the knee faster. If the strength is below 65%, there is a risk of swelling and soreness: the patient is allowed to begin sport-specific activities with more emphasis on strengthening than functional activities (isokinetic testing is repeated every 2 months). A return to competitive sports is allowed according to the improvement in strength and confidence. These are the results after ACL reconstruction followed by accelerated rehabilitation in 806 patients (76% of the total) at a mean follow-up of 4 years (range 2 to 9.1 years, SD 1.6):

1. Mean ROM 5°/0°/140° (contralateral 6°/0°/140°)
2. Stability. Mean manual maximum KT1000 arthrometer difference 2.0 ± 1.5 considering the period 1990–1993 in 93% of chronic reconstructions. In 92% of acute reconstructions, the difference was ≥ 3 mm

3. Quadriceps muscle strength. Cybex II dynamometer isokinetic strength test at 180°/s revealed in chronic and acute reconstruction means of 94% and 91% of muscle strength, respectively, in comparison with the contralateral side
4. International Knee Documentation Committee (IKDC) evaluation form. Normal or nearly normal in 89% of acute and 85% of chronic cases, radiographically no joint space narrowing in 94% of acute and 89% of chronic reconstructions. Moreover, no patients had more than 50% joint-space narrowing
5. Return to sport-specific activities 1990–1993: 76% by 2 months after surgery

Shelbourne states that accelerated rehabilitation programs do not increase graft failure: evaluation showed that before 1987 (when accelerated rehabilitation was started), 4.4% of the patients tore their grafts while after this, the percentage dropped to 2.6%.

Howell

Dr. Howell [42–44] prescribes an "aggressive" rehabilitation program after ACL reconstruction with double-looped semitendinosus and gracilis tendon. After surgery, the knee is not braced and discharge from the hospital is on the same day of reconstruction. Weight bearing is as tolerated with crutches, usually until the third postoperative week. By the first 7–10 days after surgery, the knee must move from 0° to 90°: the patient performs active motion with heel slides and prone stretching as tolerated. During the first 2 weeks, muscle strengthening exercises are performed (straight leg raises, isometric hamstring and quadriceps contractions, hip muscle exercises). The patient is instructed about wound care. During the third and fourth postoperative weeks, he can use the stationary bicycle (10–15 min two times a day) without wheel resistance and moreover can walk and swim as tolerated: knee flexion should be at least 120°. Open and closed kinetic chain exercises are allowed without restriction (suggested time 1 h/day at least three to five times a week) starting from the fourth postoperative week (lower weight and higher number of repetitions are prescribed to build endurance). At the end of the eighth postoperative week, the patient should feel his knee well enough to start light jogging, golf, basket shooting, and agility training such as forward and backward running and side-to-side crossovers. From the eighth to the 16th postoperative weeks, weight and resistance on the exercise machine are increased. Long bikes rides are encouraged on a level surface, first increasing distance and then speed. A return to full and unrestricted sports activities is usually at 4 months after evaluation of Lysholm score, stability, ROM, thigh circumference, and ability to perform a single-leg hop-test. The patient is taught about the fact that regaining full confidence in the reconstructed knee may take 6 months to a year.

At follow-up 4 months after surgery, the difference from contralateral performance of the manual maximum test was less than 3 mm in 90% of knees (no significant increase at a follow-up of 2 years). The hop index was between 95% and >105% at 2-year follow-up. The author places great importance on the method of graft fixation for maximizing results regarding stability and early return to sports activities with "aggressive" rehabilitation.

Our Experiences

DSTG ACL Reconstruction with Mitek Ligament Anchor

Valid fixation is fundamental to avoid the increase in laxity after ACL reconstruction, especially using hamstring tendon as graft. Our group [36] reported the results of ACL reconstruction using DSTG fixed on the femur with a 25-mm Mitek ligament anchor with the two tendons looped around the slot in the anchor in 47 patients with isolated complete ACL injury. The average patient age at ACL reconstruction was 28 years (range 17–48) and average injury-surgery interval 19 months (range 1–156). Sixty-five percent of patients were involved in IKDC class I and II activities. Fixation of the graft in the tibia was performed with an RCI screw (Rounded Cannulated Interference screw; Donjoy, Carlsbad, CA, USA) supplemented with a spiked washer and bicortical screw.

At 24-month follow-up, we clinically reviewed 43 patients (two patients did not present to follow-up examinations, one with an ACL reinjury and the other with fracture due to an accident). Rehabilitation was without braces. Partial weight bearing was allowed immediately with two crutches (in the first 3 days after surgery only for bathroom visits) and full weight bearing after 1 month. Return to sports activities were after 6 months from ACL reconstruction. We clinically evaluated all patients with the IKDC evaluation form. Tests using KT1000 for joint stability and Cybex II for concentric isokinetic muscle strength were performed in 40 patients with normal contralateral knees.

At 12 months, knee pain was referred by 6 patients. Nobody reported giving-way episodes. The KT1000 side-to-side difference (ssd) was 2.2 mm at 30 lbs (range 0–5 mm) and 58% of patients had less than 3 mm, apart from one case with 6 mm after reinjury playing soccer. Quadriceps deficits were 5%, 6%, and 5.5% and flexor deficits were 5.5%, 7%, and 5% at angular speeds of 60°/s, 120°/s, and 180°/s, respectively, in comparison with the opposite normal sides.

At 24 months, 98% of the patients were subjectively satisfied with the results of the ACL reconstruction (final IKDC grading: 93% satisfactory). No patients complained of swelling or giving way. Pain attributed to soft tissue irritation around the fixation devices was reported by 2%. Nonpainful patellofemoral crepitus was present in 24%. Joint stability was the same as at the previous follow-up. Quadriceps deficits were 2% at all velocities, flexors deficits were 5% at 180°/s and 4% at 120°/s and 60°/s. Eighty-five percent of patients returned to preinjury levels of activity.

Many studies with various periods of follow-up reported similar values (deficits ≤10%) of flexion torque after ACL reconstruction using hamstring tendon as graft [2, 4, 5, 48, 49, 51, 87, 88]. Other authors [19, 52] described higher flexion torque deficits.

These good results in the recovery of flexor strength after tendon harvesting can be explained with their regeneration potential [29]. Furthermore, it could be interesting to measure not only concentric but also eccentric isokinetic torque to find a more functional index, such as the ratio of eccentric hamstring to concentric quadriceps moments for extension or that of concentric hamstring to eccentric quadriceps moments for flexion [1].

DSTG ACL Reconstruction with Bone Mulch Screw

To obtain strong and stiff femoral fixation closer to the joint when performing ACL reconstruction with DSTG, we now use the bone mulch screw in which both tendons are looped around the nose of the screw. Tibial fixation and the rehabilitation program are the same as previously described.

At a follow-up of 12 months, we reviewed 101 patients of a total of 102. (One refused to participate). The average age at ACL reconstruction was 27 years (range 16–50) and the injury-surgery interval was 25 months (range 1–180). We used the IKDC form, KT1000 evaluation (30-lb ssd), and Cybex II isokinetic concentric test.

The results at 12-month follow-up show a 95% satisfactory final IKDC grading. Tibial translation was within 5 mm in 96% of patients (average KT ssd at 30 lb was 2.4 mm, with 67% of patients within 3 mm). No patient complained of activity-restraining symptoms. Patellofemoral crepitus was symptomatic in one patient. Isokinetic evaluation showed a deficit of 7% for quadriceps and hamstrings at 60°/s, and an 8% average deficit of internal rotation strength was found at 30°/s. This measurement is important because hamstrings are involved not only in knee flexion but also internal rotation [79]. Radiographically, the femoral tunnel was not identifiable in the sagittal plane in most cases, while tunnel widening was found in 46% of the tibias.

We can state that ACL reconstruction with DSTG

fixed proximally using bone mulch screws gives excellent results in terms of subjective evaluation, knee stability, and muscle strength recovery. Furthermore, graft fixation close to the joint and the use of bone graft in the tunnel decrease tunnel widening.

Prospective Study: BPTB Versus DSTG

In 1994 we published a prospective study [2] to report the results after 28 months of follow-up (range 22–39) in 63 patients with chronic ACL injuries surgically treated in strictly alternating manner using either BPTB or DSTG grafts (interval from injury to surgery: at least 6 months). The STG grafts were double-looped (four strands). Proximal fixation was achieved by securing the proximal loop of the tendons with a cortical screw and spiked plastic soft tissue washer; tibial fixation was obtained by tying the sutures over a cortical screw and washer. The BPTB was fixed distally with an interference screw, while in femur fixation it was with a press-fit locking of the patellar bone fragment and four nonabsorbable sutures tied over a cortical screw and washer.

The rehabilitation program was a bit slower in progression and less aggressive than that in use today: after surgery, patients wore splints for 1 month and began ROM exercises from the second postoperative day (0°–90° before discharge from the hospital), full weight-bearing was allowed by the end of the second postoperative month, stationary bike with short crank and proprioceptive exercises started during the second postoperative month, exercise against resistance in the 0°–45° ROM was avoided until the sixth month, running started after 4 months, and the return to sport activities occurred between 6 and 8 months postoperatively. We could not review three patients at follow-up, so each of the two groups was composed of 30 patients.

After 28-month follow-up, there was no significant difference in symptomatology. Return to sports participation was more frequent in the BPTB group (80% vs. 43%, $p < 0.01$), but an extension loss ($\leq 3°$) was present more often in this group (47% vs. 3%, $p \leq 0.001$).

The KT1000 arthrometer side-to-side difference of >5 mm at 30 lb was present in 13% of the BPTB group patients and in 20% of those with DSTG grafts (no significant difference). Patellofemoral crepitus was more frequent in the BPTB group (17% vs. 3%). No significant differences were found measuring extension and flexion concentric torque deficits with a Cybex II isokinetic machine: the average deficits were less than 10% and slightly higher (peak extension torque deficit at 60°/s 10.7%) in the DSTG group.

A new evaluation of the same groups was performed at an average follow-up of 5.7 years (range 5.2–6.2) [3]. Two significative differences between the groups were recorded: (1) no giving way was present in the patellar tendon group, while it was reported in 13% ($p = 0.03$) of

the patients in the DSTG group, and (2) recovery of hamstring strength was lower in the DSTG group at both 60°/s (93% vs. 102%, $p = 0.03$) and 180°/s (90% vs. 103%, $p = 0.07$). Return to sport, objective stability, ROM, and patellofemoral symptoms (asymptomatic crepitus was present in 10% of patients in both groups) were not significantly different. KT1000 arthrometer stability testing showed an average ssd of 3.1 mm at 30 lb for the BPTB and 4.0 for the DSTG groups. Decrease in stability (DSTG group in comparison with previous evaluation at a follow-up of 28 months: 3.2 mm vs. 4.0 mm) was lower (3.2 mm vs. 3.4 mm) if we excluded patients whose distal graft fixation was made with sutures (ssd 5.2 mm) and not very different compared with the BPTB group (3.4 mm vs. 3.1 mm). In conclusion, we can state that much of the translation recorded in the DSTG group was due to nonoptimal fixation.

We are now performing a new prospective study to compare the clinical and functional results of ACL reconstruction in isolated chronic ACL injuries using DSTG and BPTB grafts fixed on the femur with the same technique: bone mulch screw for the hamstring tendons and blunt nose screws for the patellar tendon. The rehabilitation program is that already described in this chapter using both BPTB and DSTG. These prospective studies are important to learning the relative importance to final results of choice of graft, surgical technique (tunnel placement, fixation devices), and rehabilitation program.

Rehabilitation Protocol

The goals of rehabilitation are: restore full ROM and regain muscle strength and motor control (proprioception) without provoking graft elongation or rupture. A written rehabilitation program is given to each ACL-deficient patient. The therapeutic exercises are detailed with clear drawings and pictures. In this way, all patients can perform the rehabilitation with satisfactory compliance and no continuous supervision. In our opinion, the best solution would be a prolonged rehabilitation in specialized centers, but these are rare and expensive, so only a small number of patients (such as high-level athletes) can attend them. Therefore, in accordance with several studies [9, 68, 82] in which no advantages were found in frequently supervised over periodically supervised home rehabilitation (observing parameters like function, activity level, anterior tibial translation, muscle strength, and subjective satisfaction), the latter solution is prescribed for most patients; the role of the periodical supervisors (orthopedic surgeon and physiatrist with the help of physical therapists) is to control, correct, and improve the exercise methods.

Our program follows both time-based and criterion-based progressions; it is the same for ACL reconstruction with BPTB or semitendinosus and gracilis. The patient's name, date, and type of surgery are entered on the first page. In particular, we also indicate ACL graft (BPTB or DSTG), combined lesions and surgical treatment if performed: medial collateral ligament (MCL), lateral collateral ligament (LCL), meniscus lesion treated with meniscectomy or suture, and area and grade of chondral lesion. This is done for quick recognition of the main information about the treated knee. We do not use CPM. A postoperative brace is prescribed only if there is combined ligamentous injury or if meniscal suture is performed.

We now describe all the information and exercises that the patients can read in their programs. It is important to remind patients that a medical control is necessary before starting each new phase of the rehabilitation program. The presence of soft-tissue swelling or effusion and the lack of expected ROM are reasons to stop the progression to the following phase.

Phase 1: Before Surgery

Psychological preparation of patients to surgery and rehabilitation is very important to obtain their maximum commitment. Moreover, the surgeon and the patient should choose together the best period to perform

ACL reconstruction (minimum 3 weeks after the injury to avoid complications like lack of knee motion after surgery). Before surgery, the patient must reach these goals:

1. Control of pain and swelling with rest, cryotherapy (ice bags for 20 min three times a day), NSAID, and dressing (not during exercises).
2. Recovery of full ROM with passive and active knee extension in supine position with the heel raised slightly (Fig. 1), passive knee extension in prone position with the leg out of the bed and the knee on the edge, active knee extension with the heel on an inclined plane (Fig. 2), and active knee flexion in supine position on a slide board (Fig. 3) or performing wall slides (Fig. 4). (Another way to perform active knee flexion is in the sitting position).
3. Reestablishment of normal gait by walking with crutches (partial weight bearing also using a mirror to note mistakes) and the knee in full extension during weight bearing and flexed during the swing phase of the gait. If there is a chronic ACL injury (more than 30 days elapsed), the patient must also regain muscle strength (quadriceps and hamstrings).

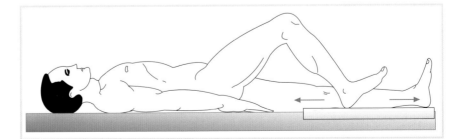

Fig. 1. Passive and active knee extension in supine position with the heel on a support such as a rolled towel

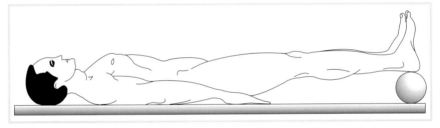

Fig. 2. Active knee extension with the heel on an inclined plane

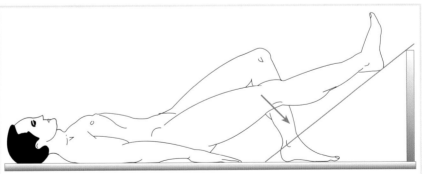

Fig. 3. Active knee flexion sliding on a board

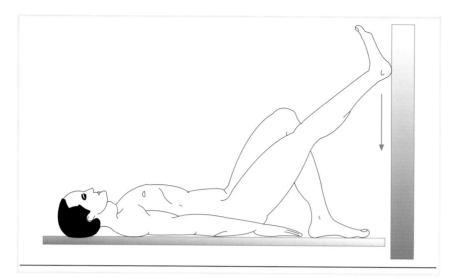

Fig. 4. Passive knee flexion (wall slides)

4. Preoperative evaluation: when in the hospital, anterior tibial translation (KT1000) and isokinetic concentric and eccentric muscle torque (Cybex) are measured. An IKDC form is filled out for every patient.

Phase 2: First and Second Postoperative Weeks

1. Cryotherapy: ice bag on the knee (20 min six times a day).
2. Active foot flexion-extension ("ankle pump" exercise 5 min every half hour).
3. Full knee extension: passive knee extension with heel on a support such as a rolled towel 5–10 min every hour, active knee extension with the heel on an inclined plane performing quadriceps contraction to low the knee toward the bed surface.
4. Isometric quadriceps contractions: placing the contralateral hand on the muscle to feel contractions 5 min/h while in the hospital and 5 min three times a day when discharged, straight leg raises with the knee fully extended without extension lag (10-min session of raising the limb 20 cm slowly, holding the contraction for 6 s, and then resting for 5 s) four to five times a day.
5. Knee flexion: active knee flexion sliding on a board (10 min every 2 h up to 90° during the first week). To achieve full knee flexion, the exercises can also be performed while sitting with the leg out of the bed or in supine position sliding down with the foot leaning on a wall (wall slides).
6. Gait: partial weight bearing with two crutches is allowed from the first postoperative day to visit the bathroom, then gradually increased as tolerated. When discharged, the patient must main-

tain full knee extension and achieve at least 100°–110° of knee flexion at home. At the end of every exercise session, 20 min of cryotherapy must be performed.
7. EMS: it is possible to perform electrical quadriceps stimulation maintaining the knee in full extension.
8. Warning: to prevent loss of extension, the patient must not place supports under the knee. To prevent graft strain, he may extend the knee actively only up to 45° (Fig. 5).

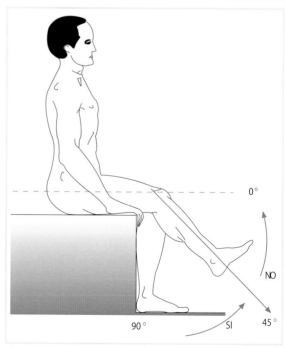

Fig. 5. Active knee extension from 90° to 45° (stopping at 45°) without resistance while sitting

Phase 3: Third and Fourth Postoperative Weeks

If there is lack of extension, a new exercise is added to the protocol: passive knee extension in prone position with the leg out of the bed and a light weight (0.5–1 kg) on the heel for 15 min three times a day (Fig. 6). The best way to check extension is to observe heel height during the exercise. Patellar mobilization must be done with the knee in full extension (5 min three times a day). Muscle exercises:

1. Straight leg raises with weight on the thigh (Fig. 7) (20 repetitions holding the contraction for 8 s four times a day).
2. Two-legged minisquat with up to 45° of knee flexion using crutches (ten repetitions slowly two to three times a day).
3. Active extension 90° to 45° (stopping at 45°) without resistance while sitting
4. Active knee flexion in standing position.
5. Active assisted flexion (more than 120°) in sitting position exerting with hands a posterior drawer at the level of tibial tuberosity.
6. Cocontractions: simultaneous isometric (60°) contractions of quadriceps and hamstrings muscles. It can be helpful to feel the muscle contractions with the hand.
7. Gait: increase weight bearing gradually as tolerated with one or two crutches. It can be useful walk in front of a mirror trying to achieve full knee extension in the weight-bearing phase and flexion during the swing phase of the gait.

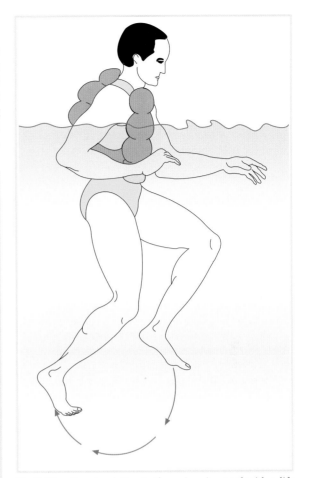

Fig. 8. Bicycling simulation in the swimming pool with a life jacket

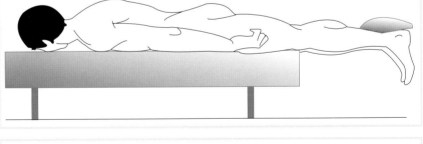

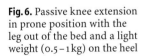

Fig. 6. Passive knee extension in prone position with the leg out of the bed and a light weight (0.5–1 kg) on the heel

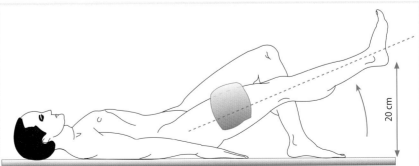

Fig. 7. Straight leg raises with weight on the thigh

8. Swimming pool. From the end of the third week, it is possible to perform the following water exercises: walking forward and backward, straight leg raises, aquajogging with a flotation life jacket, adductor/abductor/flexor exercises, and bicycling simulation with a life jacket (Fig. 8).
9. Stationary bicycle for 10 min two to three times a day slowly, without wheel resistance, and pedaling with the forefoot.

Cryotherapy must be performed at the end of any session of exercises and in the evening.

Phase 4: Second Postoperative Month

1. In comparison with the contralateral knee, extension lag must be obtained. If necessary, the patient continues stretching exercises and can apply a hyperextension device during the night.
2. Flexion must be more than 120° and gradually reach the contralateral level (full ROM).
3. Gait: the patient can walk without crutches and gradually returns to activities of daily living and light work. Climbing and descending stairs is forbidden until the end of the second postoperative month.
4. Stationary bicycle: 15 min three times a day with low wheel resistance (50 W) simulating a slow ride on level road, pedaling with the forefoot.

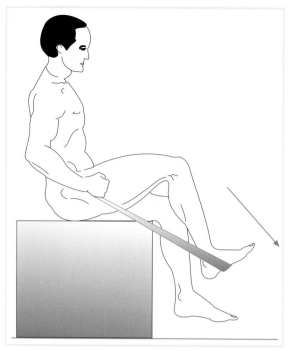

Fig. 9. Active knee extension with elastic tubing resistance (leg press), stopping at 45°

Muscle strengthening exercises with elastic tubing are useful because they allow gradual resistance: leg press stopping at 45° (Fig. 9), knee flexion while sitting with the plantar surface of the foot sliding on the floor (Fig. 10), half squat in the 45° – 90° ROM (Fig. 11), "duck

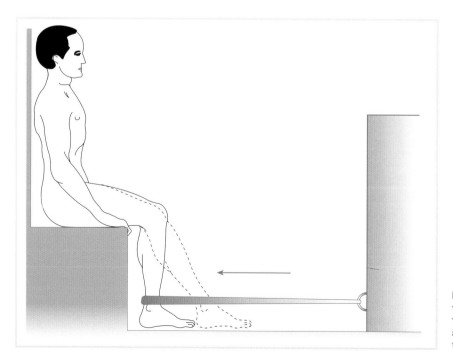

Fig. 10. Active knee flexion with elastic tubing resistance while sitting with plantar surface of the foot sliding on the floor

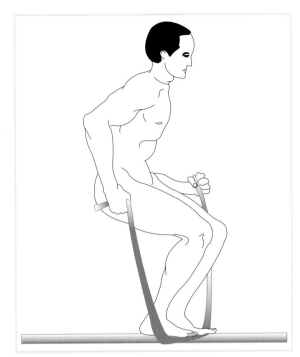

Fig. 11. Half squat with elastic tubing resistance in the 45°–90° ROM

walk" with the knee flexed and the trunk bent forward (Fig. 12), and hip muscle (adductors, abductors, flexors, extensors) strengthening exercises first without and later with elastic resistance. Exercises to be performed in the swimming pool are: walking into the deep water, straight leg raises, adduction and abduction, frontal and lateral climbing and descending stairs, underwater stationary bicycle, and aquajogging with a life jacket. Swimming the breaststroke is forbidden. Moreover, the knee may not be flexed more than 30° while swimming.

Cryotherapy must be performed at the end of all exercise sessions and in the evening.

Phase 5: Third Postoperative Month

The exercises described previously must be continued. Other exercises are added: eccentric quadriceps strengthening exercises like two-legged squatting up to 90° (on land and in a swimming pool), climbing and descending stairs into the water (20–40 cm, gradually increasing), two-legged jumping into the water, concentric quadriceps strengthening exercises (active full knee extension-flexion without resistance), and one-legged proprioceptive exercises on unstable surfaces (5 min three to four times a day) for balance and coordination to regain dynamic control of the knee joint, first on a simple board with only one axis of instability

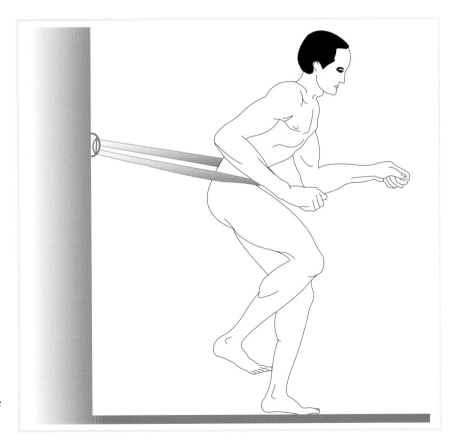

Fig. 12. "Duck walk" with the knee flexed and trunk bent forward

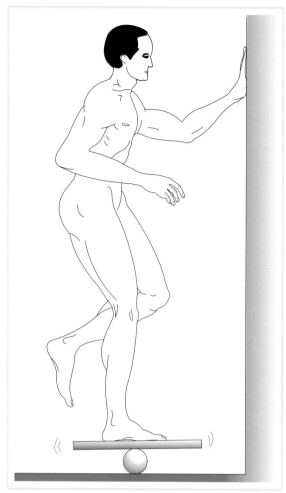

Fig. 13. Proprioceptive exercise on unstable surface

(flexion-extension or pronation-supination of the foot) and then with instability in all axes (hemispherical base) with the knee flexed at 30° (Fig. 13). The patient

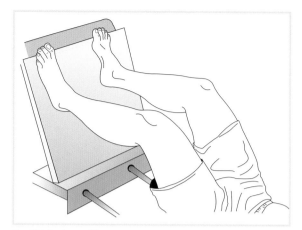

Fig. 15. Horizontal leg press

starts proprioceptive exercises in sitting position, then with the hands against a wall, and then balancing on one leg. Jogging is allowed on a straight course for 10 min/day. Bicycling can be started for brief periods (10 – 15 min) on a level road. Jumping on springboards is useful for enhancing proprioception without overloading the knee joint. Attending a gym, it is possible to use some devices:

1. Nordic skiing simulator 10 – 20 min after a good muscle warmup
2. Rowing simulator (Fig. 14) to be performed with erect spine, flexing first the leg and then the arm for 10 – 20 min after a good muscle warmup
3. Horizontal leg press (Fig. 15) for 10 – 20 min cautiously with a resistance of 5 – 10 kg and after a good muscle warmup
4. Slide board (Fig. 16), sliding alternately on the left and on the right
5. Step machine or stair climbing simulator, to be performed cautiously and briefly with low loads.

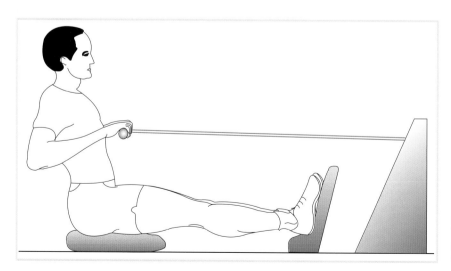

Fig. 14. Rowing simulator, to be performed with erect spine, flexing the leg first and then the arm

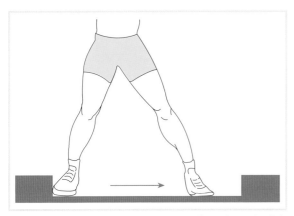

Fig. 16. Sliding alternately to the left and to the right on the slide board

Phase 6: Fourth Postoperative Month

Tests are done for joint stability (KT1000), isokinetic muscle torque at 60°/s, 120°/s, and 180°/s (Cybex), and functional index (Hop test).

Subjective assessment and clinical condition are recorded according to IKDC guidelines. After the measurements, jogging time and distance may be increased, adding change of direction (drawing "o" and "8" figures) and running uphill and downhill. Bicycling is possible with increased distance and also uphill and downhill. The swimming pool should be attended, performing freestyle and jumping into the water. Proprioceptive exercises are continued. Concentric quadriceps strengthening must be performed (active full knee extension-flexion with or without resistance applied below the patella but not on the ankle). Isokinetic training at an angular speed of 180°/s can be useful (resistance applied proximally with dual pad antishear device).

Starting from the fifth postoperative month, the patient can practice running with acceleration, deceleration, and "stop and go" if there is good coordination and muscle strength. Moreover, a return to sport-specific activities can begin after a medical control.

Return to sports is allowed starting the sixth postoperative month. Twelve months after surgery, clinical condition (IKDC), joint stability (KT1000), and isokinetic muscle torque (Cybex) are tested again.

Conclusion

The goals of rehabilitation after ACL reconstruction are: joint stability (protection of the healing graft), full ROM (including hyperextension at levels of the uninvolved side), muscle strength (both concentric and eccentric), proprioception, and preinjury levels of activity. Both grafts used in most ACL reconstruction (BPTB,

STG) allow one to achieve these targets if the surgical technique has been well performed.

Rehabilitation programs must be continually modified and improved by means of basic research (histological and biomechanical studies) and clinical studies. The patient must follow time-based and criterion-based progressions in the postoperative period. To obtain good exercise compliance and strong personal motivation (active and passive exercises are the major rehabilitation tool), patients must be informed that technical devices such as continuous passive motion, cryotherapy, electrical muscle stimulation, biofeedback, and braces are not effective alone. The rehabilitation program must be individualized according to the combined lesions, preinjury sport-specific activities, and activity levels of each patient.

References

1. Aagard P, Simonsen EB, Magnusson SP, Larsson B, Dyhre-Poulsen P (1998) A new concept for isokinetic hamstring:quadriceps muscle strength ratio. Am J Sports Med 26: 231–237
2. Aglietti P, Buzzi R, Zaccherotti G, De Biase P (1994) Patellar tendon versus doubled semitendinosus and gracilis tendons for anterior cruciate ligament reconstruction. Am J Sports Med 22:211–218
3. Aglietti P, Zaccherotti G, Buzzi R, De Biase P (1997) A comparison between patellar tendon and doubled semitendinosus/gracilis tendon for anterior cruciate ligament reconstruction. A minimum five year follow up. J Sports Traumatol 19:57–68
4. Aglietti P, Buzzi R, Zaccherotti G, Simeone AJV, Puddu GF (1998) Recupero della forza muscolare dopo ricostruzione del LCA: Confronto tra tendine rotuleo e semitendinoso-gracile. Ital J Ortop Traumatol 24 (S):368–376
5. Anderson AF, Snyder RB, Lipscomb A (1994) Anterior cruciate ligament reconstruction using the semitendinosus and gracilis tendon augmented by the Losee iliotibial band tenodesis. A long term study. Am J Sports Med 22:620
6. Arvidsson I, Arvidsson H, Eriksson E, Jansson E (1986) Prevention of quadriceps wasting after immobilization: An evaluation of the effect of electrical stimulation. Orthopedics 9:1519–1528
7. Barber FA, McGuire DA, Click S (1998) Continuous-flow cold therapy for outpatient anterior cruciate ligament reconstruction. Arthroscopy 14:130–135
8. Bassett FH, Kirkpatrick JS, Engelhardt DL, Malonne TR (1992) Criotherapy-induced nerve injury. Am J Sports Med 20:516–518
9. Beard DJ, Dodd Ca (1998) Home or supervised rehabilitation following anterior cruciate ligament reconstruction: A randomized controlled trial. J Orthop Sports Phys Ther 27:134–143
10. Beard DJ, Dodd CAF, Trundle HR, Simpson AHRW (1994) Proprioception enhancement for anterior cruciate ligament deficiency. J Bone Joint Surg 76-B:654–659
11. Beynnon BD, Howe JG, Pope MH, Johnson RJ, Fleming BC (1992) The measurement of anterior cruciate ligament strain in vivo. Int Orthop 16: 1–12
12. Beynnon BD, Johnson RJ, Fleming BC, Renstrom PA, Nichols CE, Pope MH, Haugh LD (1994) The measurement of elongation of anterior cruciate ligament in vivo. J Bone Joint Surg Am 76-A: 520–531

13. Beynnon BD, Fleming BC, Johnson RJ, Nichols CE, Renstrom PA, Pope MH (1995) Anterior cruciate ligament strain behavior during rehabilitation exercises in vivo. Am J Sports Med 23:24–34

14. Beynnon BD, Johnson RJ, Fleming BC, Peura GD, Renstrom PA, Nichols CE, Pope MH (1997) The effect of functional knee bracing on the anterior cruciate ligament in the weight-bearing and nonweight-bearing knee. Am J Sports Med 25:353–359

15. Beynnon BD, Johnson RJ, Fleming BC, Stankewich CJ, Renstrom PA, Nichols CE (1997) The strain behavior of the anterior cruciate ligament during squatting and active flexion-extension. Am J Sports Med 25:823–829

16. Buzzi R, Zaccherotti G, Giron F, Aglietti P (1999) The relationship between the intercondylar roof and the tibial plateau with the knee in extension: Relevance for tibial tunnel placement in anterior cruciate ligament reconstruction. Arthroscopy 15: 625–631

17. Bynum EB, Barrack RL, Alexander AH (1995) Open versus closed chain kinetic exercises after anterior cruciate ligament reconstruction. Am J Sports Med 23:401–406

18. Caraffa A, Cerulli G, Proietti M, Aisa G, Rizzo A (1996) Prevention of anterior cruciate ligament injuries in soccer. Knee Surg Sports Traumatol Arthrosc 4 :19–21

19. Carter TR, Edinger S (1999) Isokinetic evaluation of anterior cruciate ligament reconstruction: Hamstring versus patellar tendon. Arthroscopy 15: 169–172

20. Casscells SW (1991) Is CPM useful following anterior cruciate ligament reconstruction? Arthroscopy 7: 38

21. Cohn BT, Draeger RI, Jackson DW (1989) The effects of cold therapy in the postoperative management of pain in patients undergoing anterior cruciate ligament reconstruction. Am J Sports Med 17:344–349

22. Dahlstedt L, Samuelson P, Dalen N (1996) Cryotherapy after cruciate knee surgery. Acta Orthop Scand 67:255–257

23. Daniel DM, Stone ML, Arendt DL (1994) The effect of cold therapy on pain, swelling, and range of motion after anterior cruciate ligament reconstructive surgery. Arthroscopy 10:530–533

24. DeVita P, Lassiter Jr T, Hortobagyi T, Torry M (1998) Functional knee brace effects during walking in patients with anterior cruciate ligament reconstruction. Am J Sports Med 26:778–784

25. Drez D, Paine RM, Neuschwander DC, Young JC (1991) In vivo measurement of anterior tibial translation using continuous passive motion devices. Am J Sports Med 19:381–383

26. Edwards DJ, Rimmer M, Keene GCR (1996) The use of cold therapy in the postoperative management of patients undergoing arthroscopic anterior cruciate ligament reconstruction. Am J Sports Med 24:193–195

27. Eriksson E, Haggmark T (1979) Comparison of isometric muscle training and electrical stimulation supplementing isometric muscle training in the recovery after major knee ligament surgery. Am J Sports Med 7:169–171

28. Eriksson E (1981) Rehabilitation of muscle function after sport injury – major problems in sports medicine. Int J Sports Med 2:1–6

29. Eriksson K, Larsson H, Wredmark T, Hamberg P (1999) Semitendinosus tendon regeneration after harvesting for ACL reconstruction. Knee Surg Sports Traumatol Arthrosc 7: 220–225

30. Falconiero RP, DiStefano VJ, Cook TM (1998) Revascularization and ligamentization of autogenous anterior cruciate ligament grafts in humans. Arthroscopy 14:197–205

31. Fitzgerald GK (1997) Open versus closed kinetic chain exercise: issues in rehabilitation after anterior cruciate ligament reconstructive surgery. Phys Ther 77:1747–1754

32. Fleming BC, Beynnon BD, Nichols CE, Johnson RJ, Pope MH (1993) An in vivo comparison of anterior tibial translation and strain in the anteromedial band of the anterior cruciate ligament. J Biomech 26:51–58

33. Fleming BC, Beynnon BD, Tohyama H, Johnson RJ, Nichols CE, Renstrom PA, Pope MH (1994) Determination of a zero strain reference for the anteromedial band of the anterior cruciate ligament. J Orthop Res 12:789–795

34. Fleming BC, Beynnon BD, Renstrom PA, Peura GD, Nichols CE, Johnson RJ (1998) The strain behavior of the anterior cruciate ligament during bicycling. An in vivo study. Am J Sports Med 26:109–118

35. Fleming BC, Beynnon BD, Renstrom PA, Johnson RJ, Nichols CE, Peura GD,Uh BS (1999) The strain behavior of the anterior cruciate ligament during stair climbing: An in vivo study. Arthroscopy 15:185–191

36. Giron F, Aglietti P, Simeone AJV, Zaccherotti G (1999) Prospective evaluation of anterior cruciate ligament reconstruction using doubled STG rigidly fixed to bone. Arthroscopy 15(Suppl):52–53

37. Haggmark T, Eriksson E (1979) Cylinder or mobile cast brace after knee ligament surgery: A clinical analysis and morphologic and enzymatic studies of changes in the quadriceps muscle. Am J Sports Med 7:48–56

38. Henning CE, Lynch MA, Glick KR (1985) An in vivo strain gauge study of the anterior cruciate ligament. Am J Sports Med 13: 22–26

39. Ho SSW, Illgen RL, Meyer RW, Torok PJ, Cooper MD, Reider B (1995) Comparison of various icing times in decreasing bone metabolism and blood flow in the knee. Am J Sports Med 23:74–76

40. Howe JG, Wertheimer C, Johnson RJ, Nichols CE, Pope MH, Beynnon B (1990) Arthroscopic strain gauge measurement of the normal anterior cruciate ligament. Arthroscopy 6:198–204

41. Howell SM (1998) Principles for placing the tibial tunnel and avoiding roof impingement during reconstruction of a torn anterior cruciate ligament. Knee Surg Sports Traumatol Arthrosc 6:49–55

42. Howell SM, Hull ML (1998) Aggressive rehabilitation using hamstring tendons. Am J Knee Surg 11:120–127

43. Howell SM, Taylor MA (1996) Brace-free rehabilitation, with early return to activity, for knees reconstructed with a double-looped semitendinosus and gracilis graft. J Bone Joint Surg 78A:814–825

44. Howell SM, Wallace MP, Hull ML, Deutsch ML (1999) Evaluation of the single-incision arthroscopic technique for anterior cruciate ligament replacement. Am J Sports Med 27:284–293

45. Kartus J, Stener S, Kohler K, Sernert N, Eriksson BI, Karlsson J (1997) Is bracing after anterior cruciate ligament reconstruction necessary? Knee Surg Sports Traumatol Arthrosc 5:157–161

46. Khalfayan EE, Sharkey PF, Alexander AH, Bruckner JD, Bynum EB (1996) The relationship between tunnel placement and clinical results after anterior cruciate ligament reconstruction. Am J Sports Med 24:335–341

47. Konrath GA, Lock T, Goitz HT, Scheidler J (1996) The use of cold therapy after anterior cruciate ligament reconstruction. Am J Sports Med 24:629–633

48. Kramer J, Nusca D, Fowler P et al (1993) Knee flexors and extensor strength during concentric and eccentric muscle actions after anterior cruciate ligament reconstruction using the semitendinosus tendon and ligament augmentation device. Am J Sports Med 21:285

49. Lipscomb AB, Johnston RK, Snyder RB et al (1982) Evaluation of hamstring strength following use of semitendinosus and gracilis tendons to reconstruct the anterior cruciate ligament. Am J Sports Med 10:340

50. Lutz GE, Palmitier RA, Chao EYS, (1993) Comparison of tibiofemoral joint forces during open-kinetic-chain and closed-kinetic-chain exercises. J Bone Joint Surg Am 75A:732–739

51. Maeda A, Shino K, Horibe S (1996) Anterior cruciate ligament reconstruction with multistranded autogenous semitendinosus tendon. Am J Sports Med 24:504

52. Marder RA, Raskind JR, Carroll M (1991) Prospective evaluation of arthroscopically assisted anterior cruciate ligament reconstruction. Patellar tendon versus semitendinosus and gracilis tendons. Am J Sports Med 19:478

53. Markolf KL, Gorek JF, Kabo JM, Shapiro MS (1990) Direct measurement of resultant forces in the anterior cruciate ligament. J Bone Joint Surg 72A:557–567

54. Markolf KL, Burchfield DM, Shapiro MM, Cha CW, Finerman GA, Slauterbeck JL (1996) Biomechanical consequences of replacement of the anterior cruciate ligament with a patellar ligament autograft. J Bone Joint Surg 78A:1728–1734

55. Mikkelsen C, Werner S, Eriksson E (1999) OKC vs. CKC knee extensor training following anterior cruciate ligament reconstruction. Knee Surg Sports Traumatol Arthrosc. In press

56. Muellner T, Alacamlioglu Y, Nikolic A, Schabus R (1998) No benefit of bracing on the early outcome after anterior cruciate ligament reconstruction. Knee Surg Sports Traumatol Arthrosc 6:88–92

57. Noyes FR, Mangine RE, Barber S (1987) Early knee motion after open and arthroscopic anterior cruciate ligament reconstruction. Am J Sports Med 15:149–160

58. Ohkoshi Y, Ohkoshi M, Nagasaki S, Ono A, Hashimoto T, Yamane S (1999) The effect of cryotherapy on intraarticular temperature and postoperative care after anterior cruciate ligament reconstruction. Am J Sports Med 27:357–362

59. O'Meara PM, O'Brien WR, Henning CE (1992) Anterior cruciate ligament reconstruction stability with continuous passive motion. Clin Orthop 277:201–209

60. Panariello RA, Backus SI, Parker JW (1994) The effect of the squat exercise on anterior-posterior knee translation in professional football players. Am J Sports Med 22:768–773

61. Paternostro-Sluga T, Fialka C, Alacamlioglu Y, Saradeth T, Fialka-Moser V (1999) Neuromuscular electrical stimulation after anterior cruciate ligament surgery. Clin Orthop 368:166–175

62. Prins J, Cutner D (1999) Aquatic therapy in the rehabilitation of athletic injuries. Clin Sports Med 18:447–461

63. Richmond JC, Gladstone J, MacGillivray J (1991) CPM after arthroscopically assisted anterior cruciate ligament reconstruction: comparison of short- versus long-term use. Arthroscopy 7:39–44

64. Rigon A, Viola R, Lonedo F (1993) Continuous passive motion in reconstruction of the ACL. J Sports Traumatol 15:187–192

65. Risberg MA, Holm I, Steen H, Eriksson J, Ekeland A (1999) The effect of knee bracing after ACL reconstruction. Am J Sports Med 27:76–83

66. Rosen MA, Jackson DW, Atwell EA (1992) The efficacy of continuous passive motion in the rehabilitation of anterior cruciate ligaments reconstructions. Am J Sports Med 20: 122–127

67. Rougraff B, Shelbourne KD, Gerth PH, Warner J (1993) Arthroscopic and histologic analysis of human patellar tendom autografts used for anterior cruciate ligament reconstruction. Am J Sports Med 21:277–284

68. Schenck RC Jr, Blaschak MJ, Lance ED, Turturro TC, Holmes CF (1997) A prospective outcome study of rehabilitation programs and anterior cruciate ligament reconstruction. Arthroscopy 13:285–290

69. Selkowitz DM (1989) High frequency electrical stimulation in muscle strengthening. A review and discussion. Am J Sports Med 17:103–111

70. Shelbourne KD, Davis JT (1999) Evaluation of knee stability before and after participation in a functional sports agility program during rehabilitation after ACL reconstruction. Am J Sports Med 27:156–161

71. Shelbourne KD, Gray T (1997) Anterior cruciate ligament reconstruction with autogenous patellar tendon graft followed by accelerated rehabilitation. Am J Sports Med 25: 786–795

72. Shelbourne KD, Nitz P (1990) Accelerated rehabilitation after anterior cruciate ligament reconstruction. Am J Sports Med 18:292–299

73. Shelbourne KD, Rask BP (1998) Controversies with anterior cruciate ligament surgery and rehabilitation. Am J Knee Surg 11:136–143

74. Shelbourne KD, Rubinstein RA, McCarroll JR, Weaver J (1994) Postoperative cryotherapy for the knee in ACL reconstructive surgery. Orthop Int 2:165–170

75. Shelbourne KD, Klootwyk TE, Wilckens JH, De Carlo MS (1995) Ligament stability two to six years after anterior cruciate ligament reconstruction with autogenous patellar tendon graft and participation in accelerated rehabilitation program. Am J Sports Med 23:575–579

76. Snyder-Mackler L, Ladin Z, Schepsis AA, Young JC (1991) Electrical stimulation of the thigh muscles after reconstruction of the ACL. J Bone Joint Surg 73A:1025–1035

77. Snyder-Mackler L, Delitto A, Stralka SW, Bailey SL (1994) Use of electrical stimulation to enhance recovery of quadriceps femoris muscle force production in patients following ACL reconstruction. Phys Ther 74:901–907

78. Snyder-Mackler L, Delitto A, Bailey SL, Stralka SW (1995) Strength of the quadriceps femoris muscle and functional recovery after reconstruction of th ACL. J Bone Joint Surg 77A:1166–1173

79. Solomonov M, Baratta R, Zhou BH (1987) The synergistic action of the anterior cruciate ligament and thigh muscles in maintaining joint stability. Am J Sports Med 15:207

80. Stuart MJ, Meglan DA, Lutz GE, Growney ES, An KN (1996) Comparison of intersegmental tibiofemoral joint forces and muscle activity during various closed kinetic chain exercises. Am J Sports Med 24:792–799

81. Tovin BJ, Wolf SL, Greenfield BH, Crouse J, Woodfin BA (1994) Comparison of the effects of exercise in water and land on the rehabilitation of patients with intra-articular anterior cruciate ligament reconstruction. Phys Ther 74:710–719

82. Treacy SH, Barron OA, Brunet ME, Barrack RL (1997) Assessing the need for extensive supervised rehabilitation following arthroscopic ACL reconstruction. Am J Orthop 26:25–29

83. Wilk KE, Escamilla RF, Fleisig GS, Barrentine SW, Andrews JR, Boyd ML (1996) A comparison of tibiofemoral joint forces and electromyographic activity during open and closed kinetic chain exercises. Am J Sports Med 24:518–527

84. Woo SLY, Debsky RE, Withrow JD, Janaushek MA (1999) Biomechanics of knee ligaments. Am J Sports Med 27:533–543

85. Wojtys EM, Kothari SU, Huston LJ (1996) Anterior cruciate ligament functional brace use in sports. Am J Sports Med 24:539–546

86. Yack HJ, Collins CE, Whieldon TJ (1993) Comparison of closed and open kinetic chain exercise in the anterior cruciate ligament-deficient knee. Am J Sports Med 21:49–54

87. Yasuda K, Tsujino J, Ohkoshi Y et al (1995) Graft site morbidity with autogenous semitendinosus and gracilis tendons. Am J Sports Med 23:706

88. Zaccherotti G, Aglietti P, Bandinelli I (1997) Long-term isokinetic evaluation of quadriceps and hamstrings strength following anterior cruciate ligament reconstruction. J Sports Traumatol 19:141–158

11 Rehabilitation After Posterior Cruciate Ligament Injuries

Enrico Giannì, Guglielmo Cerullo, Giancarlo Puddu

Introduction

The nonoperative or surgical management of posterior cruciate ligament (PCL) tears is still very much a matter for discussion. In fact, the symptoms are slight in most cases, while the quality of the results offered by surgery is uncertain. The clinical progress of the natural history of the lesion is not clear [1–10]. Insufficient understanding of modern rehabilitation practices after nonsurgical and surgical treatment is another cause of poor clinical and functional results.

Joint instability due to PCL damage is often tolerated by patients, since it does not cause the giving-way associated with anterior cruciate ligament (ACL) tears. Good long-term results and resumption of sport, often at the previous level, have been reported after nonoperative management, though many patients eventually present patellofemoral and medial compartment arthrosis [1–10] because the extensors are anomalously required to constantly resist posterior translation of the tibia. The patellofemoral joint is thus exposed to wearing-down stresses. Young subjects with severe laxity, clinically significant instability and radiographical evidence of a posterior tibial translation exceeding 10 mm should be reconstructed when the onset of degeneration is foreseen. A PCL tear is followed by gravity-induced posterior translation of the tibia. Incomplete and intrasubstance PCL and neo-PCL lesions must thus be protected against posterior stretching of the tibia. This is essential to prevent elongation of the healing fibres. Absence or reduction of the force of gravity promotes the formation of good-quality repair tissue with well-oriented fascicules and cells that produce large-diameter collagen fibrils. Limitation of the effects of gravity is also the rule after reconstruction with autograft or allograft. In the second week, a neoligament goes through a process of cell necrosis that results in a loss of strength. In the eighth week, there is revascularisation with recolonisation by fibroblasts from the vascular apparatus. Subsequent differentiation leads to cells that produce type I and III collagen, similar to the normal ligament and with more glucoamine glycans. The graft is reshaped over the course of about a year by a biological prcess known as ligamentisation [11].Offsetting of gravity gives a ligament tissue with a modulus of elasticity and a tensile strength similar to those of a healthy ligament. Immobilisation is a well-known impediment to joint ligament healing. Knee mobilisation is essential to promote the formation of good-quality collagen and correctly oriented fibres of sufficient diameter [12–13]. When employed in cases of PCL damage or reconstruction, it must counteract lengthening of the ligament or graft due to gravity.

Rehabilitation rests on three concepts:

1. Opposition to the force of gravity, which tends to lengthen the new or the scarring ligament by keeping the tibia in the posterior drawer position
2. Slow re-establishment of complete knee flexion
3. Late commencement of open-kinetic-chain knee flexor exercises, since they subluxate the tibial plateaus posteriorly

Anatomy and Biomechanics of the PCL

The PCL originates from the lateral aspect of the medial femoral condyle and inserts on the posterior aspect of the tibia, 1–1.5 cm distal to the joint line. According to the position of their anatomic insertions, the PCL is composed of two components:an anterolateral (AL) and smaller posteromedial (PM) bundle. In addition, there are two variable lateral bundles called meniscofemoral ligaments. They originate from the posterior horn of the lateral meniscus and insert anteriorly (ligament of Humphry) and posteriorly (ligament of Wrisberg) on the lateral aspect of the medial femoral condyle near the the PCL insertion [14].The anterolateral component is twice the size of the posteromedial component in cross-sectional area, and its structural properties (stiffness, ultimate strength) are approximately 150% of those of the posteromedial bundle.

Functionally, the anterior fibres (AL) are slack in extension and progressively tighten as the knee flexes. The posterior fibres, on the other hand, are taut in extension and relax as the flexion proceeds. In biomechanical terms, the PCL provides 95% of the tibia's resistance to posterior translation with respect to the femur in the same way as the anterior cruciate ligament

(ACL) prevents its anterior translation. The posterior stabilisers are the arcuate popliteal ligament and the posteromedial and posterolateral capsules.The exact role of the Humphry and Wrisberg ligaments is unknown.The quadriceps is also a powerful dynamic stabiliser of posterior instability, since its contraction during knee extension produces an anterior vector that reduces posterior translation of the tibia. It is important to distinguish between isolated tears and associated tears of the PCL, because there are significant differences in treatment.

Frequency and Causes of PCL Tears

PCL tears are often overlooked due to their association with leg, femur and hip fractures. Apart from the objective difficulty of diagnosis in cases of this kind, priority is naturally given to bone injuries. PCL injuries represent 3%–20% of all the knee ligament injuries, of which 30% are isolated and 70% are combined with other ligamentous injuries [15–16]. Four traumatic mechanisms are likely:

1. Direct anterior-posterior trauma sustained by the tuberosity or middle third of the tibia with the knee flexed. This is the most common and typical of road accidents.
2. A fall with the knee flexed and the foot in equinus extension. This is typical of sports injuries.
3. Forced hyperflexion of the knee resulting in stretching of the PCL and its tearing by the shape of the roof of the intercondylar notch.
4. Sudden, violent hyperextension of the knee may damage first the ACL and then the PCL. A multicentre European study of 167 patients found the initial injury was sport-related in 26% of cases and due to a road accident (usually a motorcycle accident) in 64% [12].The American literature cites road accidents as the cause in 50%–90% of cases [17–18] and sports accidents in 40%–50%. As can be seen, other causes are rare[3–19].

PCL injuries are more likely in contact sports involving a direct blow to the tibia with the knee flexed (e.g. a football goalkeeper coming out for a save).
They are none the less recorded in other sports, such as baseball, as the outcome of a fall on the flexed knee with foot in plantar flexion.

Clinical Examination and Imaging

The severity of the injury can be graded on a scale from 1 to 3. The clinical examination is based on the posterior drawer test. Normally the medial plateau is 1 cm an-terior to the medial femoral condyle at 90° of flexion. Grade 1 injuries have 0.5-cm less step-off than the controlateral uninjured side. Grade 2 injuries have from 0.5 to 1 cm of posterior tibial translation and it is seen clinically as a loss of the entire step-off (the medial tibial plateau and the medial femoral condyle are flush). In Grade 3 injuries the medial tibial plateau is displaced posteriorly bejond the medial femoral condyle (reverse step-off). Other tests for isolated PCL insufficiency include the quadriceps active test and the gravity test.

Magnetic resonance imaging (MRI) and radiography also are used to diagnose and assess posterior knee instability. MRI distinguishes:

1. Incomplete lesions
2. Intrasubstance lesions
3. Complete lesions [20]

These are joined by avulsion of the tibial attachment bone block and femoral disinsertion. The diagnostic accuracy of the MRI for PCL injuries ranges from 96 to 100% depending on the series[21].

The irreversible plastic deformations that occur along the PCL in these two cases can only be detected by MRI. Incomplete and intrasubstance tears diagnosed by MRI that display no more than 10 mm posterior displacement during radiography under stress as advocated by Staubli [22] and, according to Puddu, [23] require non-operative management; those with a greater displacement can be treated with surgical reconstruction. If the PCL substance is intact but avulsed from the tibial or femoral insertion with an attached osseous fragment (or femoral 'peel off') primary surgical repair is performed.

In chronic cases, standard weight-bearing radiographs in anteroposterior and lateral view should be obtained [24].

General Principles of PCL Rehabilitation

The importance of joint mobilisation has already been mentioned. Caution, however, is mandatory with regard to flexion. When this exceeds 90°, increased tightening of the ligament or graft will result in its elongation. Recovery of flexion must thus proceed by degrees, both in patients with recent incomplete or intrasubstance tears and those with reconstructions.

As already stated, the PCL and ACL control translation of the tibia during knee flexion and extension. This is done via a biomechanical system with four linking bars. The ligaments of the central pivot act as a brake on joint movement caused by physiologically excessive dynamic accelerations and angular movements.

Biomechanical research has drawn on mechanics to devise a four-bar linkage model of knee joint kinematics. This model is confined to the sagittal plane. It consists of two components represented by the reciprocally moving joint surfaces (femoral and tibial epiphyses). The other two components, namely the ACL and the PCL, are represented by two bars that start from their attachments to connect these surfaces. The femoral surface slides and rolls on the tibial surface. The data provided by the model also show that:

1. The instant-by-instant centre of rotation coincides with the intersection point of the ACL and PCL at all degrees of flexion.
2. Posterior rotation of the femoral condyle is due to the restraining action of the cruciates, and that its posterior displacement increases in function of the degree of flexion.
3. The ACL and PCL resist the anterior and posterior drawer movement imposed by the joint surfaces. Exaggerated posterior translation of the tibia tears the PCL and must thus be avoided during rehabilitation of reconstructed knees and those with acute, incomplete and/or intrasubstance PCL lesions. Studies of the joint shifts imposed by the various types of exercises have illustrated the effects of muscle contraction on the position of the joint and the accessory movements to which it is subjected [25]. Investigation of the effects of closed-kinetic-chain and open-kinetic-chain exercises on the reaction forces at the patellofemoral joint, translation of the femorotibial joint and joint stresses, has shown that they have very different effects on the patellofemoral joint. Patients with posterior instability and those with PCL reconstructions often complain of patellofemoral disturbances. Open-chain exercises allow freedom of movement of the distal segment of the leg, which can solely perform flexion and extension of the knee.

Flexion is the result of contraction of the flexors. Extension is the result of isolated contraction of the quadriceps. It requires greater tension on the part of the quadriceps and patella with an increase in the reaction forces on the patellofemoral, which peak at about 36° flexion. During extension, the area of the patellofemoral contact diminishes. This increases the contact stress per unit of joint surface area [25].

Rehabilitation of patients with PCL tears and reconstructions must include both open-chain and closed-chain exercises. Open-chain extension must be between 0° and 75° of flexion. Care must be taken to avoid patellofemoral stress. Exercises requiring greater flexion should not be used, since they evoke posterior translation forces [9]. Closed-chain exercises are more commonly employed because they train the knee for the specific recovery of PCL function. The distal seg-

ment of the leg is fixed and movements of one articulation are matched by foreseeable movements of the other articulations in the kinetic chain. In squatting exercises, for example, the lower limb works in closed chain with the foot fixed on the ground, and movements of the hip, knee and ankle joints are interrelated. Lever arm of the knee increases during flexion thus augmented quadriceps tension is needed to counteract this increase. The reaction forces of the patellofemoral increase during knee flexion, but are spread over a larger joint surface, which decreases the contact stress per unit of joint surface area. Compression on the loaded joint surfaces stabilises the joint and reduces tibial translation [9].

Closed-chain exercises are indicated to reduce tibial translation and patellofemoral stresses by means of combined contraction of the quadriceps and flexors [9, 25, 26]. The rectus femoris lengthens at the hip and shortens at the knee, whereas the flexors lengthen at the knee and shorten at the hip. There is thus a 'pseudo-isometric' eccentric and concentric contraction at the opposite ends of the rectus. This type of contraction is used during walking, going up and down stairs, running and jumping. It cannot be reproduced in open-chain exercises.

Proprioceptive Rehabilitation

This is employed during PCL rehabilitation to promote recruitment of the quadriceps for dynamic reduction of posterior translation of the tibia. Proprioceptive training improves a patient's static and dynamic equilibrium. The static proprioceptive re-education is begun when patients proceed to weight bearing without crutches and consists of six stages:

1. Recovery of sense of body position, muscle contraction and joint movement.
2. Transition from bilateral to unilateral activities.
3. Transition from eyes-open to eyes-closed activities.
4. Transition from activities on a stable support, such as the ground, to unstable surfaces, such as a soft mattress, a trampoline and Freeman's boards, or more modern equipment, such as the kinesthetic ability trainer (Fig. 1).
5. Throwing and catching a football to take the patient's mind off active control of his balance.
6. Balance recovery exercises are carried out in different joint positions to evoke different responses from the tendon and muscle receptors.

The dynamic proprioceptive re-education is indicated for patients needing to resume sports that involve running, jumping, landing, sudden changes of direction

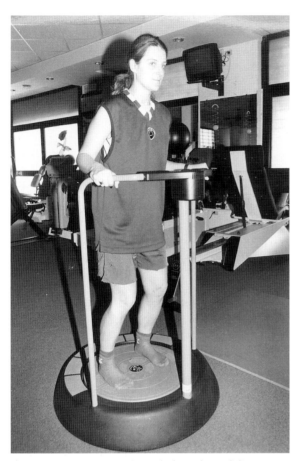

Fig. 1. Proprioceptive exercise on the kinesthetic ability trainer

and twisting movements. During such sports, athletes are obviously able to lose and then regain balance, and avoid falls and accidents that might occur by adjusting their posture so as to execute harmonious movements in a necessarily brief space of time. This brief execution is typical of athletes. It is achieved through ultra-quick muscle recruitment in co-ordinated sequences. Constant repetition of the movements specific to a given sport results in the learning of appropriate movements and acquisition of a particular ability that initially requires a conscious effort, but eventually results in automatic performance. The dynamic proprioceptive re-education programme complies with these promises. It is executed in such a way as to guide rehabilitation towards the recovery of movements specific to a given sport. It consists of seven stages:

1. Slow exercises followed by quicker movements
2. Exercise with limited effort followed by exercises requiring greater strength
3. Exercises requiring volition, followed by exercises done freely
4. Progress from walking to jogging

5. Running and sprinting
6. Jumping and changes of direction
7. Twirling and twisting around the injured or operated knee

Rehabilitation After Reconstruction of an Isolated PCL Tear

As already stated, reconstruction is indicated for young patients with an isolated PCL lesion and more than 10 mm symptomatic posterior instability to reduce such instability to prevent patellofemoral and femorotibial arthrosis.

There are many adequate grafts for the PCL reconstruction. Surgeons should choose the one they are most confortable using. Graft choices include the autograft bone patellar tendon bone, quadrupled hamstrings (gracilis and semitendinosus) and quadriceps tendon. For an allograft, most authors suggest bone patellar tendon bone, achilles tendon and quadriceps tendon.

Use is primarily made of the middle third of the patellar tendon with bone-to-bone attachment at each end and biomechanical fixation over the course of 5 weeks. Reconstruction with the semitendinosus, quadriceps or achilles tendons employs a tendon-bone anchorage with fixation in 8–10 weeks.

Ligamentisation is less successful than after ACL reconstruction for three reasons: (1) posterior translation of the tibia due to the force of gravity [27–28]; (2) overstretching of the new ligament by the flexors [9, 26, 28–30]; (3) the slant of the femoral and tibial graft tunnel, especially the latter. Precautions must thus be taken to protect the knee against gravity and the action of the flexors. Rehabilitation thus requires:

1. Immobilisation and bed rest
2. Recovery of range of motion (ROM)
3. Recommencement of weight bearing
4. Muscle strengthening
5. Proprioceptive exercises

Immobilisation and Bed Rest

The knee is immobilised in extension with a jointed brace [27–32]. Tension on the transplant is greatly reduced in extension and increased in flexion. Bed rest is in dorsal decubitus with the brace and a pillow under the triceps to prevent gravity-induced posterior translation of the tibia (Fig. 2). Brace and pillow must be used for 4 weeks.

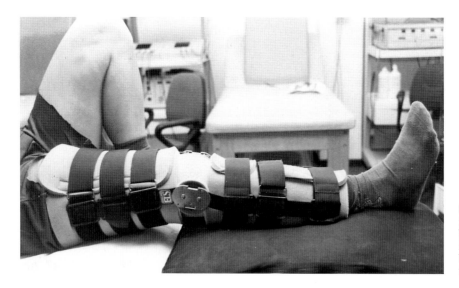

Fig. 2. The operated knee is immobilised with jointed brace. The patient must rest in dorsal decubitus with the brace and a pillow under the triceps

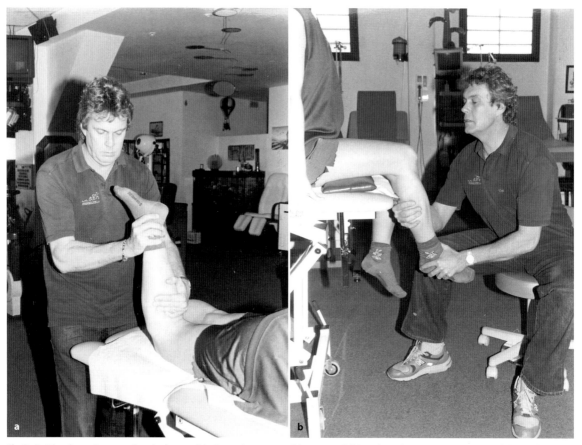

Fig. 3a,b. The therapist must flex the knee with the patient prone (**a**) or seated (**b**) and apply counterpressure with his or her hand on the triceps

Recovery of the ROM

Since the knee is immobilised in extension, recovery obviously relates to flexion. The flexion increases tension on the graft and must be regained slowly over periods varying from one study to another in the literature:

1. De Lee et al. [33], 8 weeks
2. Harner and Irrgang [27], 12 weeks
3. Jackson [29], 12 weeks
4. Noyes and Barber-Westin [30], 14 weeks
We aim to recover complete flexion in 8 weeks [32].

Manual kinesitherapy and eccentric contraction of the quadriceps are widely employed. The powered continuous passive motion (CPM) apparatus is excellent for recovery of flexion [12–30], though some workers are against it because they feel the knee is subjected to the force of gravity[9–27]. It is thus essential that the web supporting the patient's leg should not be as slack as for patients with ACL reconstruction, but very taut to prevent posterior translation of the tibia. The CPM is used for 15 days to bring flexion up to 90°. The therapist then employs passive flexion with the patient prone or seated, and applies counterpressure on the triceps (Fig. 3a,b). The patient can also improve flexion actively through eccentric and concentric contractions of his quadriceps from 0°–60° and vice versa (Fig. 4). This acts as an anterior drawer. The flexion in excess of 75° results in posterior translation. Contraction of the flexors must also be strictly avoided for the same reason. Active flexion by the patient must be accompanied by counterpressure on the proximal third of the leg (Fig. 5a,b).

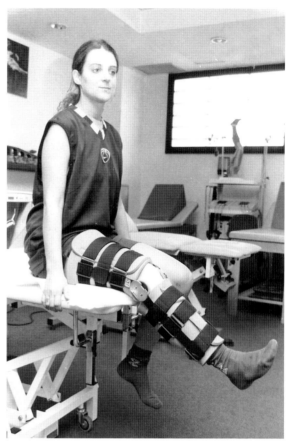

Fig. 4. The patient can improve flexion by eccentric and concentric contraction of the quadriceps from 0° to 60° and vice versa

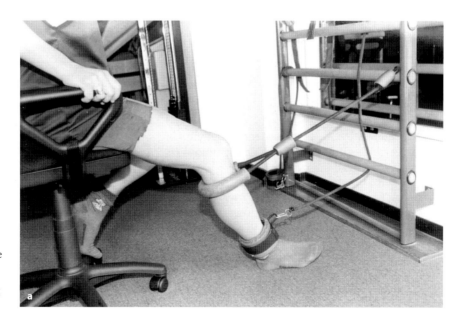

Fig. 5a,b. Active flexion by the patient must be accompanied by counterpressure on the proximal third of the leg (elastic or ball)

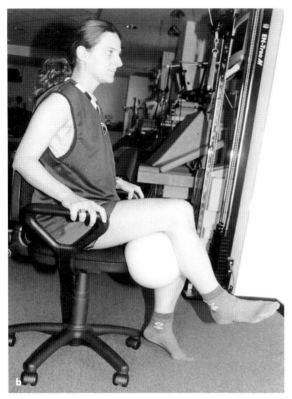

Fig. 5b

Recommencement of Weight Bearing

Early recommencement is not contraindicated, though there are wide differences of opinion in the literature:

1. De Lee et al. [33], immediate resumption
2. Clancy et al. [34], 2 weeks with walkers
3. Jackson [29], 5 weeks with walkers
4. Harner and Irrgang [27], 8 weeks with walkers
5. Noyes and Barber-Westin[30], 10 weeks with walkers

Walking can be regarded as an exercise carried out in closed-kinetic-chain with reduction of anterior and posterior translation forces. Immediate resumption of partial weight bearing can be obtained with walkers and the brace locked in extension. Walkers are abandoned when good quadriceps tone and trophism are restored. The brace is removed after 6 weeks. In the presence of peripheral knee injuries, weight bearing is deferred and immobilisation with the brace is prolonged.

Muscle Strengthening and Proprioceptive Exercises

The quadriceps can work without prejudice to the reconstructed PCL from 0°–60° in open chain[25], since it produces an anterior translation force in this range, and beyond 60° in closed chain, because the translation forces are now reduced as a result of: compression forces, changes in the angles and point of application of the forces, and combined contraction of the quadriceps and flexors[9].

One can thus begin with a bilateral semi-squat (Fig. 6). As performance improves, one can move on to step-machine and leg-press exercises. The exercise bicycle is also a closed-chain apparatus that improves lower limb muscle strength with no risk to the operated knee. To prevent flexor contractions, the foot is placed well forward on the pedal and its tip is left free (Fig. 7). The hamstrings balance the line of action of flexion, so that their posterior translation of the tibia at the knee is counterbalanced by the quadriceps.

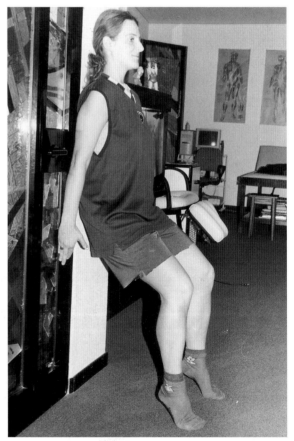

Fig. 6. The semi-squat is a closed-kinetic-chain exercise for the quadriceps and the flexors. It must be performed with the pelvis retroverted, and on tiptoe to distend the flexors

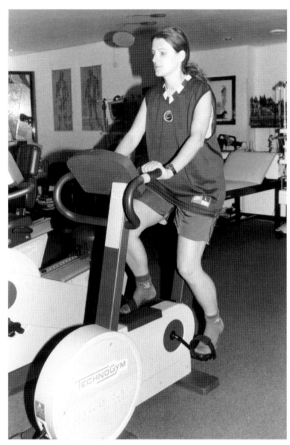

Fig. 7. The exercise bicycle

The reasons given with respect to the quadriceps also apply to closed-chain work by the flexors. They cannot work in open-chain, however, because they cause harmful negative posterior translation [9, 26, 28 – 31]. It is not yet possible to determine when a patient can start active knee flexion exercises.

Harner and Irrgang [27] maintain that the flexors can work actively 12 weeks after surgery. They can work safely when the patient is prone with his hip and knee extended (Fig. 8). Early use can safely be made of the hip and ankle joints. Proprioceptive exercises are important because they allow re-education of the damaged mechanoreceptors. They must be performed statically and dynamically in the closed-kinetic-chain mode as already explained.

The Seven Rehabilitation Stages

First Stage (First 15 Days After Surgery)

1. Knee brace locked in extension with pillow under triceps during bed rest
2. CPM set between 0° and 90°. Mobilisation is begun from 0° to 40°, 48 h after surgery and gradually increased over the next few days
3. Isometric exercises for the quadriceps (patient supine) and glutei (patient prone)
4. Partial weight-bearing with walkers and brace locked in extension

Second Stage (15th – 30th Day)

1. Medical examination and removal of stitches
2. Commencement of daily physical therapy at a rehabilitation centre
3. Knee brace locked in extension with pillow under triceps during bed rest
4. Gradual attainment of full weight bearing
5. Electrotherapy of the quadriceps

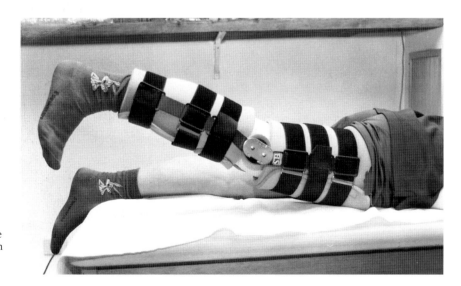

Fig. 8. The knee flexors can work when the patient is prone with the hip and knee extended, since this position eliminates the negative action of the force of gravity

6. Massage
7. Knee flexion by physiotherapist to reach 0°–90° ROM
8. Isometric exercises for quadriceps and all lower-limb muscles except knee flexors
9. Semi-squat
10. Closed-chain proprioceptive exercises

Third Stage (30th – 60th Day)

1. Medical examination (30th Day)
2. ROM attained must be 0°–90°
3. Removal of brace and pillow under triceps during bed rest
4. Abandonment of walkers if good quadriceps control achieved
5. Brace articulated at 0°–120° for another 2 weeks
6. Electrotherapy of the quadriceps
7. Massage
8. Knee flexion by physiotherapist
9. Isometric exercises for all lower-limb muscles
10. Semi-squat

11. Endless belt
12. Closed-chain proprioceptive exercises

Fourth Stage (60th – 90th Day)

1. Medical examination
2. ROM obtained must be complete
3. Physical therapy continued on alternate days
4. Isometric gymnastics continued
5. Tapis roulant (Fig. 9)
6. Swimming. Avoid breast stroke and knee flexion
7. Exercise bicycle with high saddle and foot forward on pedal to minimise knee flexion
8. Semi-squat
9. Endless belt
10. Horizontal leg-press
11. Proprioceptive exercises

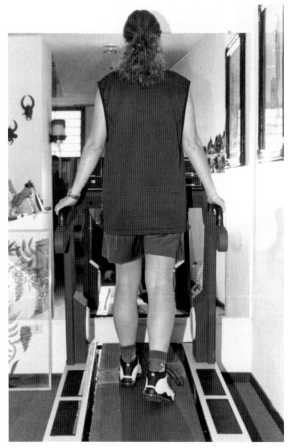

Fig. 9. Tapis roulant

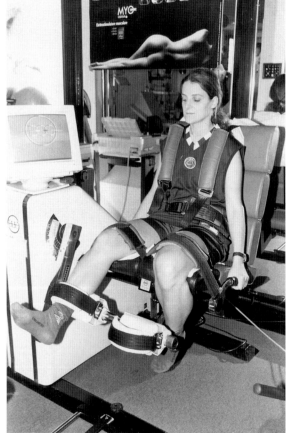

Fig. 10. Isokinetics

Fifth Stage (3rd – 6th Month)

1. Medical examination
2. Personal continuation of rehabilitation. Fortnightly contact with physiotherapist (daily if professional athlete)
3. Swimming (not breast stroke)
4. Exercise and ordinary bicycle
5. Leg press
6. Stairs climber
7. Endless belt
8. Start running
9. Start of active work for flexors
10. Proprioceptive exercises

Sixth Stage (6th – 8th Month)

1. Medical examination
2. Clinical evaluation of knee stability, and possibly radiography (under stress or according to [23])
3. Bicycle
4. Running
5. Running uphill
6. Vertical jumps
7. 'Home cross-country skiing'
8. Isokinetics (Fig. 10)
9. Dynamic proprioceptive exercises

Seventh Stage (8th – 10th Month)

1. Medical examination
2. Resumption of sport, including contact sport

Nonoperative Management and Rehabilitation

of Patients with Acute PCL Tears
Rehabilitation is the same as for surgical patients. Resolution of inflammation is the prime aim of treatment in the acute stage. Oedema and pain are best reduced by raising of the limb, application of ice, administration of anti-inflammatory drugs, immobilisation with a brace and the use of crutches for walking.

Immobilisation

A brace is applied with the knee in extension. It is removed during physical therapy and retained when walking for about a month until good quadriceps control is regained.

Recovery of Complete ROM

Resolution of inflammation is followed by active and passive mobilisation of the knee. A sliding surface under the foot is a simple and effective means of starting mobilisation. In more complex cases where movement of the joint is difficult, CPM can be usefully employed. Complete recovery of flexion must be achieved gradually over the course of a month. Open-chain mobilisation must be avoided, since contraction of the flexors produces posterior translation of the tibia and stretches the ligament fibres. Undue stretching in patients with incomplete intrasubstance tears would result in an elongated PCL at the end of the healing process [13].

Muscle Strengthening and Proprioceptive Exercises

Quadriceps and flexor strengthening is the same as after surgical reconstruction. Isometric exercises to prevent quadriceps atrophy begin on the first day. When normal joint movements become possible, closed-chain exercises can commence (exercise bicycle, semi-squat, step machine, leg press) with movements according to co-ordinated motor schemes. Proprioceptive re-education started in this way will lead to the resumption of sport after 2 or 3 months.

The Five Rehabilitation Stages

First Stage (1st – 15th Day After Injury)

1. Knee brace locked in extension with pillow under triceps during bed rest
2. Cryotherapy
3. Non-steroidal anti-inflammatory drug (NSAID) as required
4. Crutches with partial weight bearing
5. Isometric quadriceps exercises

Second Stage (15th – 30th Day)

1. Medical examination
2. Start walking with brace but without crutches
3. Remove brace for physical therapy
4. Electrotherapy of the quadriceps
5. Massage
6. Isometric exercises for all lower limb muscle
7. Recovery of ROM 0° – 90°

Third Stage (30th – 60th Day)

1. Medical examination
2. Complete weight bearing
3. Recovery of complete ROM
4. Electrotherapy of the quadriceps
5. Massage
6. Isometric gymnastics
7. Endless belt
8. Proprioceptive exercises

9. Semi-squat
10. Swimming (not breast stroke)
11. Exercise bicycle

Fourth Stage (30th – 60th Day)

1. Medical examination
2. Physical therapy on alternate days
3. Swimming
4. Exercise bicycle
5. Road cycling
6. Leg press
7. Semi-squat
8. Endless belt
9. Start running
10. Isokinetics
11. Dynamic proprioceptive exercises

Fifth Stage (90th Day Onwards)

1. Medical examination
2. Resumption of training and gradual return to specific sport

Conclusions

The correct principles regulating the rehabilitation of patients with PCL tears and reconstructions lag behind those for the ACL. Uncertainties in the diagnosis of incomplete and complete PCL injuries account for differences of opinion concerning the indications for nonoperative and surgical management. PCL reconstrucion is also far less frequently described than ACL reconstruction, and more time has been needed to perfect techniques and ensure the correct, unequivocal assessment of the clinical outcome.

Dissimilar results have long appeared in the literature. The cautious functional recovery protocols drawn up by surgeons have generated indecision on the part of physiotherapists. The results of MRI lacked precise interpretation for several years. This examination has now led to the differentiation of incomplete, intrasubstance and complete PCL tears. It also illustrates tibial bone block avulsion and femoral detachment. These data have constituted a sound basis for elaborating the rationale of operative or rehabilitative management. Progress has also been made through clinical employment of the findings of studies of knee anatomy and biomechanics, primarily with regard to the extent of the shifting of the joint surfaces during movement, especially in the sagittal plane.

Physical therapy has exploited these advances to avoid manoeuvres that would prejudice the integrity of the PCL during rehabilitation after nonoperative and operative management. Particular mention must be made of the action of the flexors, which translate the tibia posteriorly and stretch the PCL fibres, especially during hyperflexion. The following aspects of PCL rehabilitation must be stressed:

1. Early weight bearing in extension
2. Quadriceps exercises between 0° and 75°
3. Closed-kinetic-chain exercises
4. Avoidance of early maximum flexion
5. Avoidance of flexor work during open-kinetic-chain exercises

Acknowledgment. We gratefully acknowledge Jacek Jaworsky, physiotherapist (Fisioélite, Roma), for his collaboration.

References

1. Boynton MD, Tietjens BR (1996) Long-term follow-up of the untreated isolated posterior cruciate ligament-deficient knee. Am J Sports Med 24:306–310
2. Chassaing V, Touzard R (1995) Histoire naturelle de la rupture du ligament croisè postèrieur. Rèsultats de l'étude multicentrique. Rev Chir Orthop 69eme Rèunion SOFCOT [Suppl. 2] 81:49–51
3. Cross M, Powell JF (1984) Long-term follow-up of posterior cruciate ligament rupture. A study of 116 cases. Am J Sports Med 12:292–297
4. Dandy DJ, Pursey RJ (1982) The long term results of unrepaired tears of the posterior cruciate ligament. J Bone Joint Surg 64B:92–94
5. Dejour H, Walch G, Peyrot J, Eberhard P (1988) Histoire naturelle de la rupture du ligament croisè postérieur. Fr J Orthop Surg 2:112–120
6. Keller PM, Shelbourne KD, McCarroll JR, Rettig AC (1993) Nonoperatively treated isolated posterior cruciate ligament injuries. Am J Sports Med 21:132–136
7. Parolie JM, Bergfeld JA (1993) Long-term results of nonoperative treatment of isolated posterior cruciate ligament injuries. Am J Sports Med 14:35–38
8. Peterson CA, Warren RF (1996) Management of acute and chronic posterior cruciate ligament injuries. Am J Knee Surg 9:172–184
9. Schutz EA, M, Irrgang JJ (1994) Rehabilitation following posterior cruciate ligament. Injury or reconstruction. Sports Med Arthroscopy 2:165–170
10. Spindler KP, Benson EM (1994) Natural history of posterior cruciate ligament injury. Sports Med Arthroscopy 2:73–79
11. Bosch U, Kasperczyk WJ, Oestern HJ, Tscherne H (1994) Biology of posterior cruciate ligament healing. Sports Med Arthroscopy 2:88–99
12. McCarthy MR, O'Donoghue PC, Yates CK, McCarthy JLY (1992) The clinical use of continuous passive motion in physical therapy. JOSPT 15:132–140
13. Woo SLY, Wang CW, Newton PO, Lyon RM (1990) The response of ligaments to stress deprivation and stress enhancement. In: Daniel D, Akeson W, Connor J, (eds), Knee ligaments: structure, function, injury and repair. New York, Raven Press, p 337–350
14. Girgis FG, Marshall JL, Al Monajem ARS (1975) The cruci-

ate ligaments of the knee joint: anatomical, functional, and experimental analysis. Clin Orthop 106:216–231

15. Miller MD, Johnson DL, Harner CD et al. (1993) Posterior cruciate ligament injuries. Orthop Rev 22:1201–1210

16. Franklin JL, Rosemberg TD, Paulos LE, et al. (1991) Radiographic assessment of instability of the knee due to rupture of the anterior cruciate ligament. A quadriceps contraction technique. J Bone Joint Surg 73A:365–372

17. Lysholm J, Gillquist J (1981) Arthroscopic examination of the posterior cruciate ligament. J Bone Joint Surg 63A:363–368

18. Trickey EL (1968) Rupture of the posterior cruciate ligament of the knee. J Bone Joint Surg 50:334–341

19. Kennedy JC, Roth JH, Walker DM (1979) Posterior cruciate ligament injuries. Orthop Digest 7:19–31

20. Puddu G, De Paulis F, Cipolla M (1995) L'IRM dans la pathologie isolée du ligament croisé postérieur. Rev Chir Orthop, 69eme Réunion SOFCOT [Suppl. 2] 81:41–45

21. Gross ML, Grover JS, Bassett LW, Seeger LL, Finerman GAM (1992) Magnetic resonance imaging of the posterior cruciate ligament: clinical use to improve diagnostic accuracy. Am J Sports Med 20:732–737

22. Staubli HU, Jakob RP (1990) Posterior instability of the knee near extension. J Bone Joint Surg 72B:225–230

23. Puddu G, Cerullo G, Franco V (1996) Patologia del legamento crociato posteriore. In: De Paulis F, Puddu G (eds), Ginocchio: Diagnostica per immagini e inquadramento clinico. Guido Gnocchi Editore, Napoli, p.143–148

24. Rosemberg TD, Paulos LE, Parker RD (1988) The forty-five-degree postero-anterior flexion weight-bearing radiograph of the knee. J Bone Joint Surg 70A:1479–1483

25. Lutz GE, Palmiter RA, An KN, Chao EYS (1993) Comparison of tibiofemoral joint forces during open-kinetic-chain and closed-kinetic-chain exercises. J Bone Joint Surg 75A:732–739

26. Malone TR, Davies GL (1992) Open and closed kinetic-chain exercises and their application to testing and rehabilitation. AOSSM Meeting Abstracts and Outlines

27. Harner CD, Irrgang JJ (1994) Isolated and combined PCL reconstruction post-op.: rehabilitation protocol. AAOS Annual Meeting, San Francisco

28. Schutz EA, Vrana N, Irrgang JJ, Harner CD (1993) Post-operative physical therapy guidelines following PCL-reconstruction. AOSSM Annual Meeting

29. Jackson DW (1993) Rehabilitation principles following posterior cruciate ligament reconstructive surgery. AAOS Annual Meeting, San Francisco

30. Noyes FR, Barber-Westin SD (1994) Posterior cruciate ligament allograft reconstruction with and without a ligament augmentation device. Arthroscopy 10:371–382

31. Gianni E, Scala A, Puddu G (1998) Rehabilitation following the surgical and nonsurgical management of posterior cruciate ligament injuries. J Sports Traumatol 20:23–40

32. Puddu G, Gianni E, Cerullo G (1995) La réhabilitation après la réconstruction du ligament croisé postérieur. Rev Chir Orthop 81 [Suppl. 2], 63–65

33. De Lee JC, Bergfeld JA, Drez D Jr (1994) The posterior cruciate ligament. In: De Lee D (eds) Orthopaedic sports medicine. WB Saunders Company, New York, p 1374–1400

34. Clancy WG, Shelbourne KD, Rosemberg TD, Gheiner IG, Wisnefske DD, Lange TA (1983) Treatment of knee joint instability secondary to rupture of the posterior cruciate ligament. J Bone Joint Surg 65A:310–322

12 Anterior Knee Pain: An Overview of Management Options

Nicola Maffulli

Introduction

The term 'anterior knee pain' includes all pain-related problems of the anterior portion of the knee, and covers terms such as chondromalacia patella, patellofemoral arthralgia, patellar pain, patellar pain syndrome, and patellofemoral pain. Therefore, after excluding anterior knee pain resulting from intra-articular pathologies, patellar tendinopathy, peripatellar bursitis, the plica syndrome, Sinding Larsen's and Osgood Schlatter's lesions, and other rarely occurring conditions, the remaining patients with a clinical presentation of anterior knee pain can be diagnosed with patellofemoral pain syndrome (PFPS). All such patients experience pain, but patients also report other symptoms, and it is therefore appropriate to talk of PFPS.

The Patellofemoral Joint

Anatomy and Biomechanics

The patellofemoral joint (PFJ) consists of the patella, the distal and anterior parts of the femur, their articular surfaces, and the surrounding structures. Three quarters of the articular surface of the patella is covered by thick hyaline cartilage.

Its shape, the femoral trochlea, and the patellar retinaculum act as passive stabilisers of the patella. The dynamic stabilisers include all the periarticular muscles of the knee. The vastus medialis obliquus (VMO) muscle has its own nerve supply and can pull the patella medially when the knee is at an angle of 65°.

The part of the patellar surface which articulates with the femur translates proximally during knee flexion. Patellofemoral compression forces increase with increasing knee angles up to 90° of knee flexion, reaching up to eight times the body weight.

Aetiology of PFPS

Anterior knee pain is the most frequent complaint in active adolescents and young adults. They often report pain while sitting and occasional weakness and catching sensations. These symptoms often prevent students from participating in physical education and sports, although no differences were found between students with knee pain and those without, in terms of joint mobility, Q angle, genu valgum and femoral neck anteversion.

Three major contributing factors are classically considered as increasing the risk of developing PFPS: namely, malaligment of the lower extremity and/or of the patella, muscle imbalance, and excessive physical activities.

Malalignment of the Lower Extremity

Malalignment of the lower extremity found in patients with PFPS include femoral neck anteversion, genu valgum, knee hyperextension, increased Q angle, tibia vara, and hyperpronation of the forefoot. However, clinical studies have shown no biomechanical or alignment differences between patients with PFPS and healthy individuals, although a high Q angle may contribute to perpetuate PFPS. However, the Q angle can discriminate between asymptomatic and runners with PFPS. Also, the term malalignment should be used judiciously, as a large part of the normal population falls into a category generally classified as 'malalignment'.

Patellar Malalignment

The three different patterns of patellar malalignment described are subluxation without tilting, subluxation with tilting, and tilting without subluxation [1]. Although patellar tracking abnormalities have been described as a major cause of patellar pain, some studies showed no difference with imaging studies between the patients' most symptomatic and least symptomatic knees. Various limits of normality are reported, but none has been shown unequivocally to be a significant factor in the aetiology of PFPS.

The biomechanics of the PFJ may induce a higher risk of overuse in some individuals, and a combination of malalignment and diminished muscle function may increase this risk.

Muscle Imbalance

Assessment of the range of motion of the hip, knee and ankle have not demonstrated significant differences between healthy individuals and patients with PFPS.

Decreased knee extensor strength is common in PFPS patients, and various patterns of weaknesses have been reported. For example, decreased eccentric muscle strength has been reported, and quadriceps electromyographic (EMG) activity can be higher and less efficient in the painful leg compared with the non-painful leg. An abnormal relationship in the activation pattern of the VMO and vastus lateralis (VL) can alter the dynamics of the patellofemoral joint.

Many rehabilitation regimens concentrate on the importance of the VMO because of its medialisation on the patella [6]. However, neither exercises purported to selectively activate the VMO muscle nor patellar taping improved the VVMO-VL ratio [11]. Patients with patellofemoral pain show reversal of the onset of VMO and VL activity, but other studies have found no differences in the onset or cessation of muscle activity [1, 11].

The significance of muscle activity in closed versus open kinetic chain exercises has not been extensively studied, and the results of the available studies are inconclusive.

Closed kinetic chain exercises have become more popular than the traditional open kinetic chain exercises in the belief that closed kinetic chain exercises are safer. However, both closed and open kinetic chain exercises are helpful in a PFPS training programme to minimise PFJ stress.

Further investigations should study the significance of muscular imbalances and clarify whether they are a cause or effect (or both) of PFPS.

Overactivity

The stimulus to develop PFPS may be increased physical activity and overload instead of malalignment of the PFJ. Patients with anterior knee pain are more involved in competitive sports than age-matched controls, and pain is associated with increased physical activity.

Symptoms

The most common symptoms in patients with PFPS are pain, crepitus, giving way, and catching, with occasional stiffness and swelling. Crepitus is not always present in patients with PFPS, and can be present without pain or other symptoms. Swelling is mild, intermittent, and rare.

Giving way in patients with PFPS results from a sudden relaxation due to pain inhibition of the quadriceps during loading of the PFJ while standing, and should be distinguished from giving way from ligamentous instability or from a meniscal lesion. Transient catching is often reported, but it is not due to intra-articular pathology.

Pain

The source of patellofemoral pain in patients with PFPS is unclear, as there are no nerve endings in the articular cartilage, although the subchondral bone is innervated. Reactive synovitis is a possible source of pain, and the patellar retinacula are a potential source of patellofemoral pain. Increased physical activity could result in peripatellar soft tissue irritation, and pain may then originate from retinacular nerve endings, with malalignment and overuse as magnifying factors.

Strength, Pain and Inhibition

Strength deficits of the knee extensor muscles are common in patients with PFPS. The decreased torque and reduction in EMG activity in patients with PFPS, especially with eccentric knee extension, may result from quadriceps inhibition at heavy patellofemoral loads, as in eccentric knee extension and single leg vertical jump. This inhibition and the ability to develop high force torque in different situations should be considered when developing treatment programmes for patients with PFPS.

Management

As basic scientific knowledge is lacking and no strong evidence-based protocols have been published on the nature and aetiology of PFPS, it is not surprising that so many treatment regimens are in use. Unfortunately, there is little scientific evidence on which to base management. Given the number of patients with PFPS, it is sad that decisions still have to be taken based on anecdotal rather than scientific evidence [3, 8, 10, 13].

In general, we suggest slow progression of rehabilitation without increasing the symptoms. Key factors in such a programme are flexibility, strength, proprioception, endurance, functional training, and a gradual progression of the musculoskeletal load. Compliance is important, and, in the long run, even in well-supervised exercise programmes compliance is poor, with most patients dropping out. Surgery is rarely indicated, and the most frequently recommended management regimen is rehabilitation, with a high chance of success. However, the effects of an exercise programme for PFPS have not been scientifically and systematically documented. Variable success rates are reported, with great variability among studies in diagnosis, physical activity level, gender and age of the patients.

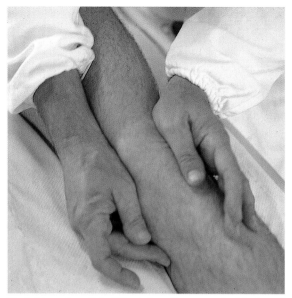

Fig. 1. Manual medial gliding of patella to stretch tight lateral structures

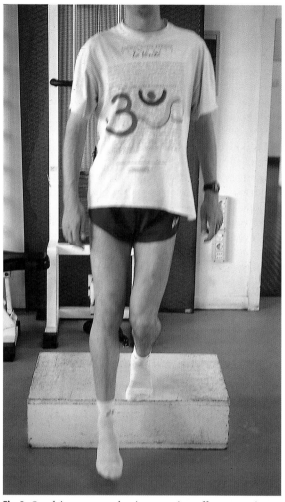

Fig. 3. Quadriceps strengthening stepping off a step trying to improve the pelvic control

In general, a rehabilitation programme should include (1) symptomatic control with relative rest (avoiding or limiting painful activities) while conditioning the other parts of the kinetic chain (upper body ergometer, cycling with the uninvolved lower limb); (2) lower extremity flexibility exercises for iliotibial band (ITB) [12], rectus femoris, gastrocnemius and hamstrings, and manual techniques to stretch the lateral peripatellar tight structures (Fig. 1); (3) progressive strengthening programme focused not only on quadriceps [2], hip adductors and flexors, but also on gluteus medius; (4) a graduated running programme; and (5) a maintenance programme.

Functional re-education should be performed also while weight bearing, as this is the most physiological position of the lower limbs in daily and sports activities. Stresses across the patellofemoral joint are reduced with closed-kinetic chain (CKC) exercises which utilise the co-contraction of quadriceps, hamstrings and gastrocnemius muscles [7] (Figs. 2, 3).

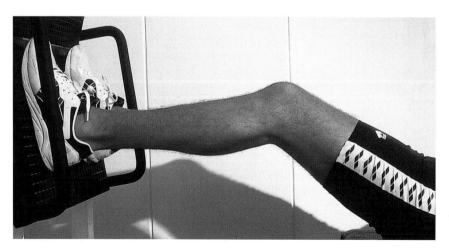

Fig. 2. CKC exercise (horizontal leg press) in terminal knee extension

Isometric training in full extension is recommended because it helps to reduce pain and can strengthen the quadriceps without a significant increase in patellofemoral joint reaction forces, as demonstrated by Kannus [9]. Strengthening of the gluteus medius muscle is also important because it causes a concurrent reduced activity in ITB muscle, so this results in a decreased pull on the patella by the lateral retinacular structures [5] (Fig. 4). Although eccentric isokinetic exercises are in fashion, there are no differences between an isometric and an isokinetic exercise programme, as both programmes show similar significant functional improvements over a control group with no treatment.

Some authors propose a comprehensive approach based on standardised information, pain monitoring, and an individually designed progressive exercise programme. Significant pain reduction and strength and physical activity level improvements are seen after

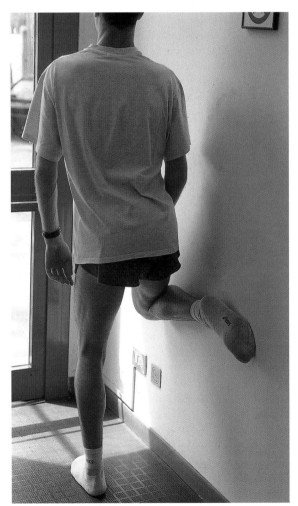

Fig. 4. Strengthening of the gluteus medius muscle in standing position. The right knee is leaning on the wall, while the left leg, in slight flexion, externally rotates the knee without moving the foot or the hip

12 weeks of treatment. Improvements may be a result of time, the standardised information, the pain monitoring system, the gradually progressive training programme, and the reduced physical activity.

The treatment effects do not seem sensitive to a particular choice of exercises. A reduction in pain after the end of the rehabilitation session may last for several hours after a session of only 10–15 min. The exercises may modify the influx of afferent signals with reduced reflex inhibition and possible increase in endorphins. Better muscle activation, with increased motor unit recruitment and a more physiological activation of the vastus medialis muscle may thus be achieved.

Training might also induce increased diffusion of nutrients to the articular cartilage through cyclical loading and unloading the PFJ, and improved nutrition to surrounding joint structures and muscles with increased vascularity. Thus, the training programme may produce beneficial effects on the PFJ, as adaptive changes can be seen in muscles, tendons, ligaments and the cartilage after regularly repeated, slowly progressing, non-strenuous rehabilitation. However, this is only speculative, with limited scientific support. Strenuous exercises may cause gradual breakdown of the musculoskeletal tissue, with deleterious effects and increased pain. The increased physical activity after treatment may contribute to the further improvements in symptoms and muscle function seen in the longer term.

Patellar Taping

Taping for patellar malalignment has now reached widespread acceptance [4]. However, patellar taping does not improve the EMG activity ratio between the

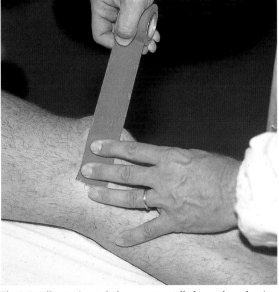

Fig. 5. Patellar taping to help correct patellofemoral mechanics

VMO and the VL muscles. Some authors suggest that there are no advantages in adding taping to a well planned rehabilitation programme. In the appropriate hands, and with the right technique, patella taping has been very successful (Fig. 5). However, more basic and clinical research, with longitudinal and randomised controlled trials, should be performed to clarify its role in PFPS.

Surgery

Although non-operative management is the first line of management for PFPS, more than 100 surgical procedures have been described. Most of these operations have not been evaluated with randomised controlled trials. They aim to treat malalignment (and are therefore called realignment procedures) or other abnormalities of the knee extensor mechanism, or the injured cartilage.

Lateral Release. In this procedure, the lateral retinaculum is sectioned longitudinally. It can be combined with other realignment procedures. Its main indications are: (1) abnormally high lateral patellar compression with tenderness and tightness of the lateral retinaculum, and lateral patellar tilt; (2) degenerative disease of the patellofemoral joint with lateral patellar tilt; and (3) persistent patellofemoral pain associated with a lateral traction osteophyte at the insertion of the lateral retinaculum into the patella. The procedure is not recommended for prepubertal patients, or in severe patellofemoral osteoarthrosis and normal patellar tracking. Results have often been unpredictable, with a reported rate of satisfactory results between 20 and 92% of patients, and the biomechanical effects of the procedure are unclear.

Proximal Realignment. Several different techniques for proximal soft tissue realignment have been described, and are indicated in patients who: (1) are skeletally immature and have a history of recurrent dislocations; (2) have an increased congruence angle with patellofemoral pain; and (3) have dysplastic femoral trochlea and poor medial patellar support of the VMO muscle, with recurrent patellar subluxations or dislocations. Satisfaction is normally high, but these procedures are now rarely used.

Distal Realignment. These procedures are most often used in patients with recurrent patellar subluxation or dislocation, and less for patellofemoral pain. They consist of transfer of the tibial tubercle. The indications are (1) persistent patellofemoral pain combined with excessive patellar tilt or subluxation or increased congruence angle; (2) lateral patellar degenerative joint disease with increased Q angle; and (3) failed lateral re-

lease procedure, especially in patients with significant lateral tilt or subluxation. Transfer of the tibial tubercle is contraindicated in skeletally immature patients, given the high risk of development of genu recurvatum in this age group. Satisfaction is high, but long-term results are unclear.

Elevation of the Tibial Tubercle. Marked decrease of patellofemoral compression forces is produced by elevation of the tibial tubercle of 1.2 – 2.5 cm. The main indication for this procedure is moderate degeneration joint disease of the PFJ unresponsive to conservative management. Results have been unpredictable, the long-term results unsatisfactory, and this procedure is now rarely used for patellofemoral pain.

Anteromedial Tibial Tubercle Transfer and Elevation. The procedure is indicated in patients with malalignment, increased Q angle, and mild-to-moderate PFJ osteoarthrosis.

Articular Cartilage Procedures. These procedures include open or arthroscopic patellar shaving, local excision of defects with drilling of the subchondral bone, facetectomy and transplantation of autologous chondrocytes. The major benefit of arthroscopic interventions might well be the dilution effect with wash-out of the debris from the knee joint. Satisfactory results are achieved in patients below the age of 25 years.

No comparative studies on these procedures are available, and the results are often satisfactory in the short term, but less is known about the long-term outcomes.

Patellectomy. Excision of the patella should be considered the last resort to treat patellofemoral diseases, as it may result in a considerable decrease in functional ability. The main indication is severe patellofemoral pain after a failed realignment in patients younger than 40 years. Contraindications are tibial-femoral disorders and patellofemoral pain of unknown origin.

Conclusion

Standardised information and reduced and modified physical activity levels will suffice in most PFPS patients with mild symptoms. Avoidance of excessive physical exercise and avoidance of prolonged sitting with knees flexed seem to be most effective. However, patients with PFPS should not completely abstain from physical activities, although they should adjust both the quantity of physical activity and the type of physical activity they undertake.

Patients with PFPS need to be patient. Improvements occur slowly, especially at the beginning, and the positive effects of rehabilitation take time. Rehabilitation should progress gradually and the success of a management regimes also depends on adjusting the exercises of the rehabilitation programme in relation to the patient's symptoms and needs.

References

1. Beaconsfield T, Pintore E, Maffulli N, Petri GJ (1994)Radiological measurements in patellofemoral disorders. A review. Clin Orthop 308:18–28
2. Boucher JP, King MA, Lefevre R, Pepin A (1992) Quadriceps femoris activity in patellofemoral pain syndrome. Am J Sports Med 20:527–532
3. Brody LT, Thein JM (1998) Nonoperative treatment for patellofemoral pain. J Orthop Sports Phys Ther 28:336–344
4. Ernst GP, Kawaguchi J, Saliba E (1999) Effect of patellar taping on knee kinetics of patients with patellofemoral pain syndrome. J Orthop Sports Phys Ther 29:661–667
5. Grelsamer RP, McConnell J (1998) Conservative management of patellofemoral problems. In Grelsamer RP, McConnell J (eds) The patella: a team approach. Aspen, Maryland pp. 119–136
6. Hanten WP, Schulthies SS (1990) Exercise effect on electromyographic activity of the vastus medialis oblique and vastus lateralis muscles. Phys Ther 70:561–565
7. Hungerford DS, Barry M (1979) Biomechanics of the patellofemoral joint. Clin Orthop 144:9–15
8. Juhn MS (1999) Patellofemoral pain syndrome: a review and guidelines for treatment. Am Fam Physician 60:2012–2022
9. Kannus P, Niittymaki S (1994) Which factors predict outcome in nonoperative treatment of patellofemoral pain syndrome? A prospective follow up study. Med Sci Sports Exerc 26:289–296
10. Natri A, Kannus P, Jarvinen M (1998) Which factors predict the long-term outcome in chronic patellofemoral pain syndrome? A 7-year prospective follow-up study. Med Sci Sports Exerc 30:1572–1577
11. Powers CM (1998) Rehabilitation of patellofemoral joint disorders: a critical review. J Orthop Sports Phys Ther 28:345–354
12. Punicello MS (1993) Iliotibial band tightness and medial patellar glide in patients with patellofemoral dysfunction. J Orthop Sports Phys Ther 17:144–148
13. Thomee R, Augustsson J, Karlsson J (1999) Patellofemoral pain syndrome: a review of current issues. Sports Med 28:245–262

13 Rehabilitation After Ankle Ligament Injury

Lars Konradsen, Per F.A.H. Renström

Introduction

The ideal goal of rehabilitation after ankle ligament injury is to restore (1) range of motion, (2) sensori-motor control, and (3) muscle strength to a pre-injury level. In the following chapter, normal requirements for each of these functions will be discussed and causes for restrictions or deficits will be addressed. The function of the foot/ankle complex during gait will be assessed and the kinematics during running presented. The scientific basis behind relevant rehabilitation modalities will be reviewed, and programs for acute and long-term ankle rehabilitation will be introduced.

Normal Requirements

Range of Motion

To be able to perform movements with ease, the movements must lie within the field of passive motion of the foot/ankle complex. Whether a loss of passive motion is perceived as a handicap depends very much on the functional requirements of each and every individual. A slight loss of ankle plantar flexion would, for example, be considered a handicap by professional dancers while it would not be of significance to most people in their everyday life. In contrast, inability to dorsiflex the ankle 10° would cause everybody to limp in each step of walking no matter how much elements like strength, coordination, and proprioception were to be trained.

Anatomically, the foot/ankle complex is usually divided into the talocrural and the subtalar joints. The range of passive motion of the talotibial joint varies from report to report mostly due to differences in methods of measurement. Maximal dorsiflexion ranges from 10° to 23° and maximal plantar flexion from 23° to 48° [1, 58]. From maximal dorsiflexion to maximal plantar flexion, all of the articular surface of the talus will at some time be contained under the tibial articular surface. The main restriction for passive dorsiflexion in the healthy subject is the Achilles tendon complex, while plantar flexion is stopped by tightened anterior tendon structures or by posterior impingement.

The subtalar joint or the talocalcaneonavicular joint complex rotates around an axis that continuously changes during movement [68]. The average axis being as described by Inman [24] with a 42° inclination in the sagittal plane and 23° of medial deviation in the horizontal plane. Again, range of motion differs, but 30° of inversion and 10° of eversion is a practical average in clinical settings [60].

When viewing the ankle from a rehabilitation point of view, it is more appropriate to consider the movement of the ankle/foot complex in a field of motion that mirrors the combination of the talotibial and the subtalar movements [37] (Fig. 1). This field is individual and changes (being reduced) with age. Injury will affect big or small areas of the field, and rehabilitation must again try to restore the sphere to what is normal for the individual.

A reduced field of motion can be caused by both mechanical and dynamic restrictions. Mechanical restrictions include bony restraints, capsular contracture and increased passive muscle/tendon resistance. In the presence of decreased dorsiflexion, contracture of the soleus complex may occur and complement the problem, and may reduce the immediate effect of a space-giving anterior procedure. Dynamic restrictions may be involuntary or voluntary. Increased muscle tone due to spinal or central nervous system diseases may involuntarily restrict ankle movement while other central nervous system or general diseases or local tendon or nerve affections may make it impossible for the subject to utilize part of the sphere of motion open to her/him. Voluntary restrictions to range of motion may be induced if pain elicited from the joint or from periarticular structures causes the subject to avoid movements in an area of the sphere that would elicit pain. Thus a subject may decide to avoid eversion movements and chose to walk with increased inversion during the stance phase as not to stress a chondral lesion lateral on the talus.

Muscle Strength

There are 32 muscles, 13 extrinsic and 19 intrinsic, that control the actions of the foot.

The extrinsic muscles of the calf are responsible for the major torque generation of the talotibial and subta-

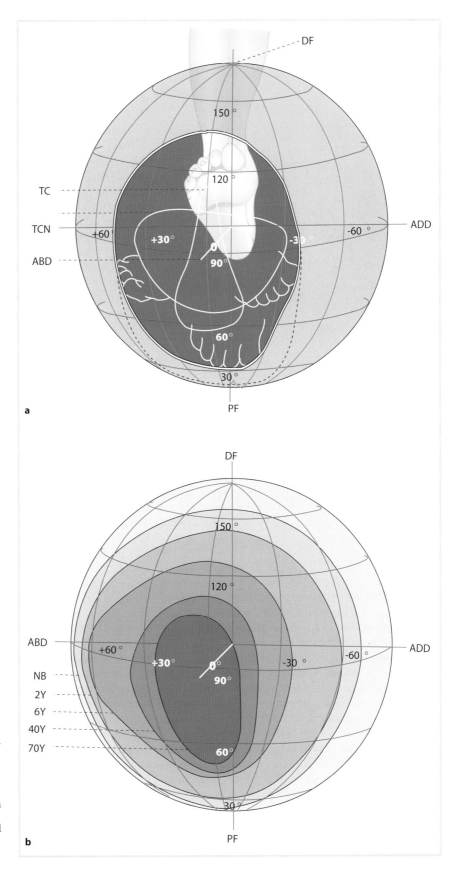

Fig. 1. Field of motion of the foot ankle complex. **a** Oval contour of the field of motion. *TC,* contribution of the talocrural joint; *TCN,* contribution of the talocalcaneo-navicular joint; *DF,* dorsiflexion; *PF,* plantar flexion; *ABD:* abduction; *ADD,* adduction. **b** Field of motion in different age groups. *NB,* newborn; *2Y,* 2 years old, and so forth. (With permission from [60])

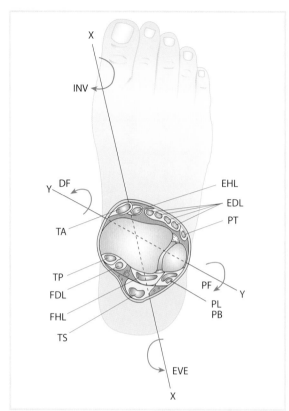

Fig. 2. Motors of the ankle and the talocalcaneonavicular joint. *XX*, axis of the TCN joint; *YY*,: axis of the talocrural joint; *INV*, inversion; *EVE*, eversion; *DF*, dorsiflexion; *PL*, plantar flexion. Invertors: *TA*, tibialis anterior; *TP*, tibialis posterior; *FDL*, flexor digitorum longus; *FHL*, flexor hallucis longus; *TS*, triceps surae. Evertors: *PL*, peroneus longus; *PB*, peroneus brevis; *EHL*, extensor hallucis longus; *EDL*, extensor digitorum longus; *TA*, tibialis anterior; *PT*, peroneus tertius. Plantar flexors: *TP, FDL, FHL, TS, PL, PB*. Dorsiflexors: *TA, EHL, EDL, PT.* (With permission from [60])

lar joints. They can be divided into antagonistic groups responsible for either dorsal/plantar flexion or inversion/eversion, but due to the oblique placement of the subtalar axis, dorsal/plantar flexors have an element of inversion/eversion action and visa versa (Fig. 2) [24]. Even the soleus muscle with its Achilles tendon attachment on the calcaneus medial to the subtalar axis acts with an inversion component. The gastrocnemius and the soleus complex have a primary propulsive function as the strongest plantar flexors of the talotibial joint. Their function is, however, mediated through the subtalar joint which requires that many of the other muscles work in combination to secure stability of the foot and ankle complex in order to produce an optimal functional base for the task of moving the body in the desired direction.

The intrinsic muscles of the foot, predominantly the flexor hallucis brevis, the extensor digitorum brevis, and the abductor digiti minimi, do not have general functions like many of the extrinsic muscles but have specific functions to the toes.

It is not possible to define required levels of strength for each of the crural muscles. But the activities of daily living require a substantial degree of force from primarily the muscles working against gravity. Peak or maximal muscle strength in both isometric and isokinetic set-ups is often used as a measurement of functional muscle ability, especially in rehabilitation situations. Maximal muscle strength will, however, only indicate whether it is within the ability of the individual to perform a specific task. If a muscle is too weak to do a necessary task, either other muscles able to create a similar torque must be recruited as seen for the tibialis posterior in the case of Achilles tendon deficiency, or another pattern of motion must be sought as in cases of peroneal nerve palsy. In either case, other structures are at risk of being injured due to overload. Other components of muscle strength must also be considered.

Often maximal strength may seem to be sufficient, but muscle endurance may be reduced, rendering the muscle too weak for the task after a number of repetitions. Finally, the balance between antagonistic muscles may have been disturbed, rendering one of the seemingly strong muscle groups too weak compared to the antagonists to be able to uphold a functional balance. Thus an overweight of ankle inversion strength compared to ankle eversion strength seems to predispose to repeated ankle distortion injuries [6].

Injury, immobilization, and reduced muscle activation will result in muscle wasting as early as 1 or 2 weeks after the onset. The degree of muscle atrophy depends on factors such as the duration of immobilization (the longer the immobilization the greater the atrophy) and the position of immobilization (tissue under tension atrophies significantly less than when placed in a relaxed position; [27]). In a number of follow-up studies after injury, persistent reduction in muscle strength has been demonstrated years after the primary injury. In healthy individuals, peak force and muscle cross sectional area correlate well, but after injury the reduction in maximal peak force is greater than suggested by the reduction in the cross sectional area. Neural factors are responsible for this discrepancy. In the injured or immobilized state, full activation might not be possible, either as an unspecific effect of disuse by a lack of optimal nerve drive, or due to reflex inhibition [63]. Inhibition of muscle activation may be present even though there is no pain or discomfort. Mild joint effusion may thus cause a significant reduction in muscle activation ability [63]. More obviously, a painful state will impede muscle activation. A summary of various treatment modalities for muscle weakness is presented in Table 1.

Table 1. Summary of various treatment modalities for muscle weakness (with permission from [19])

Treatment	Main indications	Advantages	Disadvantages/ limitations
Isometric exercise	Limited joint mobility or pain free range of motion	Easy to implement; choice of specific angles	No training of full range of motion; nonfunctional except at certain position
Dynamic exercises Constant resistance	Basic or home training programs	Concentric and eccentric training exercise; simple equipment	Inefficient matching of muscle and load torque; does not accommodate to pain
Variable resistance	Neurogen and muscle volume training	Exercise through full range of motion; concentric and eccentric exercise	Eccentric exercise cannot be avoided; does not accommodate to pain
Isokinetic concentric	Specific effects at high and low speed; muscle volume training	Voluntary maximum load through range of motion; accommodates to pain; reduced joint compression force at high speed with maintained motor unit recruitment	No load at the end of movement
Isokinetic eccentric	Muscle volume training at relatively good muscle strength	High force development	Muscle soreness when unaccustomed; difficult to accommodate to pain

Sensori-Motor Control

There are numerous receptors for motion and position in the capsule and ligaments of the ankle joint [50] together with muscle/tendon receptors of the muscles that bypass the area and cutaneous receptors in the surrounding skin and subcutaneous tissue [47]. Afferent information from these receptors constitutes the basis for classical term proprioception – the sensation of limb position and limb and joint movement [61]. When the proprioceptive information is collected and processed in cortical centers, resulting in a motor action, the term sensori-motor control is preferred.

The ability to sense limb position and movement is very accurate. Slow movements of about 1° are detectable and reproduction of joint angles can be done within 2° of accuracy [16, 26].

Ankle proprioception is primarily based on input from the ankle area. It is, however, not only receptors in ankle ligaments and capsule that supply the necessary information, as experiments with injections of local anesthetics in these areas do not affect movement threshold detection or postural stability [9]. A total stop of afferent information from the ankle/foot area by an ankle block results in decreased ankle angle reproduction abilities [32]. If the crural muscles are, however, allowed to be active, mechanoreceptors here are able to supply input that can quite accurately judge ankle position.

Loss or gross deterioration of proprioception as seen in degenerative neuropathic diseases can cause destruction of the joints, as in Charcot feet. However, acute injury to the ankle, as in ankle distortions, may also result in a proprioceptive deficit [30, 33, 38], and in subjects with repeated inversion injuries, a sensori-motor defect can be measured as impaired postural control [67], as an increased reaction time for the peroneal muscles to sudden inversion [28, 31], as increased detection threshold to ankle movement [15], and as an increased error in ankle angle reproduction [26].

Motion Patterns

When repeating known sequences of movement like walking, running, and balancing, we usually rely on preprogrammed patterns [11, 45, 61]. Each pattern can then again be altered or modified based on afferent input [11]. New tasks will often be approached using patterns that have proven successful from previous experience in similar situations combined with markedly increased activity of all muscles that may be needed for the task. With increased experience, fewer and fewer muscles will be recruited and the muscles that are involved will show decreasing activity towards a safe and economic solution [10]. In cases of functional impairment of the ankle joint due to changed mechanics or painful states, a new pattern of gait may be chosen by the subject. With time, a crossover effect will be seen, also affecting the pattern of the normal limb. Relieving the initial mechanical or pain problem by surgery will often not change the pattern of movement to normal. This has to be relearned, often in the beginning with the over-recruitment of muscle activity as seen when learning new tasks.

Locomotion

The Gait Cycle

Walking requires constant maintenance of the body equilibrium while achieving forward propulsion. For the body to stay in equilibrium, the gravitational force acting in the center of gravity, should pass through the supporting surface of the foot or through the support base defined by both feet joined anteriorly and posteriorly by a double tangent [25]. During walking there is a coordinated movement of all the major parts of the body and the displacements occur in the three planes of space, which must not be forgotten when thinking about rehabilitation. The pelvis and the lower extremities move in phase, whereas the upper back, shoulders, and upper extremities move out of phase relative to the lower segments. The support phase of walking occupies approximately 60% of the cycle with the swing phase occupying the rest (Fig. 3).

Rotational Movements. The pelvis, the femur, and the tibia rotate inward from heel-strike to 20% within the walking cycle and then rotate externally from this point and until toe-off (Fig. 3). The total range of rotational motion being: pelvis average 8°, femur 15°, tibia 19°. Distally, the transverse rotation is transmitted to and absorbed by the ankle-foot complex. Due to the obliquity of the talocrural joint axis, a limited degree of transverse rotation can be absorbed by concomitant dorsi/plantar flexion. The major transmission of tibial rotation occurs at the level of the subtalar joint. At heel strike, the subtalar joint is slightly inverted, followed by eversion which peaks at foot-flat and is maintained during the major portion of the stance phase. Just prior to heel-off, the subtalar joint is inverted, followed by eversion close to a neutral position during swing phase. The motion of the subtalar joint during the stance phase averages approximately 6° [70]. According to Mann, the internal rotation of the lower extremity is initiated distally through the subtalar eversion during weight-bearing and is transmitted to the proximal joints [44]. The external rotation of the weight-bearing extremity is initiated proximally through the swinging opposite lower extremity, producing the external rotation of the pelvis of the stance leg. This external rotation is transmitted distally and is further enhanced by the obligatory external rotation of the leg through its anterior flexion during the stance phase. Additional external rotation of the leg occurs through the metatarsal break along the

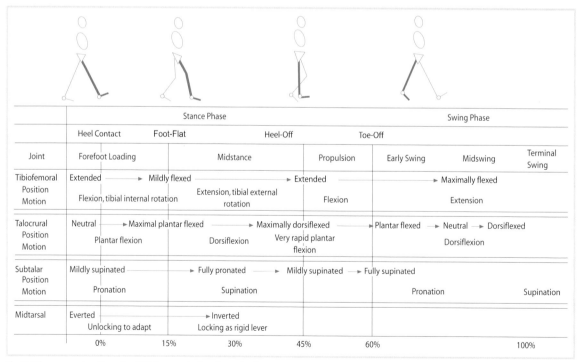

Fig. 3. The normal gait cycle. (With permission from [53])

oblique axis oriented posterolaterally at the time of heel-rise [44].

Sagittal Plane Motion. During the stance phase the ankle goes from a 10° dorsiflexed position to a 25° plantar flexed position [60]. In the swing phase, the ankle is initially plantar flexed, followed by dorsiflexion to neutral to clear the toes of the ground.

Stability of the Foot During Gait. At heel-strike, the heel is minimally inverted. From heel-strike and 20% into the cycle, the tibia rotates internally, the os calcis is everted at the subtalar joint and the forefoot is relatively supinated. As a result, the foot is in low arch, close-packed stable status, acting as an efficient structure to support the body weight. The stretching of the plantar ligaments helps them store elastic strain energy, that can be returned in the latter part of the stance phase during toe-off [70]. The following external rotation of the tibia during the progression of the stance phase induces the high-arch remodeling with the inversion of the os calcis and the relative pronation of the forefoot. The tension of the plantar soft-tissue structures is now maintained through the anterior flexion of the leg or the relative dorsiflexion of the foot. Thus, the continuum of remodeling ensures stability during locomotion from foot-flat to toe-off.

Forces on the Ankle During Gait. Forces are imparted to the ground by the body in motion through the contact surface of the foot. In the beginning of the stance phase, at heel strike, the decelerating foot comes down and the heel cushion strikes the ground with an initial shock wave, which travels in the lower extremity with impulses of up to 100 Hz [14]. The initial vertical spike force is approximately 80% of the body weight. A second force peak occurs at the middle of the cycle, surpassing the body weight by 10%. The magnitude of the force varies with the speed of the gait. Slow walk diminishes peak forces and rapid walk increases them.

Electromyographic Activity During Gait. Some muscles, like the soleus complex and the anterior tibial muscle show very consistent cyclic patterns that seem to express primarily preprogrammed strategies, while other muscles like the tibialis posterior and the peroneal muscle group show variable activity both intra- and inter-individually, suggesting a pattern that relies more on afferent input registering immediate foot/ankle balance.

Kinematics of Running

Compared with walking, running implies a floating phase consuming 20% of the cycle time for jogging, and 40% for running [25]. The support portion of the running stride is generally broken down into the impact phase, the mid-stance phase, and the push-off phase. The initial impact usually begins at the lateral aspect of heel and with the foot in slight inversion. In mid-stance, defined as the time during which the entire foot is on the ground, the subtalar joint passes from an inverted to an everted position. Eversion continues to about 85% of the support phase with maximum values ranging from 5° to 25°, depending also on factors like footwear. Seen in the sagittal plane following initial footfall, the leg rotates forward resulting in about 20° of ankle dorsiflexion. In mid-stance the ankle begins to plantarflex, reaching a maximum of 20° shortly after toe-off.

Rehabilitation Modalities and Science

Improving Range of Motion and Flexibility

Stretching. The effectiveness of different stretching techniques has been attributed to neurophysiological and mechanical factors [23, 64]. The neurophysiological foundation of muscle/tendon stretching is based on neural inhibition of the muscle undergoing stretch. A decreased reflex activity results in reduced resistance to stretch, which results in further gain of range of motion [23]. The biomechanical aspect relates to the viscoelastic properties of the connective tissue. The viscoelastic properties can be defined as two components of stretch [34, 35, 59]. The elastic component allows for an elastic temporary stretch, while the viscous component allows for a plastic stretch with a more permanent tissue elongation after the load is removed. The various stretching techniques can be summarized into ballistic stretching, static stretching, contract relax stretch, and contract relax-agonist contract [13, 23, 42, 52]. The last two are commonly referred to as proprioceptive neuromuscular facilitation (PNF) stretch techniques. A single stretch cycle has been shown to reduce passive torque at a given joint angle by about 20% [42]. A plateau in torque decline is reached after up to 45 s of stretching. Using a PNF technique, an improvement in joint range of motion compared with a static stretch can be accomplished [7, 17]. One hour after a single stretch cycle, no measurable stretch effect remains. Repeated stretches are necessary to produce an effect that can last more than 1 h [42]. Taylor et al. [64] found that four stretch cycles seemed to be the threshold for producing maximal effect, but scientific support for this is still lacking. We propose that stretching should be repeated regularly, e.g., every 6–8 h for a lasting effect.

When stretching, it remains important to remember that it is the movement sphere (for an explanation, see Fig. 1) that must be restored and not only movements in the usually defined anterior/posterior and lateral planes.

Joint Mobilization. This addresses the accessory motions of a joint (called roll and glide) using joint distraction and oscillations of varying amplitudes. Mechanical effects include stretching capsular restrictions and breaking adhesions, distracting impacted tissue, providing movement of articular surfaces and maintaining fiber distance for an orderly disposition of collagen tissue [21]. There are several reports of subtle subluxations of both the talocrural and the subtalar joints treated with success with joint mobilization. Well-documented and controlled trials are, however, lacking. This is probably due to the difficulty of objectively measuring the 'subluxations' and thus documenting the effect of treatment. Menetrey and Fritschy [49] reported 25 cases of subtalar subluxations in ballet dancers. The mechanism of injury was well established due to the superior motor control of this group. Clinical findings were primarily examiner-felt restrictions of dorsalflexion and hypomobility of the subtalar joint. In some cases, subluxations could be identified on X-rays. In all cases manipulation could reduce the subluxations and relieve pain symptoms.

Friction Massage. This is performed over an area of soft tissue adhesions perpendicular to the direction of the fibers. The technique is believed to encourage the longitudinal orientation of the scar tissue instead of allowing a disorganized connective tissue healing pattern [34]. This increases the strength of the tendon or ligament involved and improves the extensibility of the tissues [21]. Friction produces significant hyperemia in the target area [21] and may stress newly injured tissue to the degree of re-injury. Therefore, application to acute injuries cannot be advised.

Improving Muscle Strength

The principal measures to consider in the choice of a postoperative treatment program would be to avoid reflex inhibition, and to increase neural activation over the first 2–4 weeks post surgery.

Prevention of reflex inhibition is primarily done by preventing both short-term and long-term postoperative pain [2]. As mentioned, a moderate degree of joint swelling without pain can induce reflex inhibition [63], so prevention of effusion also becomes important throughout the rehabilitation period.

Increase of neural activation is achieved by functional oriented training and dynamometer training [19]. In functional training, the patient is required to activate his/her musculature in normally occurring activities. Dynamic stability, including proprioceptive information, motor control and appropriate muscle force development will be enforced by the training. Schedules may start with walking and two-leg jumping and progress to different levels of balancing, jumping, jogging and running. Strength, as measured with a dyna-

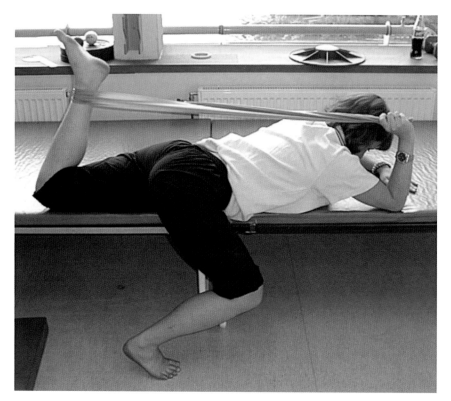

Fig. 4. Training with a towel sling to improve passive and active range of motion

mometer, has been found to improve with this functional approach [64a].

In the early phases of dynamometer training, with either isokinetic or variable resistance modalities, the increased neural activation plays a dominant role [12a, 30a, 30b]. Here it seems that training at high speeds will increase high speed maximal activation while not affecting low speed maximal activation, and visa versa [65].

If reflex inhibition is avoided or overcome, a major effect of training on muscle structure (muscle hypertrophy) can be expected over the following weeks. It does not seem that important whether dynamometric training is done isokinetically or with variable resistance.

Summary. Three post-injury/post-surgical periods can be identified [20].

The *first phase* with immobilization requires prevention of reflex inhibition and the maintenance of muscle structure. This is usually from day 0 to 1 week after surgery.

In the *second phase* with *activation,* weight is put on neural activation through functional training, and several training principles may be employed. Dynamometer training will in this phase allow training of maximal effort with a stabilized joint, but should never dominate over functional training. This is usually from week 2 to 4.

In the *third phase* with adaptation to *function,* the specific needs of the patient have to be considered. The training regime should include activities similar to the ADL functions of the specific person. The need for not only muscle strength but also for muscle endurance should be kept in mind (Fig. 4). The third phase usually starts after 4 – 6 weeks.

Improving Sensori-Motor Control

Treatment of a sensori-motor ankle deficit consists of a progressive series of coordination exercises to re-educate the ankle. Though the idea of rehabilitating sensori-motor control seems well established, not very much research has been done to establish the effect of training on ankle specific proprioceptive functions. Tropp [67] found a significant improvement in balance during single limb stance in functional ankle unstable subjects after 10 weeks of balance board exercises. The same group reported a decrease in the frequency of inversion injuries and ankle giving-way feelings when compared with an untrained ankle unstable control group. Tropp [67] also found that the subjects in question showed a change in their strategy of single limb stance, going from a broken chain strategy before training to the normal inverted pendulum strategy after completed training. So it may well be as suggested by Glencross and Thornton [16] that sensori-motor rehabilitation is as much a re-learning program as it is a physical recovery after surgery. Often the subjects themselves have a clear feeling of a perception/proprioception deficit in the ankle joint area – they can't 'feel' the ankle as they used to. And when this feeling returns it seems to coincide with complete rehabilitation. Leandersson et al. [38] found that return of single limb balance to normal values coincided with a subjective feeling of full rehabilitation in dancers. It can, however, be argued that in this group balance during single limb stance was as much a specific functional test as an unspecific test for ankle proprioception.

Summary. Training sensori-motor control through coordination exercises using unilateral balance boards, uniaxial and multiaxial teeter boards and jumping ropes relies primarily on empirical data but produces very favorable results. Restitution of normal function relies primarily on the individual's subjective feeling of a return to normal sensation, and the major effect of training seems to be achieved within 6 – 10 weeks with a 10-min effort 5 days a week.

Concomitant Modalities

External Compression

External compression using inflatable splints reduces blood flow and edema in the compressed area [3, 54]. If the external pressure of an elastic bandage can reach approximately 80 mm Hg, oozing of blood in the tissues during the acute phase is practically stopped [66].

Cryotherapy

Cold is delivered to the target tissue by conduction. The primary objectives being reduction of hemorrhage, inflammation, edema, and pain.

Physiologically, the reduced temperature will result in arteriolar vasoconstriction, slowing the local inflammatory process and increase the pain threshold [22]. There is an optimum temperature in terms of vasoconstriction, as excessive cryotherapy causes vasodilatation [5, 29]. With appropriate cooling, blood flow is reduced to two thirds after a period of 10 – 15 min [66].

The method of cryotherapy is important. Ice chips are superior to frozen gel packs, chemical ice and cool sprays [48]. Maximal contact can be achieved with cooling systems like the Cryocuff, used by many in the postoperative and rehabilitation phase.

While achieving short-term effect, cold therapy does not seem to alter the outcome of tissue regeneration [22].

Superficial Heat Application

Like cold, heat is transmitted to the body by conduction. When superficial heat is applied to the skin, internal temperatures rise slowly and do not exceed 40 °C and the duration of the peak is relatively short [39]. The heat-induced increase in blood flow primarily occurs in vessels of the skin and subcutaneous tissues, while deeper tissues seem unaffected [51]. The vasodilatatory effect causes increased vessel permeability with concomitant intercellular fluid outflow and edema. Though the neurological mechanism by which it occurs is unknown, it seems well established that superficial heating agents relieve pain [40, 51]. Finally, the heat application decreases connective tissue stiffness [71].

In conclusion, topical application of heat is indicated where increased speed of healing, mild increase in blood flow, partial relief of pain, relaxation of muscles and decrease of joint stiffness is desired.

Ultrasound

Ultrasound is thought to have a thermal, a non-thermal, and a neural effect. The thermal effect is caused by the absorption of energy in the given tissue. Depending on the frequency, ultrasound can penetrate 5 – 10 cm in-

to tissue and cause 5° – 6° of temperature increase in bone after just 2 – 20 s of application [12]. The non-thermal effects include the ability to drive large externally applied molecules deep into tissue. Topically applied medications have thus been found up to a tissue depth of 10 cm after 5 min of ultrasound treatment [18]. Vibration of gas bubbles within the tissues and changes in cell permeability inducing alterations in sodium, potassium and calcium diffusion are other non-thermal effects [12]. The neural effect is primarily an analgesic effect. This effect is reported in numerous clinical reports but the mechanism of the pain relief is not clear [18].

In rehabilitation, the ability of ultrasound to heat up deep structures still remains the prime indication. The sessions should not last more than 5 – 7 min with constant movement of the ultrasound transducer to avoid overheating [57].

Practical Rehabilitation

A graded rehabilitation program after ankle injury is suggested in Table 2.

Practical ways of applying the excercises and modalities in the program are presented below.

Table 2. Rehabilitation after ankle arthroscopic surgery or injury (adapted with permission from [53])

Phases Parameter	Acute Immobilization	Subacute Post-immobilization	Terminal	Return to activity
Goals	Protect joint integrity; control inflammation; control pain, edema and spasm	Maintain and increase soft tissue and adjacent joint mobility	Functional progression of closed chain activities; Proprioceptive retraining; Correct and control abnormal biomechanics	Preparation for return to ADL requirements
Weight-bearing status	Non- to touch weight bearing	Crutch partial weight bearing progressing towards full weight-bearing	Full weight-bearing	Full weight-bearing
Modalities	Ice; compression, elevation	Ice-ROM-ice-ROM.	Ice-ROM-ice-ROM; Manipulative treatment	Ice after functional stress
External support	Orthosis/splint	ROM orthosis	ROM-orthosis	Support if necessary
Range of motion flexibility	Early pain-free mobilization	Manipulative joint mobilization	Achilles tendon stretching	Muscle stretching
Open kinetic chain excercices	Pain-free isometrics	Alphabet ROM; Toe curls; marble pick-ups. Surgical tubing exercises in all planes	Full arch isokinetics	Ensure normal inversion/eversion strength ratios
Closed kinetic chain exercises		Low-weight bearing heel raises; soleus pumps; body weight transfers	Heel raise progression; Body weight transfers with elastic tubing resistance	Body weight transfers in inversion/eversion with tubing resistance
Proprioception, agility, balance drills; Functional programs	Low-weight bearing tilt board	Partial weight bearing Tilt board; Stork stands	Full weight-bearing on tilt board; Jumping rope	Tilt board with weight-bearing overload; Hopping
Alternative exercises	Gluteus medius strengthening	Stationary cycling	Minitramp; stationary cycling	Stair climber and lateral step-ups

Range of Motion

Active range of motion exercises are started after a few days. Traditionally, doing 'alphabet exercises' – drawing the letters of the alphabet with the foot – encourages movements in all planes. Progressing at a pace where swelling and pain are not provoked, stretching of areas of reduced movement can be achieved with extra force using a towel sling (Fig. 4). As motion in the joint improves, gentle Achilles tendon and ankle dorsiflexion stretches can be allowed (Fig. 5). If possible, this should be done with pre-warmed muscles. Based on the research mentioned previously, the stretch has to be held up to 45 s and be repeated at least four times every 6 – 8 h.

Joint mobilization using manual distraction and A-P glides can also start in this phase, progressing to a full program if pain free.

Strength Training

If pain free, strengthening exercises can be initiated early. Isometric exercises can usually be started fairly quickly in the dorsi/plantar flexion direction, primarily as toe raises with an increasing part of the body weight. Like for the range of motion exercises, strength exercises must be performed in the combined planes of motion. For this, elastic tubing is perfect (Fig. 6). Weights and machines utilizing weights are often difficult to control for the ankle and should be kept for the final progression of the rehabilitation program. Soleus pumps, full arch isokinetics and heel raise progression also belong at the end of the program. Finally, the strengthening program must take the type of functional demand the individual may have into account (fast versus slow, eccentric versus eccentric, endurance versus high load).

Proprioception and Sensori-Motor Control

Proprioceptive exercises usually begin as simple standing and balancing on one leg. This is followed by a progression of exercises using some type of balance board, that easily can be manufactured by the patient her/himself (Fig. 7). Tropp [67] found adequate effect on chronically unstable ankles using the balance board 10 min a day five times a week for 2.5 months. Rebman [56] noted a reduction in sprains using the balance board only 2 min twice a day. Usually, however, the patients themselves have a very definite feeling of when they have regained full sensori-motor control. In the final phase of rehabilitation, functional progression is instituted to restore agility and confidence. If the patient is an athlete, functional exercises must be sports-

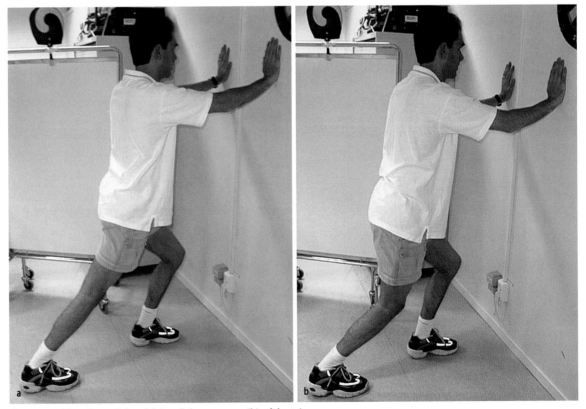

Fig. 5. Stretching the peripheral (**a**) and deeper parts (**b**) of the triceps surae

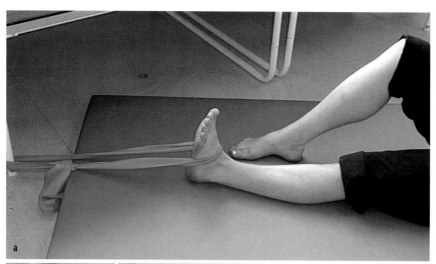

Fig. 6. Rubber tubing exercises promoting strength and endurance of **a** dorsiflexors, **b** everting, and **c** inverting muscles

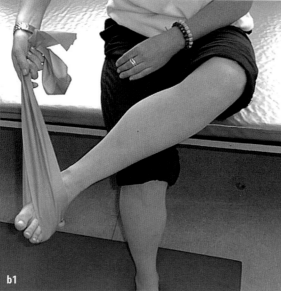

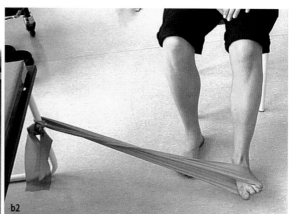

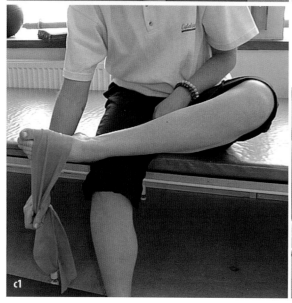

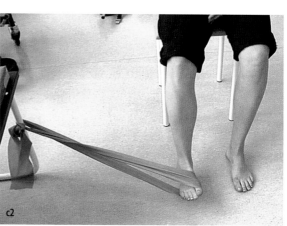

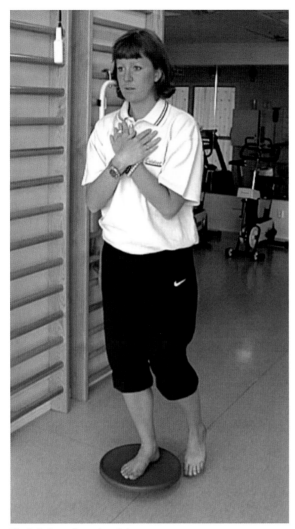

Fig. 7. Balance board training

specific. In most cases letting the subject run in figures of eight will give them a clear sensation of whether they are properly rehabilitated.

References

1. American Academy of Orthopedic Surgeons (1965) Joint motion – method of measuring and recording. Chicago, AAOS, pp 69–85
2. Arvidsson I, Eriksson E, Knutsson E, Arner S (1986) Reduction of pain inhibition on voluntary muscle activation by epidural analgesia. Orthopaedics 9:1415–1419
3. Ashton H (1975) The effect of increased tissue pressure on blood flow. Clin Orthop 113:15–26
4. Baker PL (1970) SACH heel improves results of ankle fusion. J Bone J Surg [Am] 52-A:1485–1486
5. Barcroft H, Edholm K (1943) The effect of temperature on blood flow and deep temperature on the human fore-arm. J Physiol 102:5–20
6. Baumhauer JF, Alosa DM, Renstrom PAFH, Trevino S, Beynnon B (1995) A prospective study of ankle injury risk factors. Am J Sports Med 23:564–570
7. Bohannon RW (1984) Effect of repeated weight-minute muscle loading on the angle of straight-leg raising. Phys Ther 64:491–497
8. Clarke TE, Frederick EC, Hamill C (1984) The study of rear foot movement in running. In Frederick EC (ed) Sports shoes and playing surfaces. Human Kinetics, Champaign, Ill
9. De Carlo MS, Talbot RW (1986) Evaluation of ankle joint proprioception following injection of the anterior talofibular ligament. JOSPT 8:70–76
10. Dietz V, Quintern J, Sillem M (1987) Stumbling reactions in man: significance of proprioceptive and preprogrammed mechanisms. J Physiol 386:149–163
11. Dietz V (1992) Human neuronal control of automatic functional movements: interaction between central programs and afferent input. Physiol Rev 72:33–69
12. Drez D (1989) Therapeutic modalities for sport injuries. Chicago, Year Book Medical Publishers
12a. Encke RM (1988) Muscle strength and its development. New perspectives. Sports Med 6(3):146–168
13. Etnyre BR, Lee EJ (1987) Comments on proprioceptive neuromuscular facilitation stretching techniques. Res Q 58:184–188
14. Folman Y, Wask J, Voloshin A, Liberty S (1986) Cyclic impacts on heel strike. A possible biomechanical factor in the etiology of degenerative disease of the human locomotor system. Arch Orthop Trauma Surg 104:363–365
15. Garn SN, Newton RA (1988) Kinesthetic awareness in subjects with multiple ankle sprains. Physical Therapy 68:1667–1671
16. Glencross D, Thornton E (1981) Position sense following joint injury. J Sports Med 21:23–27
17. Godges JJ, MacRae H, Longdon C, Tinberg C, MacRae P. The effects of two stretching procedures on hip range of motion and gait economy. J Orthop Sports Phys Ther 350–357, 1989.
18. Griffin JE, Karselis TC (1982) Physical agents for physical therapists, 2nd ed, Charles C Thomas, Springfield, IL
19. Grimby G (1992) Clinical aspects of strength and power training. In Komi PV (ed) Strength and power in sports. Blackwell, Oxford
20. Grimby G, Thomee R (1988) Principles of rehabilitation after injuries. In Knuttgen HG, Tittel K (eds) Olympic book of sports medicine, vol. 1, Blackwell, Oxford, pp 489–508
21. Hertling D, Kessler RN (1990) Management of common musculoskeletal disorders, 2nd edn., JB Lippencott, Philadelphia
22. Hurme T, Rantanen J, Kalimo H (1993) Effects of early cryotherapy in experimental skeletal muscle injury. Scand J Med Sci Sports 3:46–51
23. Hutton RS (1993) Neuromuscular basis of stretching exercise. In Komi PV (ed) Strength and power in sports. Blackwell, Oxford pp 29–38
24. Inman VT (1976) The joints of the ankle, Williams and Wilkins, Baltimore, p 37
25. Inman VT, Ralston HJ, Todd F (1981) Human walking., Williams and Wilkins, Baltimore, p 22
26. Jerosch J, Hoffstetter I, Bork H, Bischof M (19959 The influence of orthoses on the proprioception of the ankle joint. Knee Surg Sports Traum Arthroscopy 3:39–46
27. Kannus P, Jozsa L, Renstrom P, Jarvinen M, Kvist M, Lehto M, Oja P, Vuori I (1992) The effects of training, immobilization and remobilization on musculoskeletal tissue. 2. Remobilization and prevention of immobilization atrophy. Scand J Med Sci Sports 2:164–176
28. Karlsson J (1989). Chronic lateral instability of the ankle joint. A clinical, radiological and experimental study. Thesis. Gothenburg University Hospital, Gothenburg, Sweden

29. Kellett J (1986) Acute soft tissue injuries – a review of the literature. Med Sci Sports Exerc 18:489–500

30. Kleinrensink GJ, Stoeckart R, Meulstee J, Sukul DMKSK, Vleeming A, Snijders CJ, Noort AV (1994). Lowered motor conduction velocity of the peroneal nerve after inversion trauma. Med Sci Sports Exerc 26:877–883

30a. Komi PV, Buskirk ER (1972) Eccentric and concentric conditioning on tension and electrical activity of human muscle. Ergonomics 15(4):417–434

30b. Komi PV (1984) Physiological and biomechanical correlates of muscle function: effects of muscle structure and stretch-shortening cycle on force and speed. In: Terjung RL (ed) Exercise and Sport Sciences. The Collamore Press, Lexington, Mass. p. 81

31. Konradsen L, Ravn JB (1990) Ankle instability caused by prolonged peroneal reaction time. Acta Orthop Scand 61:388–390

32. Konradsen L, Ravn JB, Soerensen AI (1993) Proprioception at the ankle: the effect of anaesthetic blockade of ligament receptors. J Bone Joint Surg [Br] 75-B: 433–436

33. Konradsen L, Olesen S, Hansen HM (1998) : Ankle proprioception and eversion strength after acute ankle inversion injuries. Am J Sports Med 26(1):1–6

34. Kessler RM (1983) Friction massage. In: Kessler RM, Hertling D (eds.) Management of common musculoskeletal disorders. Harper & Row, Philadelphia

35. Kottke FJ, Pauley DL, Ptak KA (1966) The rationale for prolonged stretching for correction of shortening of connective tissue. Arch Phys Med Rehabil 47:345–352

36. Lambert KL (1971) The weight bearing function of the fibula: A strain gauge study. J Bone Joint Surg [Am] 53(3):507–513

37. Lang J, Wachsmuth W (1972) Paktische anatomie: Ein Lehr- und Hilfsbuch der anatomischen grundlagen ärtzlichen handelns. Vol 1, Part 4, Bein und Statik. Springer, Berlin, p 370

38. Leandersson J, Eriksson E, Nilsson C, Wykman A (1996) Proprioception in classical ballet dancers: A prospective study of the influence of an ankle sprain on proprioception in the ankle joint. Am J Sports Med 24:370–374

39. Lehmann JF (1982) Therapeutic heat and cold. 3rd ed. Williams & Wilkins, Baltimore

40. Licht S (1965) Therapeutic heat and cold. 2nd ed. Waverly Press, Baltimore

41. Lynch AF, Bourne RB, Rorabeck CH (1988) The long term results of ankle arthrodesis. J Bone Joint Surg [Br] 70-B:113–116

42. Magnusson SP, Simonsen EB, Aagaard P, Gleim GW, McHugh MP, Kjaer M (1995) Viscoelastic response to repeated static stretching in the human hamstring muscle. Scand J Med Sci Sports 5:342–347

43. Magnusson SP, Simonsen EB, Aagaard P, Dyhre-Poulsen P, McHugh MP, Kjaer M (1996) Mechanical and physiological responses to stretching with and without preisometric contraction in human skeletal muscle. Arch Phys Med Rehabil 77:373–378

44. Mann RA (1991) Overview of the foot and ankle biomechanics. In Jahss MH (ed): Disorders of the foot and ankle. Medical and surgical management, 2nd edn, WB Saunders, Philadelphia, pp 385–408

45. Mann RA, Moran GT, Dougherty SE (1986) Comparative electromyography of the lower extremity in jogging, running, and sprinting. Am J Sports Med 14:501–510

46. Mazur JM, Schwartz E, Simon SR (1979) Ankle arthrodesis, long term follow-up with gait analysis. J Bone Joint Surg [Am] 61-A:964–975

47. McCloskey DI, (1978) Kinesthetic sensibility. Physiological Reviews 58:763–820

48. McMaster WC, Liddle S, Waught TR (1978). Laboratory evaluation of various cold therapy modalities. Am J Sports Med 6:291–294

49. Menetrey J, Fritschy D (1999). Subtalar subluxation in ballet dancers. Am J Sports Med 27(2):143–149

50. Michelson JD, Hutchins C (1995) Mechanoreceptors in human ankle ligaments. J Bone Joint Surgery [Br] 77-B:219–224

51. Michlovitz S (1986) Thermal agents in rehabilitation. FA Davis, Philadelphia

52. Moore MA, Hutton RS (1980) Electromyographic investigation of muscle stretching techniques. Med Sci Sports Exerc 12:322–329

53. Mulligan E (1991) Lower leg, ankle, and foot rehabilitation. In Andrews JR and Harrelson GL (eds) Physical rehabilitation of the injured athlete. WB Saunders Company, Philadelphia, p 217

54. Nielsen HV (1983) External pressure-blood flow relations during limb compression in man. Acta Physiol Scand 119:253–260

55. Ouzouian TJ, Kleiger B (1991) Arthrodesis in the foot and ankle. In Jahss MH, ed. Disorders of the foot and ankle, 2nd ed, vol 3. WB Saunders, Philadelphia

56. Rebman L (1986) Suggestions from the clinic: Ankle injuries: Clinical observations. J Orthop Sports Phys Ther 8:153–156

57. Rivenburgh DW (1992) Physical modalities in the treatment of tendon injuries. In Renström and Leadbetter (eds.) Tendinitis I: Basic concepts, Clinics in sports medicine, vol 11(3). WB Saunders, Philadelphia, pp 645–660

58. Sammarco GJ, Burstein AH, Frankel VH (1973) Biomechanics of the ankle. A kinematic study. Orthop Clin North Am 4:75–96

59. Sapega AA, Quedenfeld TC, Moyer RA, Butler RA (1981) Biophysical factors in range of motion exercise. Physician Sportsmed 9:57–64

60. Sarrafian SK (1993) Anatomy of the foot and ankle, 2nd edn. JB Lippincott Company, Philadelphia, pp 508–513

61. Sherrington CS (1906) On the proprioceptive system, especially in its reflex aspects. Brain 29:467–472

62. Shiavi R, Bugle HJ, Limbird T (1987) Electromyographic gait assessment, part 1: Adult EMG profiles and walking speed. J Rehab Research Development 24:13–23

63. Stokes M, Young A (1984) The contribution of reflex inhibition to arthrogenous muscle weakness. Clinical Science 67:7–14

64. Taylor DC, Dalton JD, Jr., Seaber AV, Garrett WEJ (1990) Viscoelastic properties of muscle-tendon units. The biomechanical effects of stretching. Am J Sports Med 18:300–309

64a. Tegner Y (1990) Strength training in the rehabilitation of cruciate ligament tears. Sports Med 9(2):129–136

65. Thomeé R, Renström P, Grimby G, Peterson L 81987) Slow or fast isokinetic training after knee ligament surgery. JOSPT 8:475–479

66. Thorsson O (1996) Muscle injuries in athletes. Dissertation, Lund University, Lund, Sweden

67. Tropp H (1985) Functional instability of the ankle joint. Thesis, Linkoping University Medical Dissertations no. 202, Linkoping, Sweden

68. Van Langelaan EJ (1983) A kinematical analysis of the tarsal joints. An X-ray photogrammetric study. Acta Orthop Scand (Suppl. 204) 54:147–269

69. Wright DG, Desai SM, Henderson WH (1983) Action of the subtalar and ankle joint complex during the stance phase of walking. J Bone Joint Surg [Am] 46(2):361–365

70. Wright DG, Rennels JC (1964) A study of the elastic properties of plantar fascia. J Bone Joint Surg 46:482–486

71. Wright V, Johns RJ (1960) Physical factors concerned with the stiffness of normal and diseased joints. Bull Johns Hopkins Hosp 106:215–231

Rehabilitation of the Foot Following Sports-Related Injuries and Surgical Treatment

Andrea Scala

Introduction

The foot is a complex anatomical entity subdivided into several bones and different articular modules, each providing distinct biomechanical patterns. These modular structures can change their spatial orientation instantly, thus adapting to the different functional requirements of the inferior limb. The foot is then able to provide both stability and flexibility.

The study of lower limb biomechanics during closed kinetic chain activities has highlighted the different functions of the foot as a: stable base of support to allow upright posture; rigid lever during the propulsion phase of gait; torque converter, allowing rotation of the pelvis and lower limb; shock absorber; balance while walking on inclined surfaces or uneven terrain. Physiological foot biomechanics is an efficient mechanism which saves metabolic energy. When the foot is injured or the biomechanics impaired, energy is dissipated in compensation mechanisms. A thorough understanding of foot biomechanics [6, 9] and pathomechanics [4, 15] is necessary in order to plan a correct rehabilitation program. The aim of rehabilitation is to restore the correct functioning of the injured or surgically repaired structure of the foot [14]. The nature and duration of the injury greatly influences the recovery process and the rehabilitation program. The acute lesion shows the greatest amount of pain, inflammation, hematoma, and edema. Healing can occur after the acute onset is resolved, with the foot held in an appropriate position, when the recovering process is respected and before compensation mechanisms occur. Normal range of motion, strength, and endurance may be obtained at the end of an appropriately timed rehabilitation program. On the other hand, when athletic participation is allowed on inflamed and strained foot structures, a chronic condition may occur [12].

The chronic lesion is characterized by tissue irritation and scarring, contraction and movement limitation, muscle atrophy, proprioceptive impairment, compensations due to muscular imbalance, and joint stiffness. The rehabilitation program of chronic and overuse injuries should accurately take into account the lesional mechanisms and the consequent maladaptations.

The forefoot, midfoot, and hindfoot present specific rehabilitation problems that are examined as follows.

Forefoot Functional Anatomy

The forefoot functional integrity is fundamental in the stance phase of gait [4, 6].

During this phase, the forefoot provides a wide weight-bearing surface formed by the metatarsals, and the metatarsophalangeal joint and toes, contributing to the stability of the entire body. The maximal pressure centers registered from the foot plantar surface during the gait cycle move quickly towards the forefoot after heel strike [2]. The pressure remains in the area of metatarsal heads for 30% – 55% of the whole cycle of gait, allowing adaptation to the ground and stability to progress, then moves rapidly towards the hallux. During the latest part of the stance phase, when the body weight is projected towards the following cycle, the forefoot is involved as a whole. When the rehabilitation of the forefoot is programmed, the role that the toes play during load bearing must be fully appreciated [11]. Toes are very delicate structures that sustain the body weight while remaining extremely flexible. Muscles and tendons of the toes must be efficient in order to assure the joint mobility and stabilization while forefoot supination and pronation movements occur.

The flexor digitorum brevis muscle (FDB) and interosseous muscles are essential for toe stabilization during the load-bearing phase.

Interosseous muscles and lumbricals stabilize metatarsophalangeal joints. Since interosseous muscle insertion is proximal to the metatarsophalangeal joints, they also stabilize the tarso-metatarsal joint, thus becoming the active stabilizers of the forefoot during the load-bearing phase.

The hallux is provided with particularly powerful muscle-tendinous units to sustain the take-off phase. About half of the body weight is sustained by the first metatarsal and hallux. Flexor hallucis brevis (FHB), flexor hallucis longus (FHL), abductor hallucis, adductor hallucis, and the gleno-sesamoid system act as active stabilizers of the first metatarsophalangeal joint during load bearing.

The proximal insertion of these muscle-tendinous units allows stabilization of the proximal joints of the foot medial column.

The stabilization mechanisms in the foot do not change from walking to running. The differences are in a marked increase in the force generated, increase range of motion of the joint of the lower extremity, and alterations of the phasic activity of the muscle of the lower extremity. The increased force of running, which can be as high as 250% of body weight, compared with 80% when walking [2], can cause exaggerated solicitations in the forefoot.

During the stance phase, the forefoot instantaneously modifies its position in order to compensate for structural or pathologic changes occurring in other structures of the foot.

These compensation mechanisms assure foot balance and generally do not result in symptoms.

When the anatomical condition which generates compensation is not corrected, the compensating capsular, ligamentous, and muscle-tendinous structures wear out.

Pathologic changes and consequent deformities of the forefoot may intervene, such as symptomatic callosities, inflammatory changes of joints and tendon sheaths, tendon retraction, toe malalignments, or painful deformities of metatarsophalangeal joints.

Before the rehabilitation program is undertaken, the forefoot anatomy and function should be fully understood in order to prevent any pathological change, limiting of function and deformation. The aims of the rehabilitation treatments are to facilitate the recovery of the injured structure and restore its functions.

Forefoot Injuries

Forefoot injuries are characterized by the great vulnerability of the soft tissues of this region and the risk related to the loss of plantigrade deambulation [10].

The skin coverage of the dorsal aspect of the forefoot does not possess a rich blood supply. The subcutaneous layer is not very thick and direct trauma may cause serious damage. Superficial bruises may cause tenosynovitis. For these reasons, forefoot injuries may be disabling and take a prolonged period of time (2–3 months) to heal.

Dorsal and plantar intrinsic muscles are often involved and are damaged when forefoot injuries occur. The result is an impaired articular function with claw toes or mallet toe deformities.

The osseous anatomy of the tarsometatarsal joint is characterized by an asymmetric arch where metatarsal bases, cuneiforms, and cuboid bone are strictly connected. The range of motion of the joint complex is very limited. The plantarflexion and the extension of the first metatarsal is 6°, while the fourth and fifth metatarsal range of motion is slightly increased relative to second and third. The relative rigidity of this bony arch prevents dorsal dislocation. The metatarsals are characterized by limited flexibility as an anatomical

unit. The pronation and supination that occurs at the subtalar joint site makes the metatarsals rotate on the frontal plane. Limitations of pronation or supination are causes of disturbance in the metatarsal region.

Injuries to the Forefoot and Toes

Injuries of the forefoot that frequently occur during sports participation are: tarso-metatarsal injuries; metatarsal arch strains; metatarsal fractures; metatarsal stress fractures; injuries of the metatarsophalangeal joints; dislocations of the metatarsophalangeal joints; fractures of the fifth metatarsal; fractures of the sesamoids; injuries of the hallux; injuries of the lesser-toes (Fig. 1a–c).

The preferred method of immobilization following an injury or surgery is to immobilize the entire joint early by firm taping. Partial weight-bearing ambulation is allowed in a firm postoperative shoe. Forefoot injuries can be both extremely painful and lingering in athletes and it is not uncommon for patients to be quite symptomatic for up to 10 weeks after the injuries.

Turf Toe

First metatarsophalangeal joint sprain may occur when the articulation is submitted to forced hyperflexion or hyperextension. Rest, ice, elevation, and TENS are used to control pain. Compression is obtained while taping the injured joint. The hallux is solidarized with the second toe. As weight bearing is allowed, a rigid orthotic under the first metatarsophalangeal joint is used in order to decrease the solicitations. When the pain subsides, active and passive motion of the joint is encouraged.

Metatarsal Arch Strains

The soft tissue of the longitudinal arch of the foot may be injured as a consequence of an excessive foot pronation and a valgus heel posture. Training errors such as a sudden increase of mileage may lead to an aggravation. Rehabilitation consists of strengthening the muscles which raise the arch of the foot (toe flexors and posterior tibialis tendon). The heel cord is also important because a tight heel cord accentuates pronation during running. Taping the longitudinal arch is performed while the toes are flexed and the ankle is extended. The use of orthosis is necessary to control hyperpronation.

Rehabilitation of Forefoot Injuries

The aim of the rehabilitation is to obtain a plantigrade foot, without painful callosities under the metatarsal heads, with correct articular functioning, without ten-

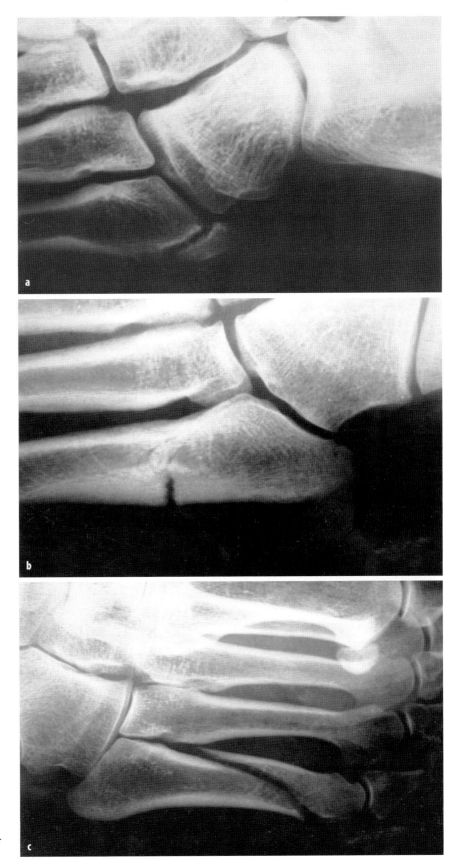

Fig. 1. a – c. Radiographs of three types of fifth metatarsal fracture which can occur during sports participation

dinous contracures or joint stiffness, and with the capacity to adapt to uneven terrain by means of immediate pronation and supination adjustments.

In order to accomplish this purpose, the anatomical structures involved should be evaluated: blood and lymphatic circulation, tendons and tendon sheaths, tarsometatarsal joints, metatarsophalangeal joints, intrinsic and extrinsic foot muscles.

When rehabilitating the forefoot after injury or post-surgery, the importance of the metatarsal cushion should be stressed. The ball of the foot is crossed by a series of sagittal septa, where the metatarsal cushion and the separately ensheathed fat bodies are located. Anteriorly, transverse lamellae and the superficial insertion of the plantar aponeurosis are found. Through this framework of supporting tissues, the tendons, vessels and nerves find their way from the deep compartments of the foot to the toes. Edema and scar tissue after injuries and surgery may alter this delicate structure. Nerve conduction and blood circulation may be impaired. The purpose of rehabilitation is to help restore the correct functioning of metatarsal cushioning.

Rehabilitation of Forefoot Injuries: Acute Phase

In the acute phase, all injuries to the forefoot are correctly treated by means of application of rest, ice, compression and elevation (RICE).

Rest is the first-aid principle in the acute phase. Shortly after the injury, the area involved needs rest to accommodate the healing process. Crutches, braces, taping, and splints are useful in maintaining the proper articular position and good anatomical alignment of the healing joints.

Ice is applied over the injured region by means of a chemical ice pack or ice pieces contained in a bag. Ice massage may be performed by the patient. The period of application should not exceed 15–20 min because of the risk of capillary circulation impairment. While ice is applied, passive stretching exercises may be performed by a cooperative patient.

Compression is obtained by means of elastic bandages and adhesive elastic bandages applied shortly after the injury. Positive pressure stockings are applied later after the removal of a splint or a cast. Stockings are useful for avoiding post-immobilization edema during the resumption of weight bearing.

Elevation of the injured foot 30–50 cm above the level of the heart is useful to prevent swelling, especially in the first 24–48 h after injury. Elastic bandages, taping, and plaster casts are very well tolerated if the limb is elevated. Elevation is of great help in controlling swelling in later phases of rehabilitation, too.

Early, gradual motion is encouraged when the affected joints are free from immobilization. Stretching and ROM exercises are performed after ice application.

Functional taping, elastic bandages, and some splints allow early mobilization. A cautious passive and active mobilization contributes to the reabsorption of the edema and swelling and leads to a less stiff scar. Adherences between the joint and surrounding tissue are prevented or minimized. Circulation is stimulated by reducing the edema.

Regaining the range of motion is a priority as soon as the pain decreases and motion of the affected joint is tolerable. Passive motion should be possible shortly after the injury or the day following the operation. Passive motion must be slow and delicate in order to prevent further inflammation and pain. The motion is performed for 5 min initially, and then extended to 30 min, six to eight times a day. Repeated series of isolated extension and flexion of the involved joint are advisable in order to avoid excessive fatigue of the injured joint. Continous passive motion (CPM) devices are very useful in rehabilitating foot and ankle injuries or after surgical repair.

Rehabilitation of Forefoot Injuries: Intermediate Phase

Physical modalities and therapeutic exercises are used with the goals of relief of pain, control of edema and inflammation, and regaining of motion, force and dexterity.

Contrast Baths. The temperature of the cold water is $10°-15°C$, that of the warm water is $40°-43°C$. The warm cycle lasts for approximately 5 min and the cold cycle 1–2 min. Treatment should continue for 20–30 min and conclude with the cold cycle; it should be repeated two or three times a day.

Pool Exercises. Active and passive movements of the injured foot are performed. A life jacket can be used to move the affected limb without weight bearing while still maintaining the heart and respiratory conditioning. The deambulation may be resumed in the swimming pool with partial weight bearing. High-voltage electrical stimulation in conjunction with a cold whirlpool is an effective modality for relieving pain and swelling and helping the athlete regain normal ambulation without limping. The use of a whirlpool is advised for 15 min followed by walking for 5 min. The treatment is repeated two to three times a day.

Transcutaneous Electrical Nerve Stimulation. Transcutaneous electrical nerve stimulation (TENS) is a useful tool in this phase of rehabilitation because it reduces the amount of pain, allowing a wider range of motion. Many other types of electrical stimulation are available. The main differences are in the patterns of the electric wave. Different patterns of electric stimulation should be used with specific indications.

Ultrasound. Ultrasound is used for different purposes: lysis of the tissue adherences; relief of pain; treatment of tenosynovitis that is often associated with forefoot injuries. Ultrasound is used underwater for 5–10 min at $1-1.5\,W/cm^2$.

Low-Level Laser. Laser therapy can be employed to offer analgesia, improve healing, or decrease edema of soft tissues.

Manual Soft Tissue Massage. Various techniques are used with the goals of relieving pain and muscular spasm, and improving local vascular flow.

Lymphatic Manual Drainage. This is used to control impairment of lymphatic flow and vascular stasis associated with injury and/or immobility.

Electrical Muscle Stimulation. Voluntary contraction of the muscles and active motion of the injured foot should be encouraged. In particular cases, electrical muscle stimulation of the ankle can be used. In severe injuries followed by prolonged immobilization, and in case of injuries of peripheral nervous branches, electrical stimulation facilitates the beginning of motion.

Continuous Passive Motion. Regaining range of motion is a priority as soon as pain decreases and motion of the affected joint is tolerable. Passive motion should be possible shortly after the injury or the day following the operation. Passive motion must be slow and delicate in order to prevent further inflammation and pain. Motion is performed for 5 min initially, and then extended to 30 min, six to eight times a day. Repeated series of isolated extension and isolated flexion of the involved joint are advisable in order to avoid excessive fatigue of the injured joint, while gaining range of motion. Continuous passive motion (CPM) devices are very useful in rehabilitating foot and ankle injuries or after surgical repair.

Strengthening. Strengthening exercises of the intrinsic foot muscles include activities such as picking up small objects using the toes and performing curl exercises. A towel is placed on a smooth surface, and the patient is seated with the injured foot on the towel. A heel lift is placed under the calcaneus to isolate motion at the phalanges. The patient flexes the toes to pull the towel towards the body. A weight is placed at the end of the towel in order to increase resistance.

Rehabilitation of Forefoot Injuries: Recovery Phase

In this phase the aim of the rehabilitation is to resume walking. Pain-free ambulation without limping is an especially important goal because limping exacerbates the inflammatory process by maintaining pressure on injured tissues. The athlete starts with slow, straight walking on flat, and then on uneven surfaces. Next, S- or 8-patterns are implemented, gradually modifying speed and type of terrain. The use of a tapis roulant is highly advisable because it allows checking of the pattern of walking, while modifying pacing and/or sloping.

Limping should be carefully evaluated, if present, and corrected. Only after walking is correctly resumed can jogging become a feasible activity. Jogging without an appropriate warm-up and stretching exercises should not be allowed. Patients are advised to gradually increase the speed, avoiding sudden stops and starts. After patients have reached the maximal controlled speed they can begin starts and stops and subsequently perform cutting maneuvers. Running a figure of eight around obstacles set out 20 m is also allowed. Then the obstacles are placed closer, at 15, 10, and finally at 5 m in order to mimic cutting movements.

Proprioceptive Exercises. Proprioceptors in articular tissues, ligaments, and tendons are especially vulnerable to disruption. The aim of proprioceptive exercises is to regain adaptive reflexes of the affected limb. Proprioceptive exercises are: balance, leaning forward and backward, bending down, touching the floor and returning to an upright position, heel raises, ball catching and throwing. Exercise begins on a hard flat surface with eyes open and weight bearing on both feet, then progresses to a soft surface and is performed with eyes closed and in a monopodalic stance with bare feet. The elastic trampoline is a very useful device to advance proprioceptive rehabilitation. The biomechanical ankle platform system (BAPS) is also generally utilized. The patient performs active flexion-extension and inversion-eversion exercises while sitting. Then active motion is allowed while standing on the disk and holding a chair-back for balance. In the final stage the patient provides his own balance standing on the disk. The proprioceptive exercises should be repeated four to six times a day for 10–15 min.

Strengthening Exercises. Isometric contractions of different groups of muscles such as invertors, evertors flexors and extensors may be performed while the foot is placed against a fixed object. Isotonics for the intrinsic and extrinsic muscles of the foot may be performed with elastic resistance. Isokinetic strengthening may begin when the patient has regained full range of motion and full weight bearing, and signs of inflammation and edema areabsent.

Stretching Exercises. stretching exercises for the musculotendinous units on the plantar side of the foot are performed by extending the hallux and the toes at the metatarsophalangeal joints and extending the ankle. Passive stretching can be performed by the physiotherapist and by the patient. An inclined plane can be utilized when the patient is standing. The heel cord exercises are useful for elongating the plantar structures of the foot. Stretching exercises for the extensors and the dorsal structures of the foot are performed by flexing the hallux and the toes at the metatarsophalangeal joint, and by flexing the ankle. Passive stretching can be performed by the physiotherapist and by the patient. Elongation should be maintained for 2–4 min, six to eight times a day. Ballistic movements should be strictly avoided.

Forefoot Overuse Injuries: Metatarsalgia and Hallux Valgus

Running and jumping submit the forefoot to an increased functional request compared with walking. In running, the range of motion of the foot increases by as much as 50%. In sports-active subjects affected by metatarsalgia and hallux valgus, forefoot biomechanics is altered.

As the first metatarsal separates from the second and goes into metatarsus varus, weight is transferred to the second and third metatarsal heads. This causes metatarsalgia of the second and third metatarsals and often causes claw-toe deformity of the second and the third toe, with the second toe overlapping the great toe. The study of progression of the center of plantar pressures in patients with hallux valgus deformity and metatarsalgia shows that the center of pressure points remain toward the heel, then rapidly progress across the metatarsal head area with little or no participation by the big toe in weight bearing [2, 6, 11]. Sports participation when forefoot functioning is impaired may lead to a chronic overuse condition. Pain and bursitis over the medial exostosis of the first metatarsal head are present in hallux valgus. Metatarsophalangeal joint subluxation, edema of the surrounding tissues, extensor tendon tightness and painful callosities under the metatarsal head are usually observed in the case of metatarsalgia [2, 4, 5, 9, 11].

These concepts should be kept in mind when considering the best treatment of hallux valgus deformity and metatarsalgia in athletic individuals. Specifically designed orthotics and temporary suspension of sport participation are advised. The rehabilitation program as outlined above for forefoot injuries should be followed for an appropriate period. When conservative treatments fail to show significant improvement, surgery is considered.

The osteotomies of the first metatarsal bone are the treatment of choice for the realignment of hallux valgus [1, 16, 17]. Distal osteotomies of lesser metatarsals are the procedure for the metatarsalgia [16, 17].

Rehabilitation After Bunionectomy and Lesser Metatarsals Distal Osteotomies

The postoperative rehabilitation program is divided into three phases: the first postoperative week; the second and third week post-surgery; the third to fourth week after the operation.

First Postoperative Week. The aim of rehabilitation is: to avoid joint stiffness, adherences between anatomical layers involved in surgical incisions, blood and lymphatic stasis; to allow immediate, gradual weight bearing.

Rest and elevation are highly recommended. The foot is maintained above chest level while resting and the knee is slightly flexed. The stability of the surgical correction allows immediate motion and partial weight bearing, utilizing appropriate postoperative shoes.

The patient performs the self-rehabilitation exercises which have been taught before surgery. These exercises must be performed from the first postoperative day even if the postoperative dressing is present. The operated foot is firmly held by the patient's hands and the forefoot is then manipulated. For self-rehabilitation of the hallux, the patient is comfortably seated on the bed or on a carpet. The operated foot is flexed to the patient's lap, where it is possible to easily manipulate the foot. The other inferior limb is slightly flexed or extended. When the right forefoot has to be rehabilitated it is held by the left hand and the right hand passively manipulates the operated forefoot. For metatarsophalangeal joint range of motion, the left hand firmly holds the forefoot and the first two fingers of the right hand slowly but firmly perform the flexion and extension movements of the first phalanx of the hallux. For the interphalangeal range of motion, the left hand firmly holds the first phalanx while the right hand gently flexes and extends the second phalanx. The aim of the self-rehabilitation of the lateral metatarsophalangeal joints is to allow the tips of the toe to touch the ground after surgical correction of the claw toe deformity. The toes are then carefully flexed at the metatarsophalangeal joint. Both the hands firmly hold the forefoot and the two thumbs flex the toes, pushing on the first phalanx. When self rehabilitation is impossible, a third person may help in performing a passive range of motion exercises. The general rules are that the exercises must be performed slowly and must gradually achieve the full range of motion. Complete flexion of the toes and flexor muscle power must be obtained. The range of motion exercises must be repeated several times a day. A set of exercises, taking 10–20 min, and repeated six to eight times per day is advised. The exercises must be continued for 2 to 3 months after the operation.

Other exercises should include non-weight-bearing active range of motion exercises, with particular care to the complete flexion, and weight-bearing exercises. Reflex antalgic extension of the operated toes while weight bearing is to be avoided. The tips of the toes should point to the ground while walking and weight bearing. Active range of motion should be repeated several times a day, trying to achieve the full range of motion.

Postoperative shoes are utilized in order to allow immediate partial weight bearing. Deambulation is allowed for periods limited to 10–15 min, five to six times daily. After the deambulation, the operated limb should be elevated above chest level.

Reeducation of walking is extremely important. While rehabilitating a forefoot operation, one should keep in mind that the patient was accustomed to keeping their weight in the posterior aspect of foot to avoid pressure over the painful portion of the foot. This attitude must be corrected to facilitate the resumption of forefoot weight bearing. The patient must learn to shift the load onto the toes.

Second Postoperative Week. After the removal of stitches, range of motion exercises are progressively increased. A series of prolonged active and passive movements are started and are more frequently repeated during the day. TENS is used to obtain mobilization without pain. Low-level laser is used to decrease the amount of inflammation and to reduce scar retraction.

To remove the edema, manual lymphatic drainage is used. Pulsed ultrasounds are used to avoid adherences between capsular structures, tendons, and subcutaneous tissues. Electric stimulations of lower leg muscles are used after a period of prolonged immobilization.

The manual therapy is based on manual lymphatic drainage, transverse massage, superficial and deep soft tissue massage. These procedures are extremely useful in order to passively remove the lymphatic and venous stasis. Surgical incisions and tissue retraction during foot surgery procedures may impair lymphatic, venous, and arterial microcirculation. Weight bearing abstention without joint mobilization worsens the peripheral circulation impairment and predisposes to edema and swelling, as during non-weight-bearing, the plantar venous network is not compressed by body weight and the powerful leg muscles pump is not efficient.

After the full active and passive range of motion is regained, exercises against resistance are performed in order to restore the power of the hallux during take-off. Rehabilitation in a swimming pool by means of gradual resumption of weight bearing while wearing a life vest is encouraged.

Third and Fourth Postoperative Weeks. Walking is allowed without restriction. Normal lifestyle, including job activities, is resumed. Comfort shoes with soft or

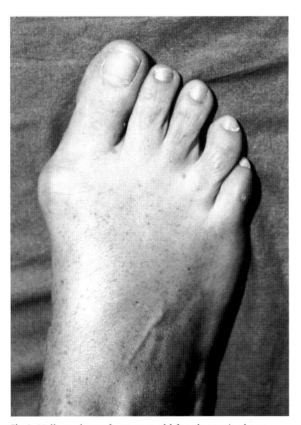

Fig. 2. Hallux valgus of a 28-year-old female tennis player

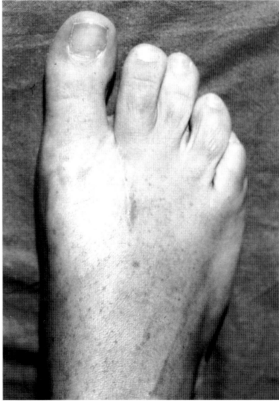

Fig. 3. Postoperative appearance of the forefoot

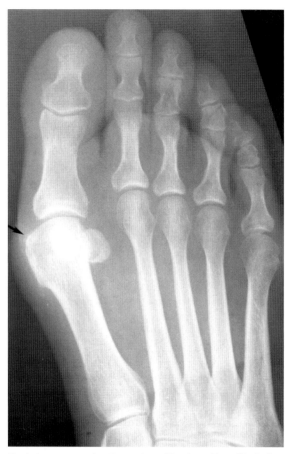

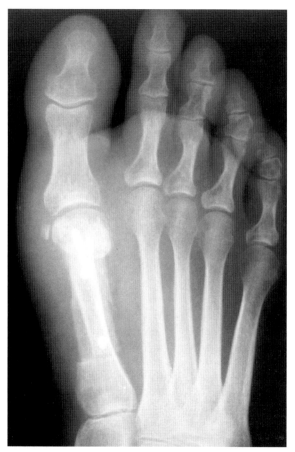

Fig. 4. Anteroposterior X-ray view of forefoot affected by hallux valgus and metatarsalgia. Note the lateral dislocation of the sesamoid bone and first metatarsal varus

Fig. 5. Postoperative X-ray that shows the realignment of the hallux and the first metatarsal bone, and the reduction of the sesamoid bone

elastic upper may be used. The leg muscles venous pump and the venous network of the foot sole are solicited by weight bearing and are very efficient in removing peripheral stasis. Elastic gradual compression stockings are used in case of persistence of edema. A regular pair of shoes may be worn at the end of this period.

Mild jogging is resumed when the normal weight-bearing pattern is recovered. Cutting exercises are allowed after the running speed reaches the pre-operative levels. Step exercises and jump training need another 10 days (Figs. 2–5).

Injuries to the Talus

Transchondral Fractures of the Talar Dome

These fractures are produced by a force transmitted from the articular surface of a contiguous bone across the joint and through the articular cartilage to the subchondral trabeculae of the fractured bone [7].

The classification system most often used for osteochondral fractures is based on the radiographic ap-

pearance of the lesion. Stage I is a compression fracture; Stage II is partial separation of the osteochondral fragment; Stage III is complete separation of the fragment without displacement; and Stage IV is a displaced osteochondral fracture. These injuries are not rare, but since they are often subtle or not visible on initial radiographs because they are either undisplaced or the X-ray projection does not allow visualization, delayed diagnosis is common. Treatment of osteochondral fractures depends on the stage of the lesion and the extent of the patient's symptoms. Asymptomatic, nondisplaced lesions do not require treatment. Symptomatic Stage I and II lesions often respond well to 6 weeks in a short-leg cast. Medial Stage III lesions also may become asymptomatic after a period of immobilization. Medial Stage IV lesions and lateral Stage III and IV lesions do not respond well to conservative management and require excision. Other lesions that continue to be symptomatic despite immobilization should also respond well to surgical excision.

After an immobilization period, both conservative and surgical treatment rehabilitation includes: contin-

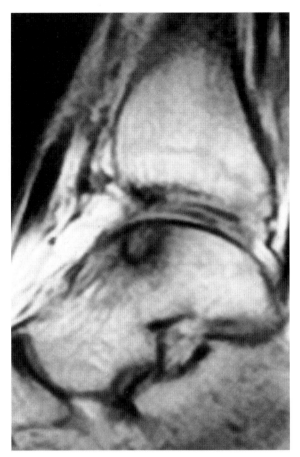

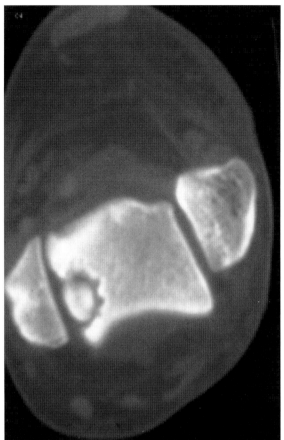

Fig. 6. MRI of Stage I of transchondral fracture of talar dome

Fig. 7. CT scan of Stage III of transchondral fracture of talar dome

uous passive motion devices, TENS for pain control, ultrasound in the case of tissue adherences, massage and manual or mechanic lymphatic drainage, and electrical stimulation of the leg muscles. Crutches should be used until full weight bearing and normal walking is possible, usually at 4 weeks, when stretching and strengthening exercises are commenced. Proprioceptive exercises are advised before mild jogging. Cutting movements are commenced when pain is completely gone (Figs. 6, 7).

Fractures of the lateral process of the talus occur following severe ankle sprains. Since the clinical presentation of lateral ligament rupture is overwhelming, the fracture may not be suspected. The plain X-rays are often negative and CT scan or MRI are necessary to detect this fracture (Fig. 8).

When surgical treatment of such fractures is not considered, an early rehabilitation program must be planned out. Rest, ice, compression, and elevation are the basic principles for controling pain and edema. TENS and nonsteroidal anti-inflammatory drugs may help in the initial phase. Continuous passive motion devices are utilized as soon as pain decreases. After

2 weeks, weight bearing can be gradually resumed. Therapy boot or ankle braces are used if there are concomitant ankle ligament disruptions. The wearing of elastic compressive stockings may be of great help in treating refractory edema. Electric stimulation of the leg muscle is used. Crutches should be used until full weight bearing and normal walking is possible, usually at 4 weeks. Stretching and strengthening exercises are commenced. Proprioceptive exercises are advised before mild jogging. Cutting movements are commenced when pain has completely gone.

Overuse Diseases and Injuries to Achilles Tendon and Related Surgical Procedures

Tendinopathy

Inflammatory diseases of the surrounding tissues of the Achilles tendon are most often due to overuse. There are several causes of the inflammation: limited extension of the ankle; decreased plantar flexion strength; abnormal pronation; rigid cavus foot; rearfoot varus; training errors; improper running, jumping

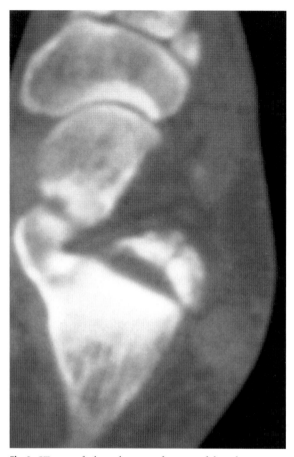

Fig. 8. CT scan of a lateral process fracture of the talus

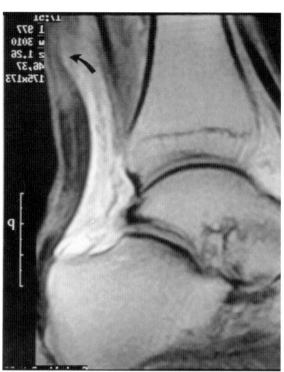

Fig. 9. MRI of chronic tendinitis of Achilles tendon. Note the enlargement of the tendon and the midsubstance degeneration

or kicking techniques; unfit shoes; uneven terrain. Stopping the tendon abuse is the most important measure. Removal of the causes is also important. Rest, stretching, and cold therapy are used.

Orthotics to elevate the heel or to control pronation are prescribed. A pain-free gait must be maintained. Range of motion exercises are performed: active extension to gently stretch the calf; passive dorsiflexion using a towel; resistive plantar flexion exercises using a towel. As symptoms improve, the routine progresses to passive stretching and resistive exercise off a step. Pool walking and backward walking are advised since the tendon is less solicited. The use of a calf machine provides appropriate exercises. The 7-day regimen consists of three sets of ten repeats at a slow speed with no pain on days 1 and 2; moderate speed with no pain on days 3, 4 and 5; and fast speed with slight discomfort allowed on days 6 and 7.

The Achilles tendon is presumably involved in the chronic inflammatory process when chronic symptoms (longer than 16 weeks) and pain associated with acceleration or exertion are observed. When prolonged conservative treatment fails to relieve pain, surgical in-

tervention is recommended. After the operation of tendon debridement, the rehabilitation program outlined above delays progress. Full recovery is obtained at the sixth or eighth month (Fig. 9)

Insertional Diseases

Several disturbances related to sport activities are localized in the distal insertion area of the Achilles tendon: retrocalcaneal and precalcaneal bursitis, paratenonitis and tendinosis, inflammation of the osteotendinous junction, Haglund's process and retrocalcanal bone spurs. An accurate diagnosis of the diseases occurring in this region is mandatory before the rehabilitation program is elaborated. In acute phase, rest, cold, decrease of mileage while the patient works on stretching and controlled strengthening exercise is usually helpful. In chronic cases the rehabilitation program is protracted since symptoms are persistent. The local reaction to overuse is blood supply impairment of the peritendinous and the tendon tissues which seems to be responsible for the symptoms.

It seems that hyperthermic therapy may solicitate a

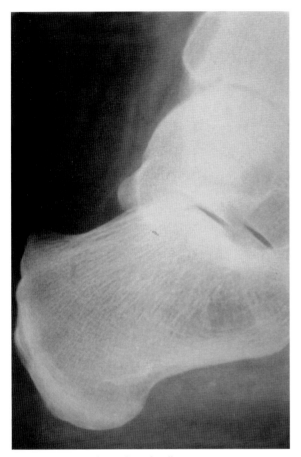

Fig. 10. Posterior calcaneal Haglund's process

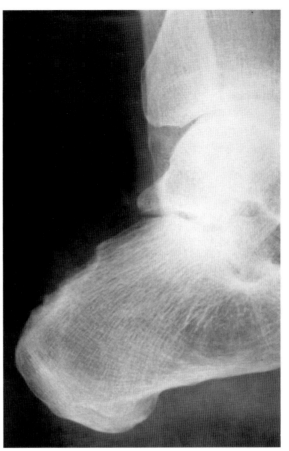

Fig. 11. Postoperative appearance of the partial calcaneal ostectomy

reactive newly formed vascular network. If rehabilitation fails to relieve symptoms, surgical debridement, with removal of Haglund's process or retrocalcaneal bony spur, is advisable (Figs. 10, 11).

Ruptures of the Achilles Tendon

Achilles tendon rupture not infrequently occurs in mature athletes. This injury is highly disabling as athletic participation is temporarily or permanently inhibited.

Nonsurgical Treatment

The conservative functional treatment is performed with a special therapy boot. The characteristics of this modified 'boxer' boot are the reducible heel pads, which allow a gradual adjustment from plantarflexion to a neutral position. A plastic tongue prevents the patient from dorsiflexion, and the lateral shaft stabilization reduces torsion. The patient has to wear the boot for 6 weeks continuously day and night and for a further 2 weeks only during the day. While wearing the boot, the patient is allowed full weight bearing. The re-

habilitation program after the removal of the therapeutic boot is as follows: stretching and strengthening exercises of calf muscles and Achilles tendon; proprioceptive reeducation; walking on a treadmill, cycling, hydrotherapy.

Percutaneous Repair

A percutaneous suture of the Achilles tendon rupture is increasing utilized as a technique of repair. The basic principle is the use of a surgical suture using a very limited surgical approach. After the procedure, partial weight bearing with a therapy boot is allowed while the foot is held flexed at 30° for 3 weeks. The square foot position is gradually assumed within the following 5 weeks. After the removal of the therapeutic boot, the rehabilitation program is the same as previously described for nonsurgical treatment.

Surgical Treatment

Open surgery of an Achilles tendon rupture allows direct approach and steady repair of the injured tendon.

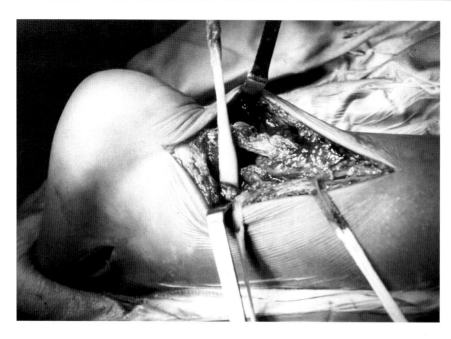

Fig. 12. In case of severely frayed Achilles tendon rupture, reconstruction is carried out using the tendon of proneus brevis as a graft. The photograph shows the harvested peroneus brevis before the suture around the disrupted Achilles tendon

When the Achilles tendon tissue is too degenerated and frayed, a graft from surrounding ankle tendons (peroneus brevis or flexor hallucis longus) are utilized for the reconstruction. The reconstruction is very solid. After the operation, during the 2 weeks of immobilization in a plaster splint or in a restricted motion brace, early plantar flexion of the ankle is possible. In the third week partial weight bearing is allowed in a therapy boot or dorsal ankle splint. In the fourth week range of motion exercises are allowed (with knee flexed as well as extended): swimming, training while wearing a floating jacket and diving in a swimming pool, stationary bicycling, isometric, isotonic and isokinetic strengthening of the calf muscle. During the fifth and sixth postoperative week low impact stress (jogging, distance running) are gradually introduced. At 8 weeks, high impact stress (sprinting, cutting, jumping) is introduced. After 3 months, return to competitive sports is allowed (Fig. 12).

Focusing Achilles Tendon Stretching Exercises

Stretching exercises are of utmost importance to assist in regaining flexibility following Achilles tendon injuries or surgical procedures. The Achilles tendon is the tendon of triceps surae, which consists of the gastrocnemius, soleus, and plantaris muscles. Gentle stretching of the triceps surae muscle group may be achieved in a non-weight-bearing position. This is appropriate for acutely injured or post-surgical patients. To stretch the gastrocnemius muscle, the patient is positioned in a long sitting position with the foot slightly elevated to allow the heel to move freely. The supination of the subtalar joint is necessary to lock the midtarsal joint and allow for ankle joint extension rather than forefoot motion. A towel is placed over the metatarsal heads, and the patient uses the towel to pull the foot into dorsiflexion until a stretch is felt at the gastrocnemius muscle. This stretch is maintained for 10–15 s and repeated 10–15 times. In order to stretch the soleus muscle, the knee is flexed 25°–30°, while the leg is held in the same position as for the gastrocnemius stretch. Stretching of the soleus is felt distally in the Achilles tendon, whereas gastrocnemius muscle stretching is felt more proximally.

The Achilles tendon stretching exercises in a weight-bearing position are performed while the patient is standing 60–70 cm from a wall. The feet are 20 cm apart and the injured leg is back.

The knee of the injured leg remains extended while the uninjured knee is permitted to flex. The patient's hands are placed on the wall for stable support. The hip of the injured side should be maintained in neutral or slight internal rotation, keeping the foot pointing straight ahead or the toes pointing inward. The heel should remain in contact with the ground and the trunk should remain in an upright, neutral position while the patient leans forward until a stretch is felt in the calf muscle. The stretch should be maintained for 20–30 s and repeated three to five times. In order to position the ankle in dorsiflexion, an inclined board may also be used. The soleus muscle may be stretched by placing the injured leg in 25°–30° of knee flexion. A stretch is obtained by squatting down and allowing both knees to bend until a stretch is felt in the lower calf or Achilles tendon area.

Heel Pain

Pain sensation in the heel derives from branches of the anterior tibial, peroneal, and posterior tibial nerves. Pain localized along the lateral aspect of the heel is principally a contact or motion sensation: it is referred to the tip of lateral malleolus or related to the peroneal tubercle area. Lateral border pain is rarely reported if compared with medial border pain. Pain of the posterior aspect of the heel may arise both at rest or during weight bearing. Pressure trigger points are the subcutaneous tissues around the Achilles tendon or the osteotendinous junction. The different clinical conditions of heel pain are classified as follows.

Plantar Pain

The plantar pain is a contact or weight-bearing sensation. Direct pressure stimulates nerve endings ramifying in the heel pad and periosteum from the posterior tibial and peroneal branches to the calcaneal zone. Plantar pain occurs very rarely at rest and it is localized along the edge of the medial or the lateral aspect. When rehabilitating the plantar aspect of the rearfoot one should consider that the heel pad of the sole acts as the first shock absorber of the body. The skin of the soles is very sensitive to touch and pressure; it has fine two-point discrimination and an acute sense of deep pressure and vibration. Withdrawal reflexes as well as postural reflexes are elicited from the soles: they are essential to balance, ambulation, and soft tissue protection.

Plantar Fasciitis

In plantar fasciitis, pain relief is based on rest and anti-inflammatory drugs. Ice massage, and massage with anti-inflammatory products may be helpful. Contrast baths and ultrasound may help relieve pain. Since extension of the toes and of the ankle stretches the plantar fascia, stretching exercises are used when pain subsides. Stretching exercises of the gastrosoleus complex are also recommended in order to restore flexibility of the heel cord [3].

Calcaneal Spur

A soft calcaneal orthotic should be used. Abnormal shoe wear, hyperpronation, limited ankle extension, technical or training errors must be reviewed and eliminated. Running on soft surfaces or grass should be advised. It is not unusual for the condition to take 2–3 months or longer to improve, even when overuse is removed.

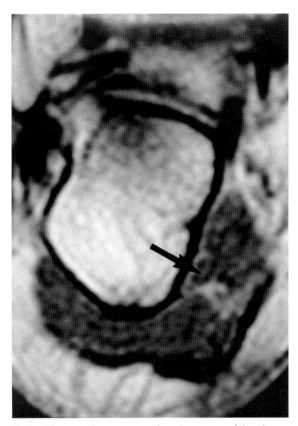

Fig. 13. The MRI demonstrates chronic rupture of the plantar fascia. Scar tissue is present among short muscles of the medioplantar surface of the foot

Rupture of the Plantar Fascia

If the plantar fascia ruptures, weight-bearing and stretching exercises should be avoided for 2 weeks. Rest and ice applications are advised. TENS is used for pain control. Soft orthotics and crutches are utilized when weight bearing is resumed. When pain subsides, stretching exercises are started. When rehabilitating sports injuries or surgery procedures of the plantar aspect of the hindfoot, the importance of the plantar soft tissue function must be considered (Fig. 13).

Medial Heel Pain

Medial heel pain is localized in the region of medial malleolus: pain in this region may arise without weight bearing and is distributed along the inner aspect of the heel. Direct involvement of the medial plantar nerve can be considered. Pain localized at the contact area of the medial border of the heel is related to the calcaneal branches of the posterior tibial nerve and is related with weight bearing [13].

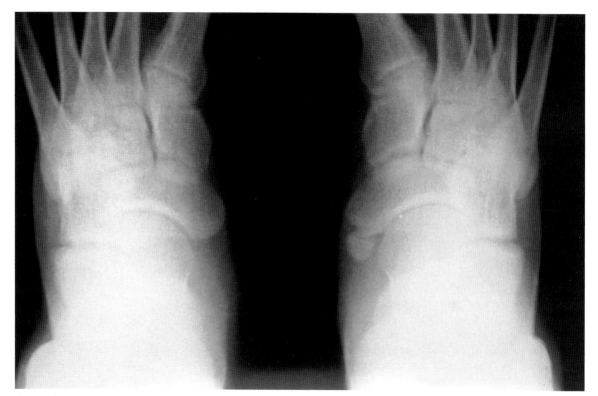

Fig. 14. The X-ray shows the detachment of the distal insertion of the posterior tibial tendon, with a bone fragment

Tarsal Tunnel Syndrome

Rest and ice massage are useful in pain control in tarsal tunnel syndrome. TENS is highly advisable. The medial arch support is prescribed and compression of the abductor hallucis must be avoided. The rehabilitation program must be prolonged for several weeks to months before surgical decompression should be considered.

Tibialis Posterior Tendon Disorders

Insertional pathology of the posterior tibial tendon (PTT) may arise acutely, following an acute ankle sprain. Chronic overuse tenosynovitis may occur, and hyperpronation can be a predisposing factor. The chronic tenosynovitis may mimic a medial heel pain condition. Accurate clinical examination and imaging findings lead to diagnosis. Appropriate orthotics for correction of the hyperpronated foot are advisable. The rehabilitation program includes rest, ice massage, and TENS. Training or technical errors should also be corrected. After the inflammation subsides, stretching and strengthening exercises of the PTT should be undertaken. When the distal insertion of the PTT is detached with a bone fragment, surgical exploration of the distal tendon and insertion is highly advised (Fig. 14).

Posterior Heel Pain

Pain of the posterior aspect of the heel may arise both at rest or when weight bearing. Trigger points in the subcutaneous tissues may be found around the Achilles tendon or the osteotendinous junction. Pain in the tendon area follows active motions of the ankle.

Calcaneal Bursitis

The insertion of the Achilles tendon is protected by two synovial bursae: the subcutaneous bursa and the retrocalcaneal bursa. These structures may become inflamed and hypertrophied in sports-related situations, due to excessive impact loading, exaggerated friction of the shoe counter on the outside of the heel, poorly constructed shoes, training errors, or excessive mileage.

Calcaneal Tendinitis

An overpronated hindfoot during the stance phase of running, rigid cavus foot, improper training with absence of stretching exercises of the Achilles tendon, excessive impact loading, and heel cord tightness are predisposing conditions of osteotendinous junction pathology of Achilles tendon (Fig. 15).

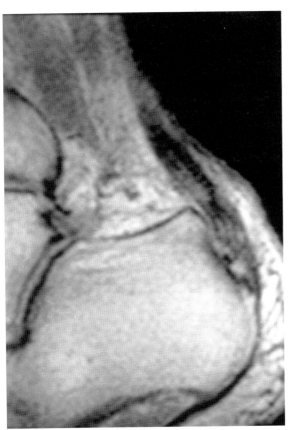

Fig. 15. The MRI shows chronic inflammation of the Achilles tendon at the distal osteotendinous junction

Calcaneal Exostoses

The calcaneal bone plays an important role in the retrocalcaneal pain condition. As a response of chronic solicitations of the distal Achilles tendon insertion, retrocalcaneal bony steps may also arise, involving tendon fibers. The condition in which the uppermost posterior corner of the calcaneum forms a sharp and prominent angle that impinges the distal Achilles tendon is also known as Haglund disease (see above). Ostectomy of the supero-posterior calcaneus angle is advised when conservative treatments fail.

Posterior Heel Pain Rehabilitation Program

Reduction of mileage and rest should be adopted in severe cases. Selection of proper shoes for training and competition is very important for athletes with significant biomechanical abnormalities. In cases of bursitis, a steroid solution may be injected into the retrocalcanal bursa, not into the tendon; TENS, ultrasound, ionophoresis and iontophoresis can be used, as well as removing or softening the counter of the shoe. For those individuals with overpronation, a rigid heel counter is mandatory in order to stabilize the subtalar joint controlling ex-

cessive pronation, but precautions against exaggerated friction must be undertaken, inserting a heel cup or a sponge pad into the shoe to protect the affected area from irritation, and using socks with soft pads in the heel area. In cases of posterior muscle tightness or retrocalcaneal bursitis, an elevated heel is advisable because the foot comes easily into neutral position, the equinus of the ankle diminishes, and abnormal stress on the osteotendinous junction is less severe.

Lateral Heel Pain

Pain localized along the lateral aspect of the heel is principally a contact or motion sensation: it is referred to the tip of the lateral malleolus or to the peroneal tubercle region. Lateral border pain is rarely reported compared with medial border pain.

Calcaneofibular Irregularity

This is the most frequent condition of lateral heel pain, followed by peroneal tendon disorders and static prob-

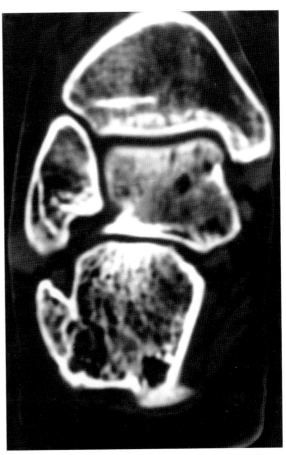

Fig. 16. The CT scan demonstrates the augmentation of the peroneal calcaneal tubercle. Peroneal tendons may be pinched between the tip of lateral malleolus and the tubercle

lems such as valgus heel. An enhancement of peroneal tubercle may arise after severe hindfoot sprains. A misdiagnosed fracture of the lateral calcaneal wall, with consequent bone callus formation, is also a cause of calcaneofibular irregularity. The peroneal tendons are pinched between the lateral bone spur and the lateral malleolus tip. Sinus tarsi pain must be also considered when treating a condition of lateral heel pain [8].

TENS, ionophoresis, phonophoresis, laser therapy, and ultrasound may be used to relieve pain. Occasionally two or three corticosteroid injections may be used. When conservative treatment fails, surgical excision of the lateral peroneal tubercle should be considered in order to prevent further damage to peroneal tendons (Fig. 16).

Complex Regional Pain Syndrome Type I

Traumatic as well nontraumatic causes are at the origin of a dysfunction of the sympathetic peripheral nervous system defined as complex regional pain syndrome type I (CRPS, formerly called reflex sympathetic dystrophy, RSD) localized at foot level. The accurate collection of the clinical history is the principal way to diagnose it. The essential features of all patients affected by RSD are pain, diffuse tenderness, vascular and trophic changes. A clinical staging of these findings is outlined as follows.

Stage I. Vasodilatation, hyperemia, hypertermia, mild to moderate edema, increased hair growth, hyperhidrosis.

Stage II. Superficial vasoconstriction with cool, pale, indurated and sometimes cyanotic skin, loss of hair, restricted motion due to pain, diffuse rarefaction of bone (radiographically assessed).

Stage III. Fixed joint contracture, fibrous ankylosis, atrophy of the skin and its appendages, advanced radiographic changes such as osteopenia, cortical bone resorption, articular erosions. The presence and persistence of pain is the resilient feature of the RSD (Figs. 17–19).

A vicious cycle is established which components are pain, emotional distress, fear to move the joints, loss of articular range of motion, acquired malalignment of forefoot or rearfoot, bony resorption, vascular impairment, trophic changes. Prevention is essential to decrease the morbidity associated with RDS. After injuries of the foot and foot surgical procedures, the use of analgesics, elevation, early joint motion in order to minimize edema and prevent joint stiffness, and avoidance of forceful passive motion are recommended.

In the early stages of the disease, the first priorities are to treat the pain and edema, then to improve the injured extremity's range of motion, third to increase strength, and finally restoring function to the limb. Anti-edema measures include elevation, compression, decongestive massage, and active ROM exercises. Most anti-edema modalities increase the interstitial hydrostatic pressure, except elevation, which decreases capillary hydrostatic pressure. Pulsed magnetic fields are an useful adjunct to control local edema and demineralization. Pain-relieving modalities include contrast baths, desensitization, fluid therapy, static splinting, and TENS. Relaxation training and biofeedback is important to control the sympathetic pain. Methods of

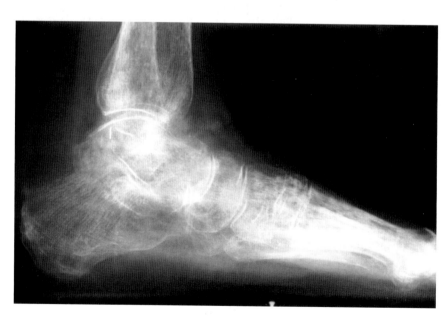

Fig. 17. Lateral X-ray of the foot that assesses a severe CRPS syndrome

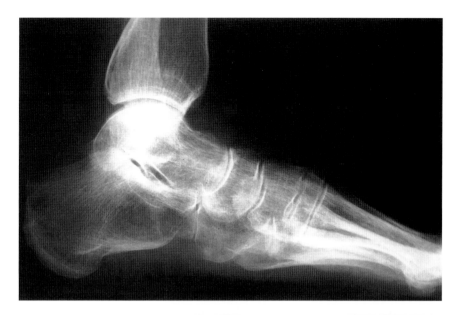

Fig. 18. Lateral X-ray of the uninvolved foot (same patient as Fig. 17)

improving the patient's ROM are ultrasound, paraffin bath, dynamic splinting, and continuous passive motion.

Medical therapy (including local anesthetic blocks, lumbar sympathetic blocks, corticosteroids, beta-adrenergic blockers, nifedipine, calcitonine, diphosphonates, and calcium tablets as a dietary supplement) are doomed to failure without the foundation of a well-planned foot therapy program.

Conclusion

Phases of Foot Injuries Rehabilitation Program

The rehabilitation program conceived for foot injuries or surgery after acute and overuse lesions of foot structures should thoroughly follow the healing process of lesions. The rehabilitation is divided into phases in order to help healing and avoid unnecessary strain on the injured structures.

Initial Phase. Aims of the initial phase are reduction of the inflammatory process, pain control, return to normal range of motion, recovery of muscle power.

Intermediate Phase. This involves a steady progression of strengthening exercises, using both open and closed kinetic chain exercises, continuing emphasis on flexibility, and initiating exercise to increase proprioception and incorporating functional activities. As strength increases, a shift is made toward improving endurance.

Advanced Phase. This focuses more on the return to full activities by emphasizing agility drills and exercises simulating work demands.

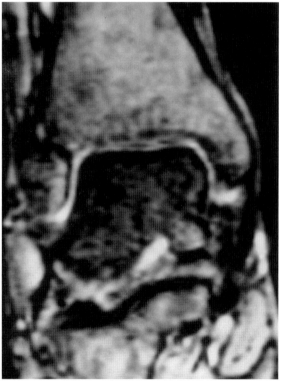

Fig. 19. MRI that shows CRPS syndrome of the talus. Although circumscribed, this form may be painful and disabling

Criteria for Return to Activity. These include: a full, pain-free range of motion; normal strength, endurance and power; full-speed painless running; ability to run a figure-of-eight pattern and to cut 90° to the left and right at full speed. Comparative isokinetic exercises of foot and ankle may be used to evaluate efficiency of the affected limb. Gait analysis may be used before returning to sports activity to detect any instability or imperfection of walking while weight bearing.

References

1. Barouk LS (1995) Scarf osteotomy of the first metatarsal in the treatment of hallux valgus. Foot Diseases 2(1):35–48
2. Betts RP, Franks CI, Duckworth T (1991) Foot pressure studies: normal and pathologic gait analyses. In: Jahss MH (ed) Disorders of the foot and ankle, 2nd edn, vol 1. WB Saunders, Philadelphia, p 484
3. Cornwall MW, McPoil TG (1999) Plantar fasciitis: etiology and treatment. J Orthop Sports Phys Ther 29(12):765–760
4. Donatelli R (1987) Abnormal biomechanics of the foot and ankle. J Ortho Sports Phys Ther 9:11
5. Hockenbury RT (1999) Forefoot problems in athletes (review). Med Sci Sports Exerc 31(Suppl 7):448–458
6. Huson A (1991) Functional anatomy of the foot. In: Jahss MH (ed) Disorders of the foot and ankle, 2nd edn, vol 1. WB Saunders, Philadelphia, p 409
7. King RE, Powell DF (1991) Injury to the talus. In: Jahss MH (ed) Disorders of the foot and ankle, 2nd edn, vol 3. WB Saunders, Philadelphia, p 2293
8. Kirk JF (1976) Sinus tarsi pain: case history. J Foot Surg 15(3):120–121
9. Mann RA (1991) Overview of foot and ankle biomechanics. In: Jahss MH (ed) Disorders of the foot and ankle, 2nd edn, vol 1. WB Saunders, Philadelphia, p 385
10. Myerson MS (1991) Injuries to the forefoot and toes. In: Jahss MH (ed) Disorders of the foot and ankle, 2nd edn, vol 3. WB Saunders, Philadelphia, p 2233
11. Nyska M, Mc Cabe C, Linge K, Klenerman L (1996) Plantar foot pressure during treadmill walking with high-heel and low-heel shoes. Foot Ankle Int 17(11):662–666
12. Omery ML, Micheli LJ (1999) Foot and ankle problems in the young athlete. Med Sci Sports Exerc 31 (Suppl. 7):470–486
13. Reinherz RP (1990) Pain along the medial arch of the foot. J Foot Surg 29(6):531–532
14. Sammarco GJ (1991) Conditioning and rehabilitation of the athlete's foot and ankle. In Jahss MH (ed) Disorders of the foot and ankle, 2nd edn, vol 3. WB Saunders, Philadelphia, p 2797
15. Tiberio D (1988) Pathomechanics of structural foot deformities. Phys Ther 68:1840
16. Valtin B (1997) (ed) Chirurgie de l'avant pied. Cahiers d'enseignement de la SOFCOT – 60. Expansion Scientifique Francaise
17. Weil LS, Borelli AH (1991) Modified scarf bunionectomy: our experience in more than 1000 cases. J Foot Surg 30:609–622

Chapter 15

Rehabilitation of Muscle Injuries

15

Donald T. Kirkendall, William E. Prentice, William E. Garrett

Introduction

Acute injuries to skeletal muscle may include such injuries as contusions, lacerations, strains, ischemia, and complete ruptures, any of which can lead to significant pain and disability, causing time to be lost to both occupational and leisure activity participation. The significance of strains, or stretch-induced injuries, is clear to the sports medicine practitioner because stretch-induced injuries can be as much as 30% of the typical sports medicine practice [13, 17, 18].

There are a variety of noncontact or indirect injuries that can affect muscle function, such as delayed onset muscle soreness (DOMS), partial strain injury, and a complete rupture of the muscle. This continuum of injuries has one thing in common: eccentric exercise – when the muscle develops tension while lengthening [2, 11, 17, 19, 21]. Unlike concentric contractions, eccentric contractions generate high forces with fewer active motor units [24].

Eccentric loading, especially during unaccustomed exercise, leads to microscopic damage to the contractile element of muscle, mostly on what appears to be random disruptions of the Z-lines in DOMS [4]. Reversible pain, weakness, and restricted range of motion are the features of DOMS. Pain usually peaks in the 1–2 days following exercise [2]. Weakness and limited range of motion can persist for over a week [11, 22]. Interestingly, there is rapid adaptation of muscle as demonstrated by successive bouts of the unaccustomed exercise produce progressively less perceived soreness and less tissue damage [2, 24].

A muscle strain injury is a disruption of the muscle-tendon unit [6]. Local pain and general weakness of the muscle are seen when an athlete attempts activity. In contrast to the protective aspects of DOMS, improper rest and rehabilitation of a minor strain of skeletal muscle can frequently proceed a more disabling injury that further increases the time lost to work and athletics.

Injury Mechanisms

Most clinicians would agree that muscle strain injuries occur when the muscle is passively stretched or activated during stretch [13, 15, 17, 18, 29]. In addition, eccentric contraction of the muscle is a frequent occurrence [6, 9, 17, 29]. Eccentric contraction is important because muscle forces can be higher during lengthening [24], adding to the forces by the passive, connective tissue element [3]. In athletics, muscle strain injuries occur to 'speed athletes' such as sprinters and participants in American football, basketball, soccer and rugby, and others. Additionally, certain muscles seem to be most susceptible to injury.

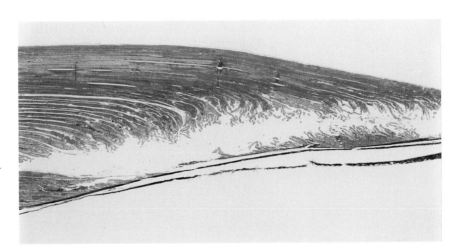

Fig. 1. Appearance of the tibialis anterior muscle of the rabbit following controlled strain injury. A small amount of muscle tissue remains attached to the distal tendon

Injury Resulting From Passive Stretch

Muscles have been stretched passively to failure from the proximal or distal tendon. Of interest is the effect of rate of strain (1, 10, and 100 cm s^{-1}), muscle pennation or the mechanical properties of muscle. Regardless of the strain rate or architecture, the muscle failed at the (distal) muscle-tendon junction (MTJ, Fig. 1) leaving a small, amount of muscle tissue attached to the tendon [5, 15, 25, 26]. The site of stretch-induced injury was near the muscle-tendon junction, but most often was not an avulsion since a variable and small amount of muscle remained with the tendon.

Injury Resulting From Active Stretch

Rabbit hindlimb muscles were isolated and stretched to failure. However, during the stretch, a muscle was stimulated tetanically, submaximally, or was unstimulated [15]. At failure the location was, as usual, the MTJ and the total strain at failure was similar among the three conditions. The force generated at failure was only 15% greater in the activated muscles. However, the energy absorbed (the difference in strain energy between passive and active conditions) was about 100% greater in the activated condition (Fig. 2). This shows that passive elements of muscle help absorb energy and that the ability to absorb energy is enhanced when the muscle is activated. This may suggest that muscles can protect themselves and joint structures from injury. The more energy absorbed, the more injury-resistant the muscle.

The increase in energy absorbed due to contraction is noted to be around 100%. Any situation that diminishes a muscle's ability to contract would reduce the muscle's ability to absorb energy making the muscle more susceptible to injury.

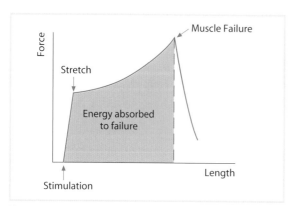

Fig. 2. Energy absorbed is shown as the area under each length-tension deformation curve

Injuries That Are Nondisruptive

The model can be modified to produce a nondisruptive injury where ultrastructural damage occurs. Histology of these injuries shows the same damage near the muscle-tendon junction with some muscle still attached to the tendon. Hemorrhaging occurs and a pronounced inflammatory response is seen 1–2 days after the injury. By the seventh day, fibrous tissue starts to replace the inflammatory reaction, leading to scar tissue [15].

This damage should reduce the ability of the muscle to develop tension. Immediately after the injury, the muscle can develop about 70% of the normal amount of tension. By 24 h later, the tension developed declines to 50% of the contralateral control muscle. Tension production slowly improves and by the seventh day, the muscle can produce 90% of the tension of the control muscle.

In contrast, when muscle with a 7-day-old nondisruptive injury was stretched and the tensile strength recorded, this tensile strength was only 77% of the control muscle [16]. This is below the 90% of tension developed just mentioned. As strains are, in part, caused by stretch, this loss of tensile strength may by why the muscle is more susceptible to a second injury; a scenario frequently seen by clinicians.

Viscoelasticity of Skeletal Muscle

Important factors in preventing muscle strain injuries include flexibility, warm-up and pre-exercise stretching. The beneficial effects of stretching are frequently attributed to stretch reflex mechanisms. An additional consideration is viscoelasticity. This can be visualized if we imagine hanging a weight on a muscle and observe its length, then watch the muscle slowly continue to increase in length with time. For tendons and ligaments, stretch the tissue to a constant length and notice that the tension gradually decreases with time. This is referred to as stress-relaxation. Perform this cyclically, and a gradual decrease in tension occurs with each successive stretch [1]. The concept of viscoelasticity applied to muscle and stretch-induced injuries has been discussed [25, 28].

Clinical Applications

It is important to take the findings of laboratory-based projects and apply them to the clinic. Do injuries in humans also occur at the muscle-tendon junction? Acute hamstring strain injuries were evaluated within 48 h of the injury in ten college athletes [8] who were examined clinically and imaged with computed tomography (CT) to determine the mechanism and location of their injury. All injuries occurred while either sprinting or kicking a soccer ball. In most cases, the injury was proximal and lateral, typically to the biceps femoris.

The mechanism involved ballistic hip flexion and knee extension. CT scanning showed the injured area as a region of hypodensity, suggesting inflammation and edema, but not local bleeding.

A larger group of athletes ($n=50$) was imaged to show injuries localized to the quadriceps, hamstrings, adductors, and triceps surae groups [23]. MRI (T2) visualized the edema, inflammation, and possible hemorrhage of muscle strain injuries. Quadriceps strains were isolated to the rectus femoris. Adductor strains were confined to the adductor longus. Of the 17 hamstring strain injuries, 11 were to the biceps femoris, 4 to the semimembraneous, and 2 to the semitendinosus. All injuries to the triceps surae group were at the distal MTJ of the medial head of the gastrocnemius. Importantly, the particular muscles susceptible to strain injuries were identified as two-joint muscles (biceps femoris, rectus femoris, gastrocnemius) or of a complex architecture (adductor longus) and occurred at the muscle-tendon junction.

There are curious, unexplained muscle injuries such as the persistent strain of the rectus femoris. Was our understanding of the nature of the strain injury consistent with our understanding of the anatomy of the rectus femoris [12]? Cadaveric dissection of the rectus femoris muscle showed a direct head originating at the anterior inferior iliac spine and an indirect head originating from the superior acetabular ridge with this tendon extending well into the mass of the rectus femoris. While laboratory work showed that most strain injuries occurred superficially at the MTJ, clinical evidence suggested a strain at the MTJ of the deep, indirect head of the rectus femoris. These injuries are different from the classically seen injury near the distal tendon because asymmetry, chronic pain, and anterior thigh masses are evident [10, 12].

A detailed study of the architecture of the rectus femoris seemed appropriate to determine if these persistent strains were related to some unique architecture [10]. The rectus femoris of cadavers was dissected and the superficial and deep tendons were confirmed. The tendon of the deep component penetrated nearly the entire length of the muscle. It originated from the superior acetabular ridge and was medial throughout its course through the muscle. The tendon began rounded, flattened out and migrated laterally and was nearly vertical in the distal third of the muscle (Fig. 3). The pennation of the rectus femoris was much more complex than the simple bipennate arrangement that is usually described. The proximal third appeared to be unipennate while the distal two-thirds were bipennate. The deep tendon and distal bipennate arrangement created a 'muscle within a muscle.'

The most common hamstring strain seen in the clinic involves one muscle, usually the biceps femoris. The more extensive injuries involve more muscles, typically at the common tendon of origin of the ham-

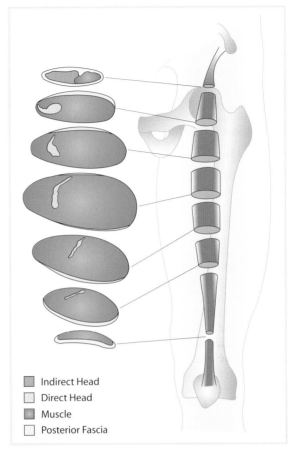

Legend:
- Indirect Head
- Direct Head
- Muscle
- Posterior Fascia

Fig. 3. Architecture of the indirect head of the rectus femoris muscle

strings. A unique hamstring strain mechanism occurs to water skiers [21]. The novice skier crouches prior to being pulled into a standing position by the boat. If the skier extends their knees too soon, the ski tip is forced down into the water and the forward momentum of the boat pulls the skier forward leading to excessive hip flexion while the knees are extended. This excessive stretch leads to either a muscle-tendon junction injury or to a more disabling avulsion injury of the tendinous origin from the ischial tuberosity. Hamstring strains to experienced skiers happen while falling forward on a single slalom ski.

Acute groin injuries are also common in sports, especially in soccer and ice hockey players [27]. Usually, the adductor longus is injured during hip abduction, yet direct and indirect hernias can also occur. There is also an abnormality in the lower abdominal wall leading to vague and poorly localized pain in the groin. This pain is felt during high intensity, ballistic motions such as kicking a soccer ball or sprinting. This is almost exclusively seen in very high caliber athletes doing intense training and competition. This 'athletic pubalgia' is associated with pain and injury in the inguinal area near the insertion of the rectus abdominis and in the adjacent internal obliques near the region noted with direct inguinal hernias without any evidence of herniation. When conservative measures fail, a herniorrhaphy procedure, reinforcing the abdominal wall musculature, can provide excellent relief.

Prevention Strategies

Repetitive Stretch and Failure Properties

The prior work cited suggests that viscoelastic properties of muscle contribute greatly to changes in muscle length and increased length can be seen to decrease strain in a muscle. A more practical question relates to the use of stretching; a commonly used method to prevent muscle strains. To study stretching, repeated stretch-release cycles were studied using the rabbit model [25]. First, the force to failure of the hind limb muscle was determined. Then the contralateral muscles were cyclically stretched to 50 or 70% of the force to failure. Ten cycles to 50% of the failure force resulted in an increase in muscle stretch at failure with no change in the force at failure or energy absorbed. When muscles were cyclically stretched to 70% of the failure force, macroscopic evidence of failure was evident even before the ten cycles were completed. Thus, cyclic stretching appears to be beneficial, and stretching that leads to forces in excess of 70% may make the muscle more, rather than less, likely to be injured.

Warm-Up

Viscoelasticity is known to be temperature-dependent and warm-up is considered to be protective against muscle strains. An attempt was made to mimic warm-up that was due to prior activity [20] as opposed to external heating. Rabbit hind limb muscle was held isometrically and tetanically stimulated for 10–15 s, which resulted in a 1 °C rise in muscle temperature. The muscle was able to stretch more prior to failure and produce more force. While the changes might be due to temperature elevation, the effects of stretch cannot be discounted in spite of the muscle being held isometrically. A constant length must still allow for some stretch of the muscle-tendon unit as the fibers contract and elastic components become stretched.

Prior Injury

There appears to be a risk of re-injury to a previously strained muscle. Clinically, patients with a major muscle strain usually describe a prior minor injury. This would suggest that after a minor injury, the mechanical characteristics of the muscle are somehow altered.

Such an alteration might precipitate a more major injury. To determine the mechanical characteristics of a muscle with a minor strain, the EDL of rabbits underwent a nondisruptive strain by stretching the muscle just short of tissue rupture [28]. Isometric and isotonic contractile properties of the control muscle were used for comparison. Finally, the muscle was passively stretched to failure at a rate of 10 cm/min. The peak tensile load and length at that load were derived for use on the experimental contralateral limb. The length change to peak load (of the control limb) was duplicated in the experimental muscle, just short of a disruptive injury. The injured muscle was then subjected to passive stretch to failure. Histology was performed on the minor injuries in a subset of rabbits. In the experimental muscles, the peak load to rupture was 63% of control and the length at rupture was 79% of control. Isotonic shortening was reduced by 51% and 6% for 100 g and 1000 g weights, respectively. The minor strain injury caused incomplete disruptions along the MTJ. Thus, a prior minor injury makes the muscle more susceptible to another injury. This suggests that early return to activity prior to complete healing entails a risk of further, more major, injury. In addition, aggressive rehabilitation designed to return an athlete to competition may be too stressful for the muscle, risking further injury. Further, injection for local pain relief while the muscle is still injured may not be appropriate because the lack of inhibition from pain could result in excessive stress on the muscle, also increasing the risk of further injury.

Fatigue

Clinical observation and the literature suggests that muscle strain injuries occur late in either training sessions or competitive settings. This leads one to conclude that fatigue must play some role in the risk of muscle injury. Mair et. al. [14] fatigued the EDL of rabbits to 25 or 50% of the force of the contralateral control using cycles of 5-s isometric tetanic contractions followed by a 1-s rest. The muscle was activated while being pulled (at 1, 10, or 50 cm/s) to failure. Similar data were collected on the unfatigued contralateral control. The force and length at failure were determined as well as the energy absorbed prior to failure. There was a trend toward a reduction in force for all groups (strain rates) tested. The rate of strain did not influence force at failure. There was no change in muscle length at any of the strain rates. There was significantly less energy absorbed in both fatigue conditions with the greatest loss occurring in the most fatigued muscle. The reduction in absorbed energy was the greatest when the muscle was pulled at 1 cm/s. The slower the rate that the muscle is stretched, the greater the energy that is absorbed. Muscles absorb energy while controlling and regulating limb movement. These data indicate that muscles become damaged at the same length regardless of fatigue. In contrast, fatigued muscle is unable to absorb energy prior to reaching the amount of stretch that causes injuries. Proper conditioning to delay fatigue is seen as a part of a rationale for the prevention of muscle strain injury.

Treatment of Muscle Strain Injuries

The pain of a muscle strain may prompt physicians to prescribe anti-inflammatories in response to the inflammatory responses known to occur following an injury. This treatment is largely empirical. Before wide use of anti-inflammatories can be accepted, the effects of such medication on muscle recovering from an injury need to be evaluated. Obremsky et. al. [16] caused a strain injury of the tibialis anterior in 50 rabbits (strain rate of 10 cm/min) that were subsequently administered piroxicam (16 mg/kg) within 6 h then 13 mg/kg every 6 h. Forty served as control and received no medications. Contractile properties and histology were determined at 1, 2, 4, or 7 days after the injury. On day 1, there was a significantly greater force in the treated animals. There was no difference between the treated and untreated animals on days 2, 4, or 7. The treated animals showed a delay in the histological repair process. These muscles showed delayed inflammatory cell infiltration, necrosis, myotube regeneration and collagen deposition. Based on these results, non-steroidal anti-inflammatory agents may be of some benefit for the early treatment of pain control and functional improvement. However, the delay in the repair process seen histologically raised concern regarding long-term treatment.

Rehabilitation of Muscle-Tendon Injuries

Rehabilitation of muscle-tendon injuries begins with an initial grading of the injury.

A strain may range from a minute separation of connective tissue and muscle fibers to a complete tendinous avulsion or muscle rupture. The severity of a muscle stain has been described with a variety of different systems of classification but strains are most typically labeled as grade 1, grade 2, or grade 3 (Table 1). It is essential for the clinician to make an initial determination as to the severity of the strain so that some estimation of the course and corresponding timelines for the rehabilitative process can be established both in the clinicians' mind and for the benefit of the patient. A full discussion of rehabilitation principles for these and other sports injuries is found in Prentice [18].

Table 1. Grading of muscle-tendon injuries

	Grade 1	Grade 2	Grade 3
Fiber damage	Fibers stretched or actually torn	Torn muscle/tendon fibers	Complete rupture of muscle belly, muscle-tendon junction, tendon insertion
Pain	Pain and tenderness with active ROM	Pain with active contraction	Intense pain that diminishes with damage to pain fibers
Deformity	None	Palpable depression in area of torn fibers	Noticeable defect in muscle belly or evidence of torn tendon
Range of motion	Full ROM possible	Less due to swelling and bleeding	Significant impairment to total loss of ROM

A grade 1 injury might leave the athlete with slight discomfort, minimal swelling, little loss of function and full range of motion. Palpation of a grade 2 injury leads to pain and a small to moderate defect. Swelling, impaired gait, and restricted range of motion lead to pain. A grade 3 injury shows a moderate to extensive defect at the site of injury and range of motion is extremely limited. There is swelling, and intense pain when palpated. Resisted range of motion may not be endured. See Table 1 for a summary of muscle-tendon injury grades.

The following section will describe rehabilitation programs for selected muscle tendon injuries according to injury grade.

Groin and Hip Flexor Strains

Grade 1. The athlete with a grade 1 groin strain may only complain of a mild discomfort and demonstrate no loss of function and have full range of motion and strength. There may be some local tenderness, little swelling and the gait will be normal.

Physical therapy modalities and pain-free stretching can begin almost immediately. These activities can include stretching the hip flexors, the adductors (seated and standing), and internal external rotators of the hip. Also, if pain-free, strengthening exercises can begin. Activities of choice include seated hip flexion, straight leg raises, hip adduction, hip internal, and external rotation. These can all be easily performed using ankle weights. More intense activities, such as standing leg adduction (straight or bent knee), and step-ups can be performed, and PNF stretching if pain-free. Slide board, plyometrics, and functional drills are appropriate if the prior activities can be performed pain-free.

Grade 2. The grade 2 injury may be painful to palpation and have some swelling. There might be some alteration to the normal gait cycle. Walking will likely be slowed with a shortened stride length on the affected limb.

The athlete with these more moderate injuries can start the rehabilitation almost immediately, too, but should begin with very mild, pain-free active range of motion. Electrical stimulation has been used to limit inflammation, pain, and muscle spasm in an attempt to increase range of motion. Use isometrics if pain is not provoked. Once pain has subsided enough, the athlete can begin stretching and strengthening exercises similar to those described in the grade 1 section above. The athlete with this grade 2 strain is likely to miss up to 2 weeks of training and competition.

Grade 3. The athlete with the grade 3 groin injury will likely need crutches to ambulate. The injured area will be painful to the touch, swelling will be evident and the range of motion will be severely restricted. The athlete will probably be apprehensive about abduction and resistance to movement will not be tolerated. Complete rest and compression may be needed for up to 3 days. Low intensity isometrics and pain-free active range of motion can begin on day 3. Crutches should be used until a normal gait has been regained. The stretching and strengthening exercises previously described should probably not begin for 7–10 days after the injury and should progress very slowly up to slide board, functional training and plyometrics. An athlete with this grade 3 strain will likely be out of training and competition for 3 weeks to 3 months.

Hamstring Strains

Grade 1. An athlete with a grade 1 hamstring strain may have a normal gait pattern, but still report some hamstring stiffness at the extremes of hip flexion.

Grade 2. The athlete with a grade 2 strain can ambulate, but with an abnormal gait. Resisted knee flexion and hip extension are painful.

Grade 3. The athlete with a grade 3 strain will probably not be able to walk without the aid of crutches. Passive hip flexion with the knee extended might be tolerated. The initial treatment is ice, compression, and elevation along with active range of motion. A reasonable program that alternates (pain-free) single-joint open chain exercises with multi-joint closed chain exercises with sufficient rest has been clinically effective; for example, stationary cycling, StairMaster, and stretching (prone hamstring and gluteal stretches, standing hamstring stretching, hamstring PNF, seated and standing hip adductor stretching, assisted hip internal and ex-

ternal rotation stretching, and piriformis stretching). This should be followed by pain-free strengthening (prone leg curls, standing hip extensions, leg press), lunges, squats (vary feet placement depending on location of strain), and PNF stretching.

It is most important to regain a pain-free gait cycle and the use of crutches may be appropriate. Ice, compression, and low intensity stretches of the hamstring are usually started soon after the injury, often as early as the first day. These stretching exercises should isolate the hamstrings by making sure the athlete maintains a normal lordotic curve when performing the exercises. Electrical muscle stimulation can help with range of motion, lessen pain, and muscle spasm. Rehabilitation during the first 3 days should be devoted to pain-free active hip and knee range of motion in the prone position. Isometric hamstring contractions should, again, be pain-free. The early re-establishment of pain-free range of motion usually lessens the time the athlete is out of training and competition. After the third day, hot packs, whirlpools, and stretching (see above) can be initiated. Once these goals have been met, usually within the first week, the athlete can begin the strengthening program described above.

Quadriceps Strains

Most quadriceps strains involve the rectus femoris. Acute pain is usually felt, particularly after the workout has been completed. There may be some swelling and loss of flexion range of motion. A rectus femoris strain can be confirmed by eliciting pain when the athlete lies prone, extends the hip and the knee is flexed.

Grade 1. Ice, compression, active range of motion exercises and isometric strengthening can begin almost immediately. After about 2 days, resistance exercises can be initiated. These exercises might include straight leg raises, isotonic leg extensions (seated and lying), hip flexion (bent knee and straight leg), leg presses and squats (rack and free weights). Stretching of the rectus femoris should be pain-free. Use some form of compression until the athlete is free of pain and is free of muscle tightness.

Grade 2. Icing and crutch walking should begin immediately and the muscle should have some form of compression 24 h a day. Electrical stimulation has been used in these first days to limit swelling, inflammation, pain, and minimize the loss of range of motion. Once the athlete is free of pain, isometric quadriceps contractions and pain-free range of motion (sitting and lying prone) should progress to increasing range of motion by lying over the edge of a table to further isolate the rectus femoris. Ice should be used along with the above exercises to regain motion.

After about a week, if the unweighted exercises just mentioned can be performed without pain, then light resistance can be added. After about a week of pain-free light resistance exercises, the athlete increases the weight for straight leg raises and adds seated and lying knee extensions. Swimming and biking can be added so long as powerful kicking is avoided and the cycle seat is high enough that pain is not produced. Passive, pain-free stretching can begin 7–14 days after the injury.

Grade 3. This serious injury puts the athlete on crutches for 1–2 weeks. Ice, compression, and electrical stimulation should be used as close to 24 h a day as possible. The athlete must have a pain-free range of motion before the compression can be removed. Once pain-free, the athlete can start *gentle* isometric quadriceps contractions and active range of motion exercises. Lying, seated and prone active range of motion should be performed. However, take care to avoid overstretching the quadriceps. Ice is helpful and heat can be used as the athlete gets closer to full range of motion. Straight leg raises can begin, but weight should not be added for 10–14 days post injury. From this point on, the athlete follows the progression outlined for grade 2 quadriceps strains. Full range of motion should be achieved by 4 weeks. Only at this time should quadriceps stretching exercises be implemented.

Table 2. Criteria for full return to sports

Injury Site	Criteria for full return to sports
Hip flexor and groin	1. Full ROM of the hip 2. Adductor strength and endurance equal to the uninvolved side 3. Ability to ambulate (walk, jog, run, hop) on the involved extremity without any compensation 4. Successful completion of a sport specific functional progression with no residual groin symptoms 5. Successful performance on functional tests (sprints, shuttle run, hop tests, etc.)
Hamstrings	1. Full ROM at hip at knee 2. Muscle strength and endurance equal to uninvolved side 3. Ability to ambulate (walk, jog, run, hop) without compensation 4. Isokinetic ratios (hamstring/quadriceps) equal to uninvolved leg 5. No residual symptoms after sport-specific functional progression exercises 6. Successful performance of functional tests (e.g., shuttle, sprints, hop tests)
Quadriceps	1. Same as hamstring
Gastrocnemius	1. Full ROM of foot and ankle 2. Gastrocnemius strength and endurance equal to noninvolved side 3. Walk, jog, run, hop on involved without compensation 4. Completion of sport-specific functional program without residual symptoms

Gastrocnemius Strains

A most important consideration in the initial management of a gastrocnemius strain is ICE with special emphasis on elevation to prevent edema in the foot. Avoiding edema is important because range of motion (ROM) can be limited and extend the rehabilitation process. Early, gentle stretching of the muscle can be followed by plantarflexor strengthening elastic bands or tubing. The athlete may bear weight using crutches, as tolerated. Dorsiflexion of the ankle, as in walking, can be painful, so the athlete may prefer crutches when holding the foot in the less painful plantarflexed position, or put heel lifts in their shoe to relieve the stretch on the muscle.

The athlete should perform gentle stretching of the calf using a towel several times a day. Active range of motion for all planes of the foot will also stretch the injured muscle. After about 7–10 days, the athlete should have a normal gait and be able to do standing calf stretches and strengthening exercises like standing double and single-leg toe raises.

The more moderate calf muscle strains may require 2–4 weeks to normalize gait due to the amount of edema in the foot and ankle. As soft tissue heals, the athlete can move from open to closed chain activities such as active plantar/dorsiflexion and inversion/eversion in a seated position plus balancing activities and resisted elastic band exercises while standing.

Evidence of a normal walking gait allows the athlete to progress to a progressive jogging program that gradually increases jogging volume and intensity. Once comfortable with jogging, plyometric exercises can be added, allowing for 1–2 days recovery to allow delayed onset muscle soreness to diminish. Sport-specific training can begin once the athlete has progressed through these steps. Most of these injuries show good healing 2–3 weeks post injury. See the criteria for full return to sports in Table 2.

Contusion Injuries

A most common form of muscle contusion is to the quadriceps and this is the example to be presented.

Grade 1. After a mild contusion, the athlete will most likely continue to show a normal pattern of gait. Swelling is unusual, but there may be some minor discomfort with palpation. Their range of motion should be normal and resisted knee extension should not cause discomfort.

Grade 2. The athlete with a grade 2 contusion also might have a normal gait. However, they may try to continue sports until the injury hinders performance. When the gait becomes abnormal, the athlete 'splints' the knee in extension to stabilize the knee and prevent the knee from collapsing and externally rotates at the hip and 'pulls the leg through' during the swing phase of gait. There is a noticeable defect, pain on palpation and a loss of 30 – 45° of prone, active range of motion. The therapist will notice quadriceps weakness with resisted knee extension.

Grade 3. Disability, severe bleeding, a marked defect, and herniation of the muscle through the fascia are common in the athlete with the grade 3 contusion. There is an extreme loss in range of motion when the athlete lies prone. Resisted knee extension may not be tolerated.

Icing and 24-h compression of the grade 1 contusion should begin immediately and the compression should continue until the absence of all signs and symptoms. Low intensity quadriceps stretching can begin on day 1 and progressive quadriceps strengthening usually starts on the second day. Strengthening exercises include straight leg raises, seated and supine leg extensions, as well as bent and straight leg hip flexion, leg presses, and isokinetics. The athlete should be carefully monitored for any loss of range of motion that would necessitate re-grading the injury to a grade 2.

Rehabilitation of a grade 2 injury begins conservatively with the use of crutches until the athlete has normal gait and is pain-free. The use of ice and 24-h compression can begin immediately and electrical stimulation may be help control swelling, inflammation and pain while promoting range of motion. Isometric quadriceps contractions can begin early, often by the third day. Ice and active, pain-free range of motion exercises (lying and sitting) continue through the fifth day. Massage and heat are not recommended as these tend to promote bleeding and the risk of myositis ossificans. Straight leg raises with resistance can begin at about day 5. Once the athlete has about 100° of active knee flexion range of motion, aquatic therapy, swimming, and cycling can begin. If the athlete has full, prone range of motion and no swelling, then heat therapy and ultrasound can be used. Progressive quadriceps strengthening (see grade 1) can begin after about 7 – 10 days. Do not rush the use of quadriceps stretching exercises; these should be delayed until around days 10 – 14.

The major difference between rehabilitation of the grade 2 and grade 3 injuries is in the initial stages. The use of crutches, rest, ice, 24-h compression, and electrical stimulation can begin immediately. However, the use of isometric quadriceps contractions does not begin until around days 5 – 7 (as opposed to day 3 for the grade 2 injury). The protocol then is similar, allowing for the initial adjustment at the outset of treatment. The timetables for both the grade 2 and 3 injuries may need to be tailored to the severity of each injury.

Myositis Ossificans

A serious direct blow to muscle can lead to tissue disruption, bleeding, and injury to the periosteum of the underlying bone that can lead to ectopic bone formation. Within 3 – 6 weeks, this ectopic bone growth can be visualized with X-rays. Proper treatment of a muscle contusion usually prevents myositis ossificans. Trying to 'play through' a grade 2 or 3 contusion, early aggressive massage, muscle stretching in spite of pain, can all lead to myositis ossificans.

One year after the original injury, surgical removal of the mass may be helpful. The condition might be aggravated if surgery is performed too soon. Rehabilitation should follow the guidelines discussed for grade 2 and 3 muscle contusions.

Summary

One of the most common injuries seen in the office of the practicing physician is muscle strain. Until recently, little data were available on the basic science of, and clinical application of this basic science for the treatment and prevention of muscle strains. Studies in the last 10 years represent action taken on the direction of investigation into muscle strain injuries from the laboratory and clinical fronts.

Findings from the laboratory indicate that certain muscles are susceptible to strain injury (muscles that cross multiple joints or have complex architecture). These muscles have a strain threshold for both passive and active injury. Strain injury is not the result of muscle contraction alone. Rather, strains are the result of excessive stretch or stretch while the muscle is being activated. When the muscle tears, the damaged is localized very near the muscle tendon junction. Following injury, the muscle is weaker and at risk of further injury. The force output of the muscle returns over the following days while the muscle undertakes a predictable progression toward tissue healing.

Current imaging studies have been used clinically to document the site of injury to the MTJ. The commonly injured muscles have been described. These include the hamstrings, the rectus femoris, the gastrocnemius and the adductor longus. Injuries inconsistent with involvement of a single MTJ prove to be at tendinous origins rather than within the muscle belly. Important information has also been provided regarding injuries with poor prognosis and which are potentially repairable surgically. These include injuries to the rectus femoris, the hamstring origin and the abdominal wall.

Data important to the management of common muscle injuries have been published. The risks of re-injury have been documented. The early efficacy and potential for long-term risks of nonsteroidal anti-inflammatory agents have been shown.

New data can also be applied to the field with respect to the beneficial effects of warm-up, temperature and stretching on the mechanical properties of muscle. These benefits potentially reduce the risks of strain injury to the muscle. Fortunately, many of the factors protecting muscle, such as strength, endurance and flexibility are also essential for maximum performance. Future studies are intended to delineate the repair and recovery process, emphasizing not only the recovery of function, but also the susceptibility to re-injury during the recovery phase.

The rehabilitation philosophy relative to inflammation and healing after injury to the musculotendinous unit is to assist the natural processes of the body while doing no harm. The course of rehabilitation chosen by the clinician must focus on their knowledge of the healing process and its therapeutic modifiers to guide, direct, and stimulate the structural function and integrity of the injured part. The primary goal should be to have a positive influence on the inflammation and repair process to expedite recovery of function in terms of range of motion, muscular strength and endurance, neuromuscular control, and cardiorespiratory endurance. The clinician must try and minimize the early effects of excessive inflammatory processes, including pain modulation, edema control, and reduction of associated muscle spasm, which can produce loss of joint motion and contracture. Finally, the clinician should concentrate on preventing the recurrence of injury by influencing the structural ability of the injured tissue to resist future overloads by incorporating various training techniques.

References

1. Abbott BC, Lowy J (1956) Stress relaxation in muscle. Proc R Soc Lond 146:281–288
2. Clarkson PM, Newham DJ (1995) Associations between muscle soreness, damage, and fatigue. Adv Exp Med Biol 384:457–69
3. Elftman H (1966) Biomechanics of muscle. J Bone Joint Surg. 48A:363
4. Friden J, Lieber RL (1992) Structural and mechanical basis of exercise-induced muscle injury. Med Sci Sports Exerc 24:521–30
5. Garrett WE Jr, Almekinders L, Seaver AV (1984) Biomechanics of muscle tears and stretching injuries. Trans Orthop Res Soc 9:384
6. Garrett WE Jr (1990) Muscle strain injuries: clinical and basic aspects. Med Sci Sports Exerc 22:436–443
7. Garrett WE Jr, Nikolaou PK, Ribbeck BM, Glisson RR, and Seaber AV (l988) The effect of muscle architecture on the biomechanical failure properties of skeletal muscle under passive extension. Am J Sports Med 16:7–12
8. Garrett WE Jr, Rich FR, Nikolaou PK, Vogler JB III (l989) Computed tomography of Hamstring muscle strains. Med Sci Sports Exerc 21:506–514
9. Glick JM (1980) Muscle strains. Prevention and treatment. Phys Sportsmed 8:73–77
10. Hasselman CT, Best TM, Hughes C, Martinez S, Garrett WE Jr, (1995) An explanation for various rectus femoris strain injuries using previously undescribed muscle architecture. Am J Sports Med 23:493–499
11. Howell JN, Chila AG, Ford G, David D, Gates T (1985) An electromyographic study of elbow motion during postexercise muscle soreness. J Appl Physiol 58:1713–8
12. Hughes C, Hasselman CT, Best TM, Martinez S, Garrett WE Jr, (1995) Incomplete, intrasubstance strain injuries of the rectus femoris. Am J Sports Med 23:500–506
13. Krejci V, Koch P (1979) Muscle and tendon injuries in athletes. Yearbook Medical Publ, Chicago
14. Mair SD, Seaber AV, Glisson RR, Garrett WE Jr (1996) The role of fatigue in susceptibility to acute muscle strain injury. Am J Sports Med 24:137–143
15. Nikolaou PK, Macdonald BL, Glisson RR, Seaber AV, Garrett WE Jr (1987) Biomechanical and histological evaluation of muscle after controlled strain injury. Am J Sports Med 15:9–14
16. Obremskey WT, Seaber AV, Ribbeck BM, Garrett WE Jr (1994) Biomechanical and histological assessment of a controlled muscle strain injury treated with piroxicam. Am J Sports Med 22:558–561
17. Peterson L, Renstrom P (1986). Sports Injuries: their prevention and treatment. In: William E. Grana (ed). Yearbook Medical Publishers, Chicago
18. Prentice WE (1999) Rehabilitation techniques in sports medicine. WCB/McGraw-Hill, Boston
19. Radin EL, Simon, SR, Rose RM, Paul IL (1979) Practical biomechanics for the orthopaedic surgeon. A Wiley Medical Publication, New York
20. Safron MR, Garrett WE Jr, Seaber AV, Glisson RR, Ribbeck BM, (1988) The role of warm-up in musclular injury prevention. Am J Sports Med 16:123–129
21. Sallay PI, Friedman RL, Coogan PG, Garrett WE Jr (1996) Hamstring injuries among water skiers. Functional outcome and prevention. Am J Sports Med 24:130–136
22. Sherman WM, Armstrong LE, Murray TM, Hagerman FC, Costill DL, Staron RC, Ivy JL (1984) Effect of a 42.2-km footrace and subsequent rest or exercise on muscular strength and work capacity. J Appl Physiol 57:1668–73
23. Speer KP, Lohnes J, Garrett WE Jr (1993) Radiographic imaging of muscle strain injury. Am J Sports Med 21:89–96
24. Stauber WT (1989) Eccentric action of muscles: physiology, injury and adaptation. Exerc Sports Sci Rev 17:157–185
25. Taylor DC, Dalton JD Jr, Seaber AV, Garrett WE Jr (l990) Viscoelastic properties of muscle-tendon units:the biomechanical effects of stretching. Am J Sports Med l8:300–309
26. Taylor DC, Seaber AV, Garrett WE (1985) Response of muscle tendon units to cyclic repetitive stretching. Trans Orthop Res Soc 10:84
27. Taylor DC, Meyers WC, Moylan JA, Lohnes J, Bassett FH III, Garrett WE Jr (l99l) Abdominal musculature abnormalities as a cause of groin pain in athletes: inguinal hernias and pubalgia. Am J Sports Med 19:239–242
28. Taylor DC, Dalton JD, Seaber AV, Garrett WE Jr (l993) Experimental muscle strain injury: early functional and structural deficits and the increased risk for reinjury. Am J Sports Med 21:190–194
29. Zarins B, Ciullo JV (1983). Acute muscle and tendon injuries in athletes. Clin Sports Med 2:167–182

16 Isokinetics in Rehabilitation

Kai-Ming Chan

Introduction

The hallmark of success in orthopaedic surgery is the quantification of functional results. As far as the patients are concerned, subjective evaluation still plays an important part in relation to relief of symptoms and disability and return to daily activities. In order to compare the results of different methods of treatment or different protocols in different centres, common quantifiable data which can correlate with the functional outcome are strongly desired. In the search for this quantification approach, the evolution of isokinetic assessment has made a significant contribution to the advancement of orthopaedic assessment and rehabilitation.

The concept of isokinetic assessment was first introduced by James Perrine in the late 1960s. While isometric and isotonic exercise still play an important role in certain stages of the rehabilitation programme, isokinetics has recently come into the lime light of the rehabilitation scene by virtue of its unique feature in providing an accommodating resistance throughout the range of motion (ROM) to allow for maximal dynamic loading.

The principal advantage of isokinetics over isometric and isotonic exercise is that it provides an accommodating resistance for muscle training and rehabilitation. Several reasons explain why isokinetic therapy is needed and isotonic testing alone is not adequate for rehabilitation and/or training. Traditional physical medicine employed isotonic testing, also known as weight training, to rehabilitate athletes to prepare them for a return to sports. Isotonic testing used weights which were increased as the limb was able to support it. There were two principal drawbacks to isotonic rehabilitation. First, the maximum weight that could be supported by the muscles was limited by the weakest point in the range of motion. Second, injury could result from falling weights or weights which exceeded the limits of the muscles. But with isokinetic therapy, the user encounters a resistance not greater than the amount of force applied to the machine. It allows the muscle to exert its own maximum strength throughout the ROM. This helps to ensure a safe and efficient treatment for the users. Besides, muscle strengthening can be instituted right

from the earliest stage of the treatment programme, thus enhancing rehabilitation by shortening the period of recovery.

Application of Isokinetic Assessment in the Sports Area

Rehabilitation of Sports Injuries

Isokinetic assessment has been extensively used as a rehabilitative tool for sports injuries in athletes. The application of isokinetics to sports medicine has made a significant contribution in the prevention, diagnosis and rehabilitation of sports injuries. Based on the principle of accommodating resistance, isokinetic devices can generate forces which can be reasonably well tolerated by joints and soft tissues. Every increase in the force applied to the lever arm will yield a proportional increase in resistance. Moreover, isokinetics can test the condition of every muscle group in the body and measure dynamic strength throughout the range of motion of a particular joint. Such variable resistance can avoid undue stress on the injured joint, and simultaneously allow maximal dynamic loading of the involved muscle throughout the exercised range of motion, thus eliminating the danger of re-injuries during early rehabilitation.

Generation of Normative Database in a Particular Population

A crucial aspect of isokinetic assessment is the development of normative databases in a particular population [4, 5, 8, 19, 20]. In most isokinetic testing devices, some computer software is included to provide convenient data collection and storage on a wide range of information on muscle characteristics (Fig. 1) More comprehensive interpretation of isokinetic testing variables can be achieved through data normalised for body weight and unilateral muscular strength ratios. The creation of such a scientifically derived normative isokinetic databank enables assessment of dynamic muscle characteristics in a variety of sedentary and athletic populations, both in males and females and

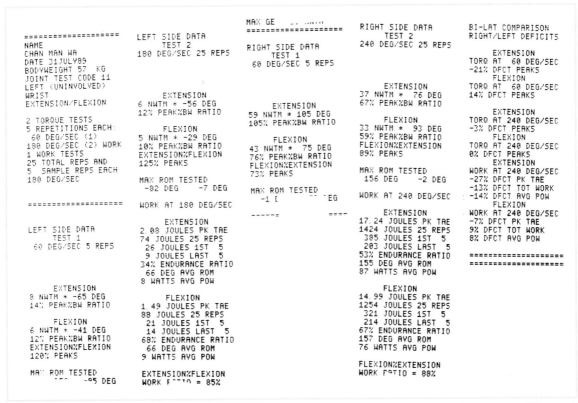

Fig. 1. Data report of a wrist test using Cybex II+ isokinetic dynamometer. (With the permission of Lippincott Williams and Wilkins)

over a range of ages and, more importantly, allows clinical evaluation and construction of well-defined training programs for a specific athletic group.

Objective Measurement of Muscle Strength

The isokinetic system excels in its ability to quantify data. It surpasses all isotonic systems in its ability to quantify variables such as peak torque and angle of occurrence, peak torque to body-weight ratio, total work, average range of motion and average power. Isokinetic assessment can provide objective assessment with provision for serial testing in the course of rehabilitation and/or training. Unlike other traditional methods such as manual muscle training (MMT), or isometric and isotonic exercises, isokinetic testing devices have shown their usefulness in providing objective quantification of muscle strength variables. The isokinetic technique quantifies changes in muscle strength at various angles in the ROM, and provides objective data on athlete's muscle performance at different stages in the course of rehabilitation and/or training. This objective information allows physicians to determine the athlete's readiness and ability to commence muscle rehabilitation after sports injuries.

Screening of Athletes

Before the concept of isokinetic exercise emerged [10], most clinicians relied on manual muscle testing and static dynamometers for measurement of muscle strength. These methods, though clinically useful in some conditions, provided little information on the dynamic qualities of muscle action. The isokinetic testing device, on the other hand, offers the possibility of objective quantification of the relative significance of muscle strength and power in specific sports. The data generated by isokinetics can also be used to compare the effects of different modes of treatment for sports injuries, or to correlate modes of exercise and training with the muscle performance of athletes.

In sports science, isokinetics plays an important role for athletic testing, rehabilitation and training. Isokinetic assessment provides an accurate, objective measurement of muscle strength for monitoring training-induced changes in muscle performance and evaluating the effectiveness of various strength-training programs. The ability to identify muscle imbalances also allows isokinetics to be used as a screening device for identifying potential talent and weakness in athletes before sports competition. Certain areas of the body are more susceptible to sports injuries, such as the external rotators of the shoulders in swimmers, the extensor muscle of the back in windsurfers and the hamstrings in runners. Identification of these areas of weakness enables physicians to gain more information about athletes' muscle performance and prevent them from potential sports injuries during a competition.

Advantages

Safety and Patient Compliance

Due to the accommodating nature of variable resistance, isokinetic assessment gives an excellent opportunity to start early rehabilitation with minimal risk of re-injury. Since the resistance is proportional to the applied force, it allows isolated muscle groups to exert maximum voluntary force throughout the entire ROM. This special feature offered by isokinetic devices can avoid pain and muscle fatigue, thus providing additional safety in rehabilitating muscle injuries.

Recent improvement in computer software also makes isokinetic devices more user-friendly. Visual display of the user-generated torque curve allows the user and the therapist to observe performance and progression during the test session. Since the assessment data are reflected on the computer monitor, users can clearly see the effort they have applied by simply referring to the shape of torque curve and the values attained for peak torque. This immediate feedback mechanism may serve as a source of motivation for the users. A past study also demonstrated the effect of visual feedback on muscle performance in isokinetic testing, as a greater increase in peak torque was found in testing sessions with visual and auditory electromyographic (EMG) feedback than in non-feedback sessions [6].

Reliability, Accuracy and Validity

The isokinetic technique, through careful validation over the years, has achieved high reliability. It allows the assessment data to be reproduced in two different units of the same type when the testing conditions and parameters are equal. Several studies have tested the reliability of isokinetic measurement and found correlation coefficients ranges between 0.93 and 0.99 [2, 9, 14, 16 – 18].

Furthermore, isokinetic testing also offers an objective, reproducible and quantifiable assessment of dynamic muscle function and provides accurate data on a range of muscle characteristics. The isokinetic assessment can be calibrated to assure accuracy in all forms of performance. Modern isokinetic dynamometers include specially designed computer software which can perform calculations on data such as torque, work and power, and provide assessment of muscle characteristics in terms of agonist/antagonist ratios, fatigue ratio,

bilateral difference, etc. Comparatively speaking, isokinetic devices generate results with higher accuracy than isometric and isoinertial exercises. The traditional isotonic and isometric modes of exercise, though widely adopted, lack the sensitivity to detect minor but significant changes in muscle strength. Isokinetic devices show their usefulness in the evaluation of muscle strength as they give a fairly precise overall assessment of the athlete's initial muscle performance and the progression made during rehabilitation and/or training.

The validity of isokinetic testing has also been shown through its wide adoption in rehabilitation of sports injuries and athletic screening. It generates relevant and meaningful quantifiable results which can correlate with functional activities with reference to a special clinical problem. The relationship between isokinetic exercise and functional activities is important for the inclusion of isokinetic exercise in rehabilitation programme to enhance muscle performance.

Disadvantages

Cost of Equipment, Availability of Time and Personnel

The use of isokinetic equipment in clinical and athletic settings requires huge capital investment. The cost of an isokinetic machine is considerable, and it may not be easily affordable for the practitioner. Also, the instrumentation of isokinetic testing also involves manpower and time. In order to compile a full set of data, isokinetic assessment usually takes quite some time to work on a joint, and therefore it cannot be used for routine assessment. Moreover, a team of experienced, specially trained personnel who are familiar with the testing procedures is also necessary for the generation of efficient, reliable and valid isokinetic results.

Functional Applicability and Standardisation of Testing Protocols

The major limitation of an isokinetic dynamometer lies in the applicability of isokinetic-derived results to functional activities. Most current isokinetic dynamometers do not exceed angular velocities of 450°/s. This test velocity becomes minimal compared with the actual dynamic sporting movements. Some scientists also argue that the force applied by isokinetic dynamometers is 'unnatural' and the motion involved is not related to that which occurs during sporting performance [11, 15]. In the field of rehabilitation and injury prevention, objective measures of muscle function are essential. However, it is also important to understand the fact that laboratory measurements do not necessarily reflect functional performance, and therefore the functional applicability of isokinetic measurement still remains questionable.

The reliability of isokinetic measurement is largely determined by the availability of carefully standardised pre-test procedures. Use of standardised testing protocols is crucial for the generation of a meaningful and accurate normative isokinetic database. In this regard, the pre-test procedures should be standardised in all testing situations so that intra-tester and inter-tester results can be compared. Factors such as subject familiarisation, patient set-up and warm-up, differences in positioning and stabilisation of the subject, as well as presence or absence of verbal encouragement may affect the reliability of isokinetic measurement. Subject reliability is even a strong confounding factor, as the patient's willingness to generate maximum effort and their tolerance of the discomfort while performing the test are always uncontrollable.

Importance of Eccentric Loading Exercise

Many dynamic movements such as lowering a heavy object, lowering the body and walking downhill involve eccentric actions [3]. Eccentric actions can produce greater muscle tension and therefore they are more effective in improving muscle strength [1]. Dean [7] proposed in 1988 that eccentric training provides more benefits to patients with limited exercise capacity because eccentric work is normally associated with lower metabolic cost and greater muscle strength compared with concentric work.

Human movements rarely involve pure forms of isolated concentric or eccentric actions. Many athletic and daily activities involve both eccentric and concentric actions. Wu et al. [21] conducted a study in 1997 on the relationship between isokinetic concentric and eccentric contraction modes in the knee flexor and extensor muscle groups using the Cybex 6000 isokinetic dynamometer (Fig. 2). All concentric and eccentric variables were highly correlated, with correlation coefficients ranging from 0.67 to 0.93. Except for two variables, all eccentric variables were greater than the concentric ones. These results suggested that in order to plan a proper rehabilitation program and prevent possible injuries, it is necessary to measure both concentric and eccentric muscle action variables.

However, until recently, most isokinetic systems offered only concentric loading to the muscle and there seems to be a lack of information on the important role of eccentric modes of exercise. Most research has centred on the effects of concentric exercise and less is known about eccentric exercise. Recognition of the importance of eccentric exercise can provide a stimulus for the integration of this measurement into the overall isokinetic assessment.

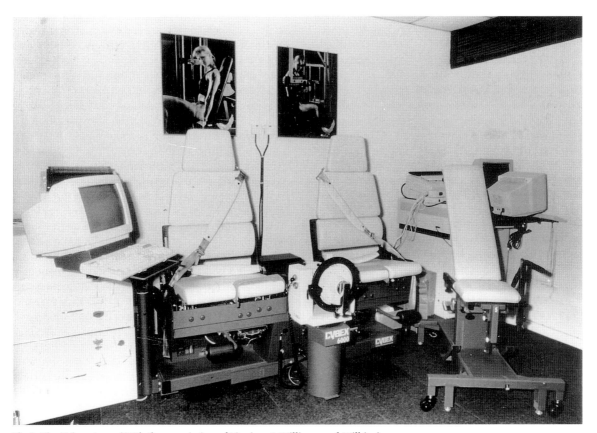

Fig. 2. The Cybex 6000. (With the permission of Lippincott Williams and Wilkins)

Illustrations of Practical Application of Isokinetics in Sports Injuries Rehabilitation

Over the past few years, the research team from the Department of Orthopaedics and Traumatology at the Chinese University of Hong Kong, conducted a series of studies on the use of isokinetics in the assessment of muscle performance of different anatomical regions such as the knee, shoulder and ankle to define statistically the span of normality among the Chinese population, and to characterise muscle performance in sports injuries. These studies have laid a solid scientific foundation for the development of isokinetic technology in the rehabilitative regimes.

Several common sports injuries encountered in Hong Kong are: meniscal injury, anterior cruciate ligament injury (ACL), chondromalacia patella, shoulder impingement syndrome, complex unstable ligamental injuries of the ankle, tennis elbow, and muscular and ligamental injuries of the back. The rehabilitation of the above injuries requires a quantitative approach utilizing isokinetic assessment and training. The following studies provided a quantitative approach in the rehabilitation of sports injuries with special emphasis on the efficacy of isokinetic assessment and training in the rehabilitation of injuries to the knee, ankle and shoulder.

Knee

Anterior cruciate ligament injury is a common and challenging problem in sports medicine. The management of ACL injury still remains highly controversial. Therefore, it is important to have an objective and quantitative assessment on the indication of surgical treatment and to assess the efficiency of the rehabilitation and/or training programme. In this study of ACL injury, isokinetics was used to define a significant correlation between an objective assessment parameter and the functional knee score.

The study hypothesised that, by increasing the hamstrings and quadriceps (H:Q) isokinetic strength ratio through strengthening the hamstrings, the functional ability of an ACL-deficient knee will improve. Forty-six recreational athletes with a completely torn off ACL were recruited to the study. The muscle performance of the subjects was measured in terms of peak torque, endurance ratio, total work and explosive power. The functional ability of the injured knee was scored using the Cincinnati rating system which grades the severity of pain and swelling; the degree of giving way (i.e., a sudden loss of instability); and the overall ability to walk, run, ascend and descend steps, and jump and twist.

The results showed that all variables involving hamstring strength have significant correlation with the functional ability score ($p < 0.01$), whereas none of the variables involving quadriceps strength were significantly correlated with the functional ability of the injured knee ($p > 0.05$) [12]. The highly significant correlation between the H:Q ratio and the functional ability of ACL-deficient knees can be used as an additional measure to guide in the decision-making process in the management of ACL-deficient knees in Chinese recreational athletes.

Ankle

In most people's minds, an ankle sprain often appears to be trivial because it is quite a common sports injury. However, athletes with sprains often report related residual symptoms. An epidemiological survey on ankle sprains was conducted among local Hong Kong Chinese athletes between June 1990 and June 1991 with a total of 380 respondents. The survey revealed that 73.5% of athletes had sustained recurrent ankle sprains, and 59% of ankle sprains had related residual symptoms. Pain and immobility which resulted from an ankle sprain would lead to secondary muscle atrophy, thus muscle weakness was often reported. This muscle weakness, especially the ankle evertor, caused a decrease in dynamic support of the ankle mortise and placed the ankle joint at risk of recurrent injuries.

In this study, isokinetic testing for ankle dorsiflexion, plantarflexion, inversion and eversion (Figs. 3, 4) at slow (60°/s) and fast (180°/s) speeds were employed to obtain a complete profile of various muscular parameters of the ankle, including peak torque, average power, total work and torque acceleration energy. A baseline study for subjects with bilateral non-injured ankles was first carried out to obtain normative data for comparison between dominant and non-dominant ankles. Isokinetic testing results revealed a generalised decrease in various muscular parameters in the injured dominant ankle and a significant decrease in various muscular parameters of ankle evertor in the injured ankles ($p < 0.05$) [22].

An isokinetic velocity spectrum training protocol was then designed for exercising the injured ankles. The protocol included a spectrum of velocities for training different types of muscle fibres for enhancing neurological and motor responses. Results in the retest indicated that the exercise protocol was effective in improving all muscular parameters of the ankle ($p < 0.05$). It also enhanced the functional performance of the injured ankles through the subjective ankle functional rating scale re-evaluation ($p < 0.05$) [22].

The findings showed that ankle sprain was never a trivial injury. Muscle weakness, especially the ankle evertor, was present through an objective isokinetic assessment of various muscular parameters of the ankle. Strengthening of the weakened ankle showed that a

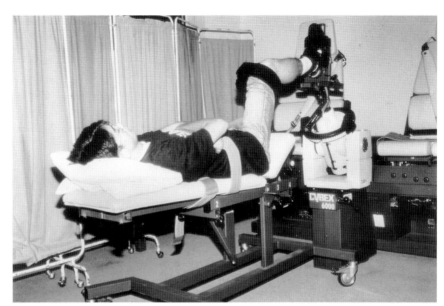

Fig. 3. Testing of ankle inversion/eversion. (With the permission of Lippincott Williams and Wilkins)

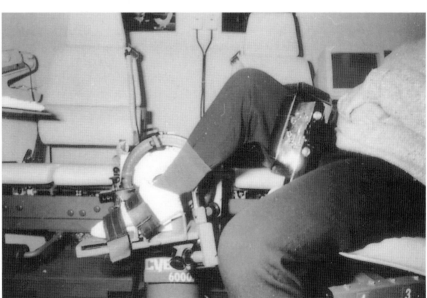

Fig. 4. Testing of ankle dorsiflexion/plantarflexion. (With the permission of Lippincott Williams and Wilkins)

positive effect in improving the functional performance of the ankle could also be attained.

Shoulder

The prevalence of shoulder impingement syndrome among elite athletes of regular upper arm sporting events could be claimed to be the result of the constant demand of bringing their arms at or above shoulder level to strive for speed and top performance. In this study, 45 athletes who were diagnosed to be suffering from shoulder impingement syndrome were examined for functional capability of their affected arm.

Twenty-seven athletes with supraspinatus tendinitis underwent an isokinetic evaluation to see if their mo-

tor performance of reciprocal flexion/extension (Fig. 5), abduction/adduction (Fig. 6) and internal/external rotation (Fig. 7) in the affected shoulders had significant difference over the unaffected sides, and whether this difference between the two shoulders was similar to that of a control group.

General results indicated that there were significant differences in all movement parameters between the two sides among impingement subjects except the endurance ratio. In comparing the impingement group with the control group, a significant difference could only be found in the endurance ratio in flexion and total work in external rotation. From the isokinetic torque graphs of the impingement subjects, it was shown that the presence of a trough at 100° of flexion

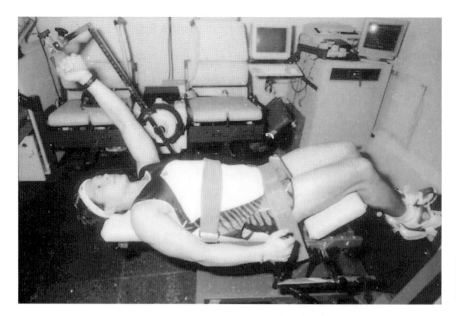

Fig. 5. Testing of shoulder flexion/extension. (With the permission of Lippincott Williams and Wilkins)

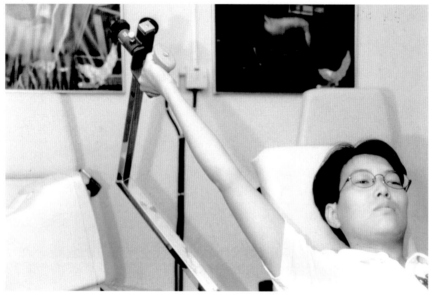

Fig. 6. Testing of shoulder abduction/adduction. (With the permission of Lippincott Williams and Wilkins)

and abduction was statistically significant ($p < 0.05$) [13]. Such a finding correlated with a biomechanical study which showed that maximal compressive stress is found at 100° in flexion and abduction, and such stress increases with internal rotation and decreases with external rotation. Despite the absence of the relative muscular force acting around the shoulder complex in the cadaver, and even though the adoption of the studied position was different from the normal functional posture, the study revealed the pattern of stress upon the supraspinatus tendon during passive arm positioning.

Elite athletes of upper arm events have greater demand for prolonged performance which induces repeated 'trapping' of the supraspinatus tendon within the subacromial space, leading to the occurrence of shoulder impingement syndrome. Further investigation on living subjects of the loading acting upon this structure may enhance the effective use of the upper arm in athletic training and the avoidance of such a shoulder problem.

Future Directions

The recent development of isokinetic technology has shown its usefulness in the rehabilitation of sports injuries and training of muscle performance in athletes. The continual modification and improvement in isokinetic devices allows sports professionals to design a

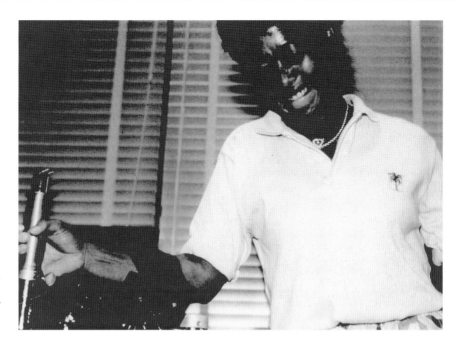

Fig. 7. Testing of shoulder internal/external rotation. (With the permission of Lippincott Williams and Wilkins)

more effective and efficient rehabilitation and/or training program.

When looking at the future direction of isokinetics development, there are several areas to consider. First, it is of paramount importance that the new isokinetic technology does not raise the cost of health care enormously. More economical and user-friendly isokinetic devices must be designed to maximise the utilisation of isokinetics in the sports field. The use of isokinetic devices in testing large muscle groups such as the hip and trunk is also another important aspect. The recent development of a trunk testing device may further enhance isokinetic assessment of muscle strength in this area. Also, the effects of isokinetic eccentric actions must also be extensively studied, as past studies have demonstrated the importance of this type of muscle action for the development of strength in relation to specific training and rehabilitation programs. In this regard, with the further improvement in isokinetic technology, new testing and training devices should include both concentric and eccentric modes so that sports professionals can have a more comprehensive understanding of their effects on muscle performance in rehabilitation and/or training. Moreover, the reliability and validity of isokinetic measurement are also important areas for further research. A consensus on reliable and valid isokinetic measures is essential for the development of meaningful databases. More sport-specific and functional patterns of movement also need to be investigated in greater depth in order to make the testing protocols.

In summary, a more comprehensive study of isokinetic technology in the current health economy is extremely important as it helps to justify the usefulness and effectiveness in the overall patient care system. Failure to weigh the relative liabilities against the potential advantages of isokinetics for patient care can cause great harm to a clinician's professionalism and the patient's treatment outcome. To strive for a balance between science and applicability, the further development of isokinetics should not simply focus on the improvements in existing testing devices, but more importantly, the interplay of solid scientific research and continuous clinical application.

References

1. Albert M (1995) Physiological and clinical principles of eccentrics. In: Albert M (ed) Eccentric muscle training in sports and orthopedics. 2nd edn. Churchill Livingstone, London, pp 23–35
2. Bemben MG, Grump KJ, Massey BH (1988) Assessment of technical accuracy of the Cybex II isokinetic dynamometer and analogue recording system. J Orthop Sports Phys Ther 7(4):12–17
3. Chan KM (1996) Introduction to isokinetics: scientific and medical aspects of isokinetics. In: Chan KM, Maffulli N (eds) Principles and practice of isokinetics in sports medicine and rehabilitation. Williams and Wilkins Asia-Pacific Ltd, Hong Kong, pp 31–69
4. Chin MK, Lo YSA, Li CT, So CH (1992) Physiological profiles of Hong Kong elite soccer. Br J Sports Med 26(4): 262–266
5. Chin MK, So CH, Yuan WY, Li CT, Wong SK (1994) Cardiorespiratory fitness and isokinetic muscle strength of elite Asian junior soccer players. J Sports Med Phys Fitness: 34(3): 250–257
6. Croce RV (1986) The effects of EMG biofeedback on strength acquisition. Biofeedback Self-Regulation 11:299–310

7. Dean E (1988) Physiological and therapeutic implications of negative work. Phys Ther 68:233–237

8. Ellenbacker TS (1996) Round table discussion. In: Chan KM, Maffulli N (eds) Principles and practice of isokinetics in sports medicine and rehabilitation. Williams and Wilkins Asia-Pacific Ltd, Hong Kong, pp 73–77

9. Farrell M, Richards JG (1986) Analysis of the reliability and validity of the kinetic communicator exercise device. Med Sci Sports Exerc 18(1):44–49

10. Hislop HJ, Perrine JJ (1967) The isokinetic concept of exercise. Phys Ther 47:114–117

11. Kannus P (1994) Isokinetic evaluation of muscular performance: implications for muscle testing and rehabilitation. Int J Sports Med 15:S11-S18

12. Li CT, Maffulli N, Chan KM, Hsu YC (1996) Isokinetic strength of the quadriceps and hamstrings and functional ability of anterior cruciate deficient knees in recreational athletes. Br J Sports Med 30: 161–164

13. Lo YP (1990) Shoulder impingement syndrome in Chinese: a functional and clinical study. Thesis, Division of Clinical and Pathological Science, Graduate School, The Chinese University of Hong Kong

14. Magnusson SP, Gleim GW, Nicholas JA (1990) Subject variability of shoulder abduction strength testing. Am J Sports Med 18(4):349–353

15. Mahler P, Mora C, Gremion G et al (1992) Isotonic muscle evaluation and sprint performance. Excel 8:139–145

16. Mawdsley RH, Knapik JJ (1982) Comparison of isokinetic measurements with test repetitions. Phys Ther 62(2):169–172

17. Moffroid M, Whipple R, Hofkosh J et al (1969) A study of isokinetic exercise. Phys Ther 49:735–746

18. Molnar GE, Alexander J (1973) Objective, quantitative muscle testing in children: a pilot study. Arch Phys Med Rehabil 54:225–228

19. So CH, Siu T, KM Chan, Chin MK, Li CT (1994) Isokinetic profile of dorsiflexors and plantar flexors of the ankle – a comparative study of elite versus untrained subjects. Br J Sports Med 28(1): 25–30

20. So CH, Siu T, Chin MK, Chan KM (1995) Bilateral isokinetic variables of the shoulder: a prediction model for young men. Br J Sports Med 29(2): 105–109

21. Wu Y, Li CT, Maffulli N, Chan KM (1997) Relationship between isokinetic concentric and eccentric contraction modes in the knee flexor and extensor muscle groups. J Orthop Sports Phys Ther 26(3):143–149

22. Yeung MS (1992) Isokinetic rehabilitation of ankle sprain. Thesis, Division of Clinical and Pathological Sciences, Graduate School, The Chinese University of Hong Kong

Chapter 17

Eccentric Exercise in the Treatment of Tendon Injuries in Sport

Nick A. Evans, Bal Rajagopalan, William D. Stanish

Introduction

Injury to the soft connective tissues is the most common disability associated with sporting activities at all levels of participation [1, 2]. Whenever these structures are subjected to forces that exceed their individual biomechanical limits, injury incites a complex healing response, necessary for successful tissue repair. For many years, sports medicine has sought to modify the reparative process, alleviate disability, and potentially expedite the return to sporting activity. Despite these intense efforts, the management of these injuries continues to pose difficulties. The extensive array of treatment options available, including chemical and physical methods, as well as surgical interventions, suggests persistent deficiencies in our understanding of the underlying pathological processes. As we proceed into the twenty-first century, the observations of ancient scientists are still relevant, and future investigators may question our current progress. Hippocrates (c 460–380 B.C.) stated that "Healing is a matter of time, but is sometimes also a matter of opportunity" [3], an observation which still applies today despite the multitude of interventions available.

The purpose of this chapter is to discuss the use of eccentric exercise as a physical method for the treatment of tendon injuries. The relevant basic science and previous scientific research will be reviewed in order to appreciate the rationale behind the development of this form of therapeutic intervention.

Tendon Basic Science

Structure

Tendon is a connective tissue band that anchors muscle to bone. Its prime function is to transmit the force generated by muscular contraction, thereby facilitating joint movement. Like all musculoskeletal connective tissues, tendon ultrastructure consists of mesenchymal cells bathed in a supporting extracellular matrix of fibrous proteins and gel-like ground substance. Healthy tendon comprises around 65–70% water, and the relative composition of its dry mass is 70% collagen, 2% elastin, and 28% proteoglycan. The physical characteristics of tendon are primarily due to the fibrous components, namely the collagen fibers which provide tensile strength, and the elastin fibers which are responsible for tendon flexibility [4]. Being a predominantly extracellular tissue with low metabolic requirements, tendon has a low blood supply compared with other tissues, which accounts for its white appearance on macroscopic inspection. Its nerve supply is mostly afferent, with neighboring nerve trunks providing Golgi organ

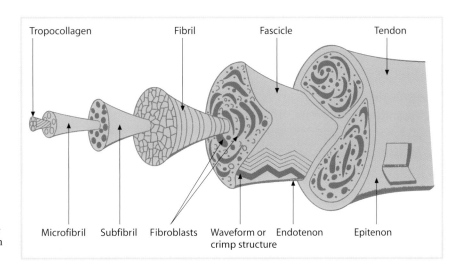

Fig. 1. Hierarchical structure of tendon. (With permission from [5])

Tropocollagen   Fibril   Fascicle   Tendon

Microfibril   Subfibril   Fibroblasts   Waveform or crimp structure   Endotenon   Epitenon

mechanoreceptors, pressure-sensing Ruffini and Pacinian corpuscles, and free nerve-ending pain receptors.

The anatomical structure of tendon exhibits a hierarchical organization of fibrillar collagen subunits of increasing size, compartmentalized within sheaths of connective tissue (Fig. 1) [5]. In order to perform its function, tendon is linked to muscle at one end, and to bone at the other. At the myotendinous junction (MTJ), the tension generated by muscle fibers is transmitted from intracellular contractile proteins to extracellular connective tissue. Despite local modifications to improve anchoring between muscle and tendon, the MTJ is the weakest link in the muscle-tendon-bone unit [6]. At the osteotendinous junction (OTJ), there is a gradual transition from soft tendon to hard bone by way of fibrocartilage [7].

Function

Tendon is the strongest component in the muscle-tendon-bone unit, exhibiting an in vitro tensile strength of between 50 to 100 N/mm² [8], approximately half that of stainless steel. Thus a tendon with a cross-sectional area of 1 cm² is capable of supporting a weight of 500 to 1000 kg.

The mechanical behavior of tendon during loading can be appreciated by considering its stress-strain curve (Fig. 2), which comprises four regions: (1) toe, (2) linear, (3) micro-failure, and (4) macroscopic failure [5]. The crimped configuration of collagen at rest disappears at 2% strain as the fibers progressively straighten during tendon loading (toe region). Beyond

this point, the tendon deforms in a linear fashion due to the molecular sliding of collagen triple helices. This deformation is reversible (elastic), and the tendon will return to its original length when unloaded, provided the strain does not exceed 4%. Under normal physiological circumstances, the strain resides within this 'safe' zone, and the tensile stress through the tendon rarely exceeds one quarter of its ultimate strength. If loading continues beyond this point into the micro-failure region, collagen fibers slide past one another, cross links fail, and the tendon undergoes irreversible plastic deformation. Macroscopic failure occurs once the tendon is stretched to 8–10% of its original length.

Tendon Injury

Injury is the loss of cells or extracellular matrix resulting from trauma, and represents a failure of cell-matrix adaptation to either sudden overload or cumulative overuse [9]. The subsequent healing response depends on whether the connective tissue injury is the result of acute macrotraumatic destruction, or chronic microtraumatic insult.

Acute Macrotraumatic Injury

Acute injury resulting from a sudden overload crisis, initiates a healing response which may be divided into three overlapping phases: (1) inflammation, (2) repair, and (3) remodeling [10]. The initial inflammatory response begins with the onset of vascular disruption,

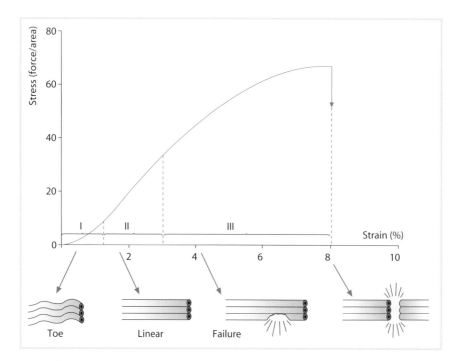

Fig. 2. Stress-strain curve of tendon. (With permission from [5])

and is characterized by the cardinal signs of redness, swelling, heat and pain. During the 3–5 days of this phase, some initial wound strength is provided, damaged tissue is removed, and reparative cells are recruited and activated. This sets the scene for the repair phase in which the damaged cells and matrix are replaced by scar tissue. During this proliferative period, the events are coordinated by macrophages, and the tenocyte, acting as a modified fibroblast, synthesizes collagen and matrix glycoproteins. This phase begins at 48 h and lasts up to 8 weeks. During the final remodeling phase, the cellularity and synthetic activity decreases, while the matrix becomes organized and collagen matures. Despite the remodeling effort, the material properties of scar tissue never match those of intact tendon. Biochemical differences in collagen, water and proteoglycan content persist indefinitely, and the final mechanical properties can be reduced by up to 30% [11].

Chronic Microtraumatic Injury

Chronic injury results from cumulative overuse and subthreshold structural damage, and is characterized by a slow, insidious onset. The inflammatory cell infiltrate and phased repair seen in macrotrauma is absent or aborted, and the distinguishing histological feature is a 'degenerative' change to a weaker, less metabolically active tissue [12, 13]. Cell atrophy and dystrophic calcification are also features of this imbalanced cell-matrix.

Chronic tendinitis can be divided into two subgroups: (1) exogenous tendinitis – which occurs as a consequence of pressure from external forces, e.g. subacromial impingement of the supraspinatus tendon; and (2) endogenous tendinitis – where the tendon itself is not of sufficient strength to meet the expectation of the applied forces, responding with microruptures within its substance.

Based on the anatomical location of the histopathological changes, it is possible to classify microtraumatic tendon injury into four types [14, 15]: (1) tendinitis – tendon strain or tear; (2) tendinosis – intratendinous degeneration; (3) paratenonitis – inflammation of the paratenon only; and (4) paratenonitis with tendinosis. This terminology is explained further in Table 1 [9].

Tendon Healing

Rest has long been advocated as a method in the treatment of tendon injuries. Indeed, if loading stresses are

Table 1. Terminology of tendon injury (after [9], [15])

New	Old	Definition	Histological findings	Clinical signs and symptoms
Paratenonitis	Tenosynovitis, Tenovaginitis, Peritendinitis	An inflammation of only the paratenon, either lined by synovium or not	Inflammatory cells in paratenon or peritendinous areolar itssue	Cardinal inflammatory signs; swelling, pain, crepitation, local tenderness, warmth, dysfunction
Paratenonitis with tendinosis	Tendinitis	Paratenon inflammation associated with intratendinosis degeneration	Same as I, with loss of tendon collagen fiber disorientation, scattered vascular ingrowth but no prominent intratendinous inflammation	Same as I, with often palpable tendon nodule, swelling, and inflammatory signs
Tendinosis	Tendinitis	Intradunous degeneration due to atrophy (aging, microtrauma, vascular compromise, etc.)	Noninflammatory intratendinous collagen degeneration with fiber disorientation, hypocellularity, scattered vascular ingrowth, occasional local necrosis or calcification	Often palpable tendon nodule that can be asymptomatic, but may also be point tender. Swelling of tendon sheath is absent
Tendinitis	Tendon strain or tear	Symptomatic degeneration of the tendon with vascular disruption and inflammatory repair response	Three recognized subgroups: each displays variable histology from purely inflammation with acute hemorrhage and tear, to inflammation superimposed upon pre-existing degeneration, to calcification and tendinosis changes in chronic conditions. In chronic stage there may be:	Symptoms are inflammatory and proportional to vascular disruption, hematoma, or atrophy-related cell necrosis. Symptom duration defines each subgroup
	A. Acute (less than 2 weeks) B. Subacute (4–6 weeks) C. Chronic (over 6 weeks)		1. Interstitial microinjury 2. Central tendon necrosisd 3. Frank partial rupure 4. Acute complete rupture	

removed from an injured tendon, symptoms usually subside. However, all musculoskeletal tissues atrophy under conditions of decreased load, and numerous studies have demonstrated the deleterious effect that rest and immobilization have on both normal and injured tendon [16–18]. After 8 weeks of immobilization, collagen degradation exceeds synthesis, thereby reducing the total collagen content. Newly synthesized collagen is immature with reduced crosslinks, making it less capable of withstanding tensile loading. Even normal ligaments, when immobilized for 8 weeks in a primate model, may take 12 months to return to normal strength [19].

Conversely, exercise loading of tendon causes both structural (hypertrophy) and material (stronger per unit area) adaptations, which increase tensile strength. Exercise accelerates collagen metabolism, increases collagen fiber density and crimp angle, producing a stronger tendon with reduced elastic modulus [16, 20–22].

Tendon injury induces an intrinsic (tendinous) and extrinsic (adjacent tissue) healing response, and the latter is responsible for the formation of peritendinous adhesions. For this reason, continuous passive motion (CPM) is superior to immobilization in its effect on tendon healing, by reducing the amount of adhesive scar tissue, and improving tendon excursion [23].

Much of the knowledge on tendon healing is derived from the study of the events following tendon laceration. The timing of biochemical and mechanical changes suggest that the healing tendon can be subjected to small forces within a matter of days. Such loading improves the strength of the healing tissue, and these observations have led to the design of early motion programs after tendon repair.

Confusion arises, however, when applying this information to tendinitis. The situation is different to tendon laceration; an initiating event may not be identifiable, and chronic pathological changes may already

exist within the tendon substance. Evaluating the healing response and its similarity to that described for complete lacerations, has been hampered by the lack of a suitable animal model for chronic tendinitis [24].

Treating Tendon Injury

General Principles

The basic principles governing clinical intervention during tendon healing are outlined in Table 2 [24]. The initial clinical assessment of the patient must include a thorough history and physical examination, identifying, in particular, any intrinsic or extrinsic factors that may be contributing to the tendon injury [25]. The exact anatomical site of the disease is located, and an estimate of the stage of healing should be made based on the degree of pain and inflammation. Imaging techniques, such as ultrasound and MRI, may be of help in this process. Establishing the stage of healing will determine the appropriate focus for initial treatment.

In general, the treatment protocol should include: the correction of existing intrinsic and extrinsic etiological factors; control of pain and inflammation, using drugs, ice, and other modalities; and instituting early motion, beginning with passive movement and stretching, then progressing to active exercises.

Principles of Exercise

The benefits of exercise in the treatment of tendon injury have a well-established scientific basis, as previously stated. Motion and tensile loading improves the material properties of collagen, enhances tendon strength and reduces the formation of adhesions and contracture.

A successful exercise program should incorporate three basic principles, namely: (1) specificity of training – the correct muscle-tendon-unit (MTU) must be

Table 2. Principles governing clinical intervention during tendon healing (after [5])

	Stage of healing Inflammatory	Fibroblastic/proliferation	Remodeling/Maturation
Time (days)	0–6	5–21	20 days and onwards. Progressive stress on tissue
Suggested therapy	Rest, ice, anti-inflammatory modalities, decreased tension	Gradual introduction of stress, modalities to increase collagen syntheses	
Physiological rationale	Prevent prolonged inflammation, prevent disruption of new blood vessels and collagen fibrils, promote ground substance syntheses	Increase collagen, increase collagen cross-linking, increase fibril size and alignment	Increase cross-linking (tendons and ligaments), decrease cross-linking(joint capsule), increase fibril size
Main aims	Avoid new tissue disruption	Prevent excessive muscle and joint atrophy	Optimise tissue healing

loaded to simulate its functional activity; (2) maximal loading – to induce strength adaptations; and (3) progression of loading – to maintain a stimulus for adaptation as the tendon becomes stronger [24].

In the case of the injured tendon, maximal loading can be defined as the force the tendon can withstand without further injury. Clinically, this is determined by the patient's pain level during exercise, as an indicator of the tendon's tolerance and potential damage.

The amount of work done by the MTU, is dependent on the three parameters: (1) load (weight); (2) distance; and (3) time. A heavier weight, moved over a longer distance, in a shorter period of time, will maximize the amount of work done. Adjustments can be made, individually or collectively, to the three parameters in order to achieve the progressive stimulus required for adaptation.

Under a given load, the tension generated across the tendon is dependent on the type of muscle contraction, which can occur in three ways (Fig. 3): (1) concentric – the MTU shortens in length resulting in positive work; (2) isometric – the MTU length remains constant while resisting force and no work is generated; (3) eccentric – the MTU lengthens in response to load, resulting in negative work [5].

The maximum tension during eccentric activation exceeds that of isometric or concentric contractions by

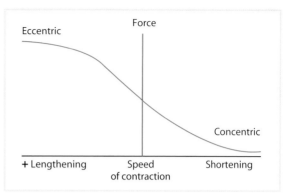

Fig. 4. Force-velocity curve for muscle contraction. (With permission from [5])

threefold [26], so the tendon is most vulnerable during this phase of activation. The tendon will disrupt partially or totally when the force exceeds its inherent tensile strength. The treatment program must therefore include strength training to render the tendon invulnerable to the stress that forced the initial disruption. If the damaging force was eccentric in type, then the tendon should be retrained in an eccentric fashion. By generating greater tension, the strength gains following eccentric exercise will be superior to those obtained by either isometric or concentric training [27].

The force generated is also dependent on the speed of contraction. Viewing the force-velocity curve shown in Fig. 4, reveals that increasing the speed of the eccentric contraction will increase the force developed [28]. Furthermore, the length of the MTU will influence the distance traveled during the contraction. Utilizing stretching will increase the resting length of the MTU, thereby enhancing its excursion (range of joint motion), and generating more elastic recoil energy which augments concentric contraction [29].

Eccentric Exercise Program

The hypothesis that tendon disruption occurs under specific conditions of eccentric loading formed the basis for the development of a graded exercise program to treat chronic tendinitis in 1979 at the Nova Scotia Sports Medicine Clinic [5]. The program employs the repetition of a movement designed to stretch the affected tendon while progressively increasing the load applied to it. To ensure adequate rehabilitation of the healing tendon, the treatment must include specific eccentric strength exercises. Although the protocol was initially developed for treating chronic tendinitis, it may be applied to any tendon injury.

The eccentric exercise program (EEP) involves five steps (Table 3) performed in the following order:

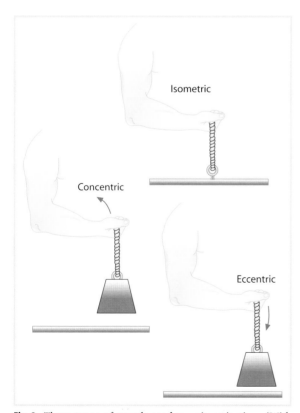

Fig. 3. Three types of muscle-tendon-unit activation. (With permission from [5])

1. *Warm up:* this is accomplished by general exercise such as cycling or jogging. It is designed to increase body temperature and circulation, and not intended to load the tendon.
2. *Flexibility:* because inflexibility is common in chronic tendinitis, it is recommended that the patient perform at least two 30-s static stretches of the involved musculotenidinous unit and its antagonist.
3. *Specific exercise:* perform three sets of 10 repetitions, with a brief rest and stretch between each set. The patient should feel pain after 20 repetitions. If symptoms are experienced earlier, then the speed or load should be reduced; if no pain is felt, then either the speed or the load should be increased (not both). Progression of the EEP is adjusted according to the flow chart (Fig. 5).
4. *Repeat flexibility exercises:* as in step 2.
5. *Ice application:* to the affected area for 10 to 15 min, to minimize inflammation provoked during the EEP.

Table 3. Eccentric exercise program (from [5][a])

1. Stretch
   a. Static stretch
   b. Hold 15–30s
   c. Repeat 3–5 times

2. Eccentric exercise
   a. Three sets of 10 repetitions
   b. Progression:
   Days 1 and 2: slow
   Days 3–5: moderate
   Days 6 and 7: fast
   c. Increase external resistance; after day 7, repeat cycle

3. Stretch, as prior exercise
4. Ice: crushed ice or ice massage applied to tender or painful area for 5–10min

[a] Reproduced with permission from [5].

The exercises are performed daily with continuing progression as guided by the flow chart (Fig. 5), until symptoms are no longer present during functional activity. Program progression can be monitored in several ways: (1) objectively – by the load applied to the affected limb and/or the speed of movement; (2) subjectively – by the patient's report of pain; and (3) functionally – by the patient's ability to successfully perform normal activities. Strength testing should not be performed until treatment is complete and the patient is asymptomatic, since generating maximum force may damage the healing tendon.

The treatment protocol is modified on an individual basis according to the degree of tendon injury, as assessed by the amount of pain and functional deficit (Table 4). Those patients who are able to participate in

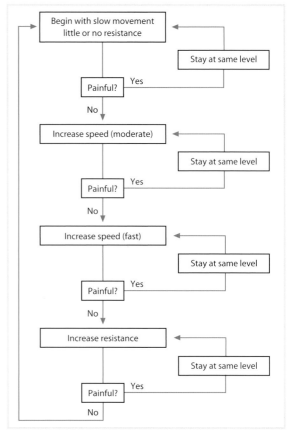

Fig. 5. Method of progression of eccentric exercise program. (With permission from [5])

athletic activity, but experience pain (mild injury) or impaired performance (moderate injury), may continue sports participation. In these cases, no change is made in daily activities, except to add the exercise program. Being allowed to continue athletic activity might be considered an advantage of the EEP over other traditional treatment plans. For patients with severe pain, modification of athletic activity will be necessary. Indeed, many of these individuals will have already reduced their activity, and some may be unable to perform. This level of pain can be interpreted as reflecting an acute inflammation, and treatment should begin at a low level of loading intensity, incorporating ice, stretching, passive movement, and other methods. Treatment is changed as healing progresses, and a gradual approach to the reintroduction of athletic involvement is adopted. The patient should be asymptomatic during non-athletic activities, and be performing the eccentric exercise rapidly. Sporting activities can then be started at about 25% of the pre-injury level, and should be done on alternate days to avoid muscle soreness, and to allow evaluation of the tendon's response to training. Whilst monitoring symptoms, progression can be made in 20% increments, until full

Table 4. Classification of tendon disorders based on pain and function (after [5])

Intensity	Level	Pain	Performance
Mild	1	None	Does not affect performance
	2	With extreme exertion only Not intense Disappears immediately when activity stops	Does not affect performance
Moderate	3	Starts with activity Lasts 1–2 h after activity	Performance may be affected
	4	With any athletic activity Increased during activity Lasts 4–6 h afterwards	Performance level significantly decreased
Severe	5	Immediately upon any activity involving tendon Sudden increase in pain of activity is continued Lasts 12–24 h afterwards	Performance markedly curtailed or prevented
	6	During daily activity	Unable to participate

training has been resumed. If pain recurs, or increases in intensity, the patient should return to the previous training level. Most patients with mild to moderate tendinitis will be asymptomatic after 6–8 weeks of the exercise program, but those with severe injury may require 10–12 weeks of rehabilitation [24].

There are several prerequisites in order for this program to be successful in the treatment of tendinitis: (1) a contemporary physiotherapy facility; (2) patient compliance and cooperation; and (3) lack of evidence of severe tendon scarring (from steroids and/or surgery) which mitigates a less than ideal result [27].

Successful completion of the EEP has been achieved when the patient is able to perform all athletic activities without pain or limitations. Lack of success is most commonly due to incorrect program progression. Either the patient is started at too high a level (and gets worse), or is not progressed to the next level of intensity (and stays the same). An increase in symptoms indicates that an inappropriate level of loading has been

chosen, or the patient is doing the exercise incorrectly. Depending on the level of symptoms, the tendinitis may now need to be treated as an acute injury. Lack of improvement using the EEP may also be due to an incorrect initial diagnosis, or an unrecognized external factor causing or perpetuating the problem. A thor-

Table 5. Eccentric exercise program for Achilles tendinitis (from [5][a])

Week	Days	Exercise	Activity level
1	1–3	Slow drop, bilateral weight support	Cannot participate
	3–5	Moderate speed, bilateral support	
	6, 7	Fast drop, bilateral support	
2	1–3	Slow, increased weight on symptomatic leg	Cannot participate in sports
	3–5	Moderate, increased weight	
	6, 7	Fast, increased weight	
3	1–3	Slow, weight supported on symptomatic leg	Pain during rapid drop; active in sports, but limited
	3–5	Moderate, weight on one leg	
	6, 7	Fast speed	
4	1–3	Slow, add 10% of body weight	Pain during vigorous activity
	3–5	Moderate, same weight	
	6, 7	Fast speed	
5	1–3	Slow, increase by 5 to 10 lb	Pain only during exertion
	3–5	Moderate speed	
	6, 7	Fast speed	
6	1–3	Slow, increase by 5 to 10 lb	Rarely experience pain
	3–5	Moderate speed	
	6, 7	Fast speed	

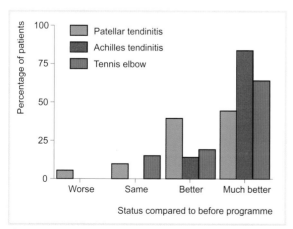

Fig. 6. Symptomatic improvement in 200 patients after 6 weeks on eccentric exercise program. (With permission from [5])

[a]Reproduced with permission from [5].

ough clinical re-evaluation of the patient may be required if there is no improvement after a 2-week period. Failure to respond to treatment should alert suspicion of non-compliance, overtraining, systemic disease, or hormonal or nutritional imbalance.

The initial success of this program was monitored during the treatment of over 200 patients with chronic tendinitis at the Nova Scotia Sports Medicine Clinic [5,

27]. Most of these patients had minimal or no symptoms after 6 weeks (Fig. 6). Since its development in 1979, the EEP has been successfully employed for the rehabilitation of tendon afflictions such as Achilles tendinitis, patellar tendinitis, tennis elbow, and rotator cuff tendinitis [5, 27, 30–32]. Examples of specific EEPs are shown in Tables 5–7.

Conclusion

Soft tissue injury during sport and exercise is common. Treatment can be frustrating, particularly if it enforces a period of rest, and there will be anxiety when resuming the same activity that caused the injury in the first place. Incorporating an eccentric exercise program (EEP), maximizes the strength of the healing tendon, enabling it to withstand the tensile loading which had previously caused damage. Treating the muscle-tendon-bone unit as a whole entity, is of paramount importance.

This chapter has discussed the scientific basis behind eccentric exercise, and the practicalities of its implementation. EEPs have been successfully used to treat athletes in our clinic for over 20 years, since its development in 1979. The protocol is designed to complement other treatment modalities, and the successful management of tendon injuries requires a multi-discipline approach, tailored to an individual basis.

Table 6. Eccentric exercise program for patellar tendinitis (after [5])

1. *Warm-up*
   a. General, whole-body warm-up
   b. Exercises not involving knee extension
   c. Sufficient when sweating is elicited

2. *Stretching*
   a. Static stretch of quadriceps and hamstrings
   b. Hold at leat 30s
   c. Repeat three times

3. *Main program*
   a. Squatting movements
   b. Focusing primarily on the rapid deceleration phase between the downward and upward movement phase
   Week 1: no added resistance on days1 and 2 (slow); days3–7 (progressively faster)
   Week 2: Add resistance (10% body weight)
   Weeks 3–6: Add 10–30lb progressively
   c. Do three sets of 10 repetitions once daily
   d. After 6weeks, three sets of three times weekly

4. *Warm-down*
   a. Static stretch in item 2

5. *Ice*
   a. Ice on patellar tendon for 5min after program

6. *Optional support*
   a. Apply tensor bandage support if desired

Table 7. Eccentric exercise program for tennis elbow (after [5])

Week	Treatment	Function
1	Forearm supported on table, 5lb (2.3kg) weight (with handle) held in hand, drop slowly into flexion, return to extension	Pain with tennis, squash, performance level 75%
2	Drop 5lb (2.3kg) rapidly	Decreased pain, performance level 75% (level 4)
3	Increase weight to 6.5lb (2.9kg)	Decreased pain, performance level 90% (level 3)
4	Increase weight to 8lb (3.6kg)	Decreased pain, performance level 90% (level 3)
5	Hang weight (2lb) (0.9kg) from racquet face, perform eccentric exercise while gripping racquet	Pain after activity, performance level 100% (level 2)
6	Increase suspended weight to 4lb (1.8kg)	No pain with activity, performance level normal (level 1)

References

1. Herring SA, Nilson KL (1987) Introduction to overuse injuries. Clin Sports Med 6:225–239
2. Jarvinen M (1992) Epidemiology of tendon injuries in sports. Clin Sport Med 11:493–504
3. Lyons AS, Petrucelli RJ (1978) Medicine: an illustrated history. Harry N Abrams, New York
4. O'Brien M (1992) Functional anatomy and physiology of tendons. Clin Sports Med 11:505–520
5. Curwin SL, Stanish WD (1984) Tendinitis: its etiology and treatment. Collamore Press, DC Heath, Lexington, MA
6. Kivist M (1991) Morphology and histochemistry of the myotendineal junction of the rat calf muscles. Acta Anat 141:199–205
7. Perugia L, Ippolito E, Postacchini F (1986) The tendons: biology-pathology-clinical aspects. Editrice Kurtis, Milanom pp 9–36
8. Elliott DH, Crawford GNC (1965) The thickness and collagen content of tendon relative to the strength and cross-sectional area of muscle. Proc Roy Soc Med 162B:137–146
9. Leadbetter WB (1992) Cell-matrix response in tendon injury. Clin Sports Med 11:533–578
10. Kellert J (1986) Acute soft tissue injuries – a review of the literature. Med Sci Sports Exerc 18:489–500
11. Amadio PC (1992) Tendon and ligament. In: Cohen IK, Diegelmann RF, Lindblad WJ (eds) Wound healing: biochemical and clinical aspects. Saunders, Philadelphia, p 384
12. Blazina ME, Akeson WH, Harwood FL et al. (1973) Jumper's knee. Orthop Clin North Am 4:665

13. Kannus P, Josza L (1991) Histopathological changes preceding spontaneous rupture of a tendon. J Bone Joint Surg 73A:1507–1525
14. Puddu G, Ippoolito E, Postacchini F (1976) A classification of Achilles tendon disease. Am J Sports Med 4:145–150
15. Clancy WG (1990) Tendon trauma and overuse injuries. In: Leadbetter, WB, Buckwalter JA, Gordon SL (eds) Sports induced inflammation. AAOS, Park Ridge, IL, pp 609–618
16. Woo SLY, Tkach LV (1990) The cellular and matrix response of ligaments and tendons to mechanical injury. In: Leadbetter, WB, Buckwalter JA, Gordon SL (eds) Sports induced inflammation. AAOS, Park Ridge, IL, pp 189–204
17. Amiel D, Akeson WH, Harwood FL et al. (1983) Stress deprivation effect on metabolic turnover of the medial collateral ligament collagen: a comparison between 9 and 12 week immobilization. Clin Orthop 172:265–270
18. Gamble JG, Edwards CC, Max SR et al. (1984) Enzymatic adaptation in ligaments during immobilization. Am J Sports Med 12:221–228
19. Noyes FR (1977) Functional properties of knee ligaments and alterations induced by immobilization: a correlative biomechanical and histological study in primates. Clin Orthop 123:210
20. Suominen H, Ritter MA, Amiel D et al. (1980) Effects of physical training on metabolism of connective tissues in young mice. Acta Physiol Scand 108:17–22
21. Woo SLY, Ritter MA, Amiel D et al. (1980) The biomechanical and biochemical proerties of swine tendons: long term effects of exercise on the digital extensors. Connect Tissue Res 7:177–183
22. Michna H (1984) Morphometric analysis of loading-induced changes in collagen fibril populations in young tendons. Cell Tissue Res 236:465–470
23. Loitz BJ, Zernicke RF, Vailas AC et al. (1989) Effects of short-term immobilization versus continuous passive motion on the biomechanical and biochemical properties of the rabbit tendon. Clin Orthop 244:265–271
24. Curwin SL (1998) The aetiology and treatment of tendinitis. In: Harries M, Williams C, Stanish WD, Micheli LJ (eds) Oxford textbook of sports medicine. Oxford, UK, Oxford University Press, pp 610–630
25. Renstrom P, Kannus P (1991) Prevention of sports injuries. In: Krauss RH (ed) Sports medicine. Saunders, Philadelphia
26. Komi PV (1979) Neuromuscular performance: factors influencing force and speed production. Scand J Sports Sci 1:2–15
27. Stanish WD, Rubinovich RM, Curwin S (1986) Eccentric exercise in chronic tendinitis. Clin Orth Rel Res 208:65–68
28. Komi PV (1973) Measurement of the force-velocity relationship in human muscle under concentric and eccentric contractions. Medicine in Sport 8:224–229
29. Fyfe I, Stanish WD (1992) The use of eccentric training and stretching in the treatment and prevention of tendon injuries. Clin Sports Med 11:601–624
30. Stanish WD, Lamb H, Curwin S (1988) The biomechanical analysis of chronic patellar tendinitis and treatment with eccentric loading. In: Müller W, Hackenbruch W (eds) Surgery and arthroscopy of the knee. Springer, Berlin Heidelberg New York, pp 493–494
31. Jensen K, DiFablo R (1989) Evaluation of eccentric exercise in treatment of patellar tendinitis. Phys Ther 69: 3
32. Alfreson H (1998) Heavy-load eccentric calf muscle training for the treatment of chronic achilles tendinosis. Am J Sports Med 26:3

18 Aquatic Therapy in Rehabilitation

Piero Faccini, Sabrina Zanolli, Dario Dalla Vedova

Introduction

The chief aim of current rehabilitation techniques is to allow the patient to re-acquire functional capacities in a shorter time, minimising disuse and/or post-surgical complications and returning the patient to normal sporting and working activity as quick as possible. Three methodology types are usually adopted:

1. Rehabilitation using passive and active closed kinetic chain
2. Rehabilitation using open kinetic chain
3. Rehabilitation in the pool

Hydrotherapy has been a part of medical treatment since Greek and Roman times. The use of water as a therapeutic technique has weathered the test of time and has repeatedly been noted for its many benefits. Even in today's era of rapidly changing technological advancements, water can still be a valuable tool in the rehabilitation of a wide variety of conditions. Hydrotherapy or aquatic therapy was first documented by Hippocrates (460–375 B.C.). Although used widely throughout the first several centuries, little was known about the effects of water as a treatment method. As time passed, all the principles relating to the physics and mechanics of aquatic exercise were often supervised by people in Europe with very little training and were surrounded by unsupported and extravagant claims. This was a major factor in preventing the widespread acceptance of hydrotherapy as a mainstay in medical treatment. In the early 1900s, there was little discussion of exercising in the water. Even until recently, hydrotherapy was thought of simply as an adjunct to treatment and not considered a separate treatment method with its own real merits.

With the proliferation of sports medicine and traumatology as disciplines, and the increasing advancements in the field of injury management, the use of swimming pools for aquatic rehabilitation has added a new dimension by hydrotherapy. Now, the use of hydrotherapy brings with it the concepts of aggressive, progressive treatment for a wide variety of diseases and orthopaedic conditions.

This chapter sets out to present an innovative pool-based rehabilitation technique prepared by the authors using kickboards as peripheral overloads ('WAT-JOB'

technique [15]). This technique, which will be described in detail, permits a faster recovery than traditional techniques, [4, 15], which is extremely important for an athlete's return to competitive activity without musculo-tendinous complications or reoccurrence of the original injury. The aim of the authors is to come up with new, more effective techniques.

The WAT-JOB Technique

One of the main tasks to be performed by physical therapists is that of continually seeking easy-to-effect therapeutic methods that conform to precise rules governing the progression of loads administered and, above all, that do not cause additional damage to a structure that has already undergone traumatic and/or surgical procedure. This methodological principle has been coupled in recent years with the concept of rehabilitation/reconditioning, namely the search for rehabilitation programmes that entail not only traditional forms of kinetic therapy but also the introduction, from the early stages part of the rehabilitation, of particular movements in keeping with the biomechanics of the movement that the patient usually performs [9]. This may, however, be difficult to achieve, for example when a patient has a complex osteo-articular pathology and gravity-based load is not possible, especially in the initial phases of rehabilitation. In such cases, modern kinesiology suggests the use of therapy techniques in water, which include the use of traditional methodologies [5, 11] (fins, antigravity objects, etc.) and the use of kickboards (WAT-JOB) which, by applying a quantifiable hydrodynamic load, make it possible to set a work schedule for the patient from the first phase of rehabilitation to the final phase of reconditioning, without subjecting the joint or injured limb to excessive loads, such as gravity-based loads, yet allowing him/her to resume specific neuro-motor functional patterns.

Theoretical Principle

Not everybody is aware that we are in daily contact with a viscous fluid, and that we live, breathe and move in a substance – air – that has its own weight and density just like any other gas or liquid [7,8]. This is because we have always been accustomed to this situation and because we move through air by our own forces at relatively low speeds.

It is not hard to discover however that air has its own 'consistency' and behaves in different ways, depending on the form of the object moving within it [12, 13].

Fluids are those substances that may be found in a gaseous or liquid state, such as air and water. This state of matter occurs when molecules do not stick closely to each other, but slide over one another quite easily.

Unlike theoretical (so-called perfect) fluids that can be found only in physics textbooks, all fluids with which we come into daily contact are viscous. The reason for this is to be sought in intermolecular forces which, although weak, as we have seen above, are ever-present in nature. Thus, if we try to place one small layer of fluid on top of another, we see that we must work continuously to keep them moving [2, 7, 8, 12]. What appears to be a 'poor' property of fluids is actually an extremely important quality: without viscosity, indeed, we would not be able to breathe, a small atmospheric disturbance would not fade away but would add to others, creating a storm, and aeroplanes would not be able to fly [1].

Fluids obviously have other correlated characteristics, such as density and kinematic viscosity, and they vary according to pressure (for aeriforms) and temperature, but in this chapter we shall not go into these aspects.

A streamlined body or one whose front section is exposed little to air offers less resistance than a stocky body with sharp edges or one with a high front section, in the same way that a smooth surface generates less friction than a rough or uneven surface [1, 8, 12].

The reason for this is the 'antipathy' (in physical terms) shown by fluids for the empty spaces they encounter: if they find one they always seek to fill it [2]. Thus, if the object is streamlined it is easy for the air or water to penetrate all over it, while if the body is uneven or stocky fluids become disorderly and turbulent, creating vortexes that re-form behind, forming a wake. To appreciate the importance of this wake, think of those dangerous clouds of water lifted up by trucks on the motorway when it is raining: sometimes they are longer and taller than the trucks that have produced them. This is useful for viewing a phenomenon that is often bigger and involves much more energy than we might imagine. For the formation of the wake and the vortexes, indeed, needed to fill the empty spaces we have mentioned, the fluid 'steals' energy from the moving body, slowing it down, before re-transforming it into pressure. To gain an understanding of the duration of a wake and of the energy involved, bear in mind that at airports some minutes must elapse between the take-offs of two normal aircraft on the same runway, or along a nearby parallel runway, because the turbulence generated by the former craft's engines and wings could even cause the second to crash. Now that we have seen what happens when moving in a fluid, it would be interesting to attempt to quantify the phenomenon so that we could predict the extent of the force needed to keep a given body moving in a given fluid. The applications of this theory are numerous and, as may be imagined, all important, ranging from a prediction of how much petrol a car consumes on the motorway to the required resistance of a bridge or a building to oppose the action of the wind, or calculation of the speed with which rehabilitation movements can be performed in order to prepare predetermined loads.

After a number of studies [4, 15], wind gallery tests [4] and theories [1, 8, 13], we have reached the conclusion that fluid dynamic forces depend on the density of the fluid in which they are generated, the speed at which one moves raised to the second power, a reference section of the body and a conventional term that we call shape coefficient, depending, as might be imagined, on the shape of the body and the way in which it meets the fluid.

The formula states:

$$F = 1/2 \varrho\, V^2\, S\, Cx,$$

where *F* is the sought fluid dynamics force in Newtons (power is obtained by considering speed raised to the third power); ϱ is the density of the fluid in which the body moves, expressed in kg/m^3, which for air is 1.2 and for freshwater 1000; both values refer to standard conditions, having seen that otherwise they would be conditioned by temperature and pressure; *V* is the speed of movement in m/s raised squared (cubed when calculating power); *S* is the reference section of the body expressed in m^2, usually the front section is taken into consideration vis-à-vis the direction of movement; and Cx is the adimensional shape coefficient which, by convention, depends only on the shape of the body at any speed and in whatever fluid it moves (this is not always true, but in most cases the difference is irrelevant).

To obtain the force expressed in kilograms, it is necessary to divide the result obtained by gravity acceleration which, for the sake of simplicity, we take to be $10\,m/s^2$ (in Rome $9.806\,m/s^2$, the simplification causing an error of 2%).

For the matter in question, attention should be paid to the final three terms of the formula, with density being an invariable: water is indeed considered in its liquid state and is thus incompressible, while for air it is difficult to work with densities other than that under standard pressure conditions (otherwise a pressurised chamber would be required). For this reason, corrections are applied to air density, owing to the difference of temperature there may be in relation to the afore-mentioned standard condition.

It should first be noted that the force depends on the square of the speed and not on its first power. This means that if a given force is required to move a body at a given speed in a given fluid, to move it at twice the speed a force not two times but four times greater is required. For power, which depends on speed to the third power, as speed increases twofold, power is eight times greater.

We should then point out that force depends on a linear basis on the surface area of the body in question [12]. This means, for instance, that a man standing up offers less resistance than the wing of a Boeing, because the latter, although it is more aerodynamic, is much bigger. By convention, the surface area is taken to be the front section, whose size is not always easy to calculate. Apart from flat shapes with straight sides, indeed, it may be necessary to measure the front section of a non-flat body whose projection may not have straight sides (think for example of the front section of one's hand or, worse still, of that of a cyclist riding a bicycle). It is possible to get round these problems by using a photograph that can be put into digital form and processed using appropriate software or, more simply but less accurately, a photograph cut into many smaller and simpler pieces in order to calculate the surface area.

The final term we are interested in is the adimensional shape coefficient.

This is so called because its conventional physical definition corresponds to the ratio between the fluid dynamics force and the semi-product of density multiplied by the speed to the second power and by the section: $Cx = F/0.5 \varrho V^2 S$. This, considering the physical size of the figures involved, i.e. the numerator and the denominator, makes it a pure number, thus without a unit of measurement, and it simply needs to be multiplied by the other terms.

Aerodynamic resistance (as well as power) varies on a linear basis according to Cx [7, 8, 12]. In this case, a problem arises when it needs to be calculated accurately. It is indeed easy to find, in books on fluid dynamics and in publications from the sector, Cx values for some standard shapes such as open-air flat sheets, cylinders or spheres. Such values are based on experimentation, having been obtained from wind tunnel tests on specially built and equipped models. It is interesting to observe how values alter according to the shape adopted by the same body, for example if the sheet or the cylinder is stretched out or not. This is because of the extent and form of the vortexes generated by bodies as they move. Clearly the bigger they are, the greater the energy they absorb and the braking effect produced at the conclusion.

Unfortunately, it is not always possible to relate the situations we are interested in to one of these hypothet-ical cases. It should indeed be remembered that the shape coefficient depends on the aerodynamic field generated around the body. This is why small changes to the shape of the body, to the distribution of volumes around it or to its speed are enough to make a significant difference to the situation. The solution to this difficulty is that of adopting semi-empirical methods to obtain acceptably accurate results in order to make correct predictions. We should stress the importance of a correct initial approach to the problem. By way of example, let us calculate the force required to move a simple object, say a flat sheet, in water at low speed. This is the case for pool rehabilitation. Let us begin by saying that the sheet is physically a flat body, that is to say two dimensions – its sides – are predominant over the third, thickness. A square sheet, whose side/side ratio is accordingly close to 1, has a shape coefficient of around 1.2. Let us assume that it is moving in the water at a speed of 1 m/s (3.6 km/h) and has sides of 20 cm (front section thus being $0.2 \cdot 0.2 = 0.04 \, \text{m}^2$).

Force is, as we have already said,

$$F = 1/2 \varrho V^2 S Cx$$

In this case:

$$1000 : 2 \cdot (1 \times 1) \cdot 0.04 \cdot 1.2 = 24 \, \text{N}$$

If we want to express this in kilograms, we must divide the sum by gravity acceleration, which we have taken as $10 \, \text{m/s}^2$. The resulting value is thus 2.4 kg.

If the speed had been 2 m/s, the value for force would have been:

$$1000 : 2 \cdot (2 \cdot 2) \cdot 0.04 \cdot 1.2 = 96 \, \text{N} \text{ or } 96/10 = 9.6 \, \text{kg}$$

which, as we have seen, is a fourfold increase in force for the doubling of speed. By way of example, let us see how much force is required to move the same sheet at 1 m/s, but in the air:

$$1.2 : 2 \cdot (1 \cdot 1) \cdot 0.04 \cdot 1.2 = 0.0288 \, \text{N},$$

or 0.00288 kg. It may therefore be seen that the fluid dynamics force required in the air in this hypothetical case is approximately 800 times less than that needed in the water. If, with the same sheet we wanted to obtain the same 24 N obtained in the water, we would have to move at a speed of

$$V = \frac{(24 \cdot 2)}{(1.2 \cdot 0.04 \cdot 1.2)} = 28.87 \, \text{m/s}$$

that is to say, 104 km/h.

These calculations refer of course to the hypothetical situation of a sheet moving uniformly in the fluid, but they are useful for offering a very clear picture of the sort of force involved in different cases. As we have seen, indeed, this makes it possible to obtain significant loads even at very low speeds, thus with the optimum control of movement.

It should not be forgotten, either, that floating in the water takes on relevant values by virtue of its high density, and that it can often be useful, reducing the weight to which a limb is subjected, and facilitating movement in accordance with given methods (as a matter of fact the principle of Archimedes also applies in the air but, since it is equal to the weight of the volume of fluid moved and, as we have seen, water is heavier than air, this phenomenon is much reduced in the air [3]).

Practical Applications

Let us move on now to the practical side of the question, namely calculation of the force needed to move a limb (e.g. the rotation of a leg around a knee) in water after a flat sheet has been firmly applied to increase resistance to forward motion.

For this purpose, special software has been developed in our Biomechanics Department, named ROSS (rehabilitation overload simulation software [16]) which considers not only fixed variables but also dependent variables, making it possible to calculate both the load applied to each movement for different kickboard surfaces and the progression of this load when increasing the speed of execution (Fig. 1).

Experimental tests carried out have confirmed figures shown in the plates for the loads obtained.

We may thus conclude by saying that the illustrated model of calculation is sufficiently accurate to describe

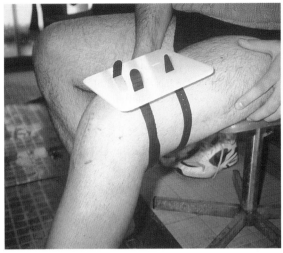

Fig. 2. Plastic kickboard

the current state of research and that, despite the existence of slight inaccuracies and the need for further investigations, it can give, quickly and using relatively simple calculations, quite a precise picture of the dynamics of the phenomenon and the nature of forces involved.

The kickboards used for this rehabilitation method are made from a plastic material. Their shape, size and placement depend on the load and on the articular areas affected (Fig. 2).

Once the surface area of the kickboard and the speed of execution of the movement is known (this can be timed quite accurately), it is thus possible to define the load to which the muscular kinetic chain affected is to be subjected or, vice versa, having established the

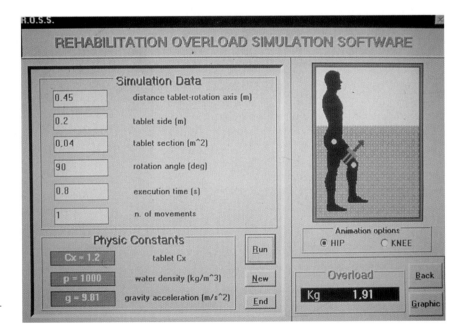

Fig. 1. ROSS software principal menu sheet

load, it is possible to specify the speed at which the movement should be performed.

For obvious reasons, this experimental model has not taken into account the floating coefficient for the human body since, in the rehabilitation phase, weights can be applied to the patient to counteract this upward force or, more usually, the patient can hold on to suitable bars [5, 6].

Description of the Work Method in the Pool

For rehabilitation purposes, a kickboard is used such as the one illustrated in Fig. 3, consisting of a quadrangular sheet of hard plastic material, with an anatomical rib underneath. The kickboard thus adapts to the shape of the muscular zone in which it is placed and is held in place using a Velcro belt.

The pool-based work method using kickboards must conform to the following methodology:

1. *Isometric dynamometry* (assessment of muscular strength)
2. *Choice of load to be applied using software* (quantity, intensity) and of the characteristics on which *movement* will be based (width of kickboard, number and speed of repetitions).
3. *Execution of the movement* (after having placed the patient in the pool in optimal conditions).

It is vitally important that the patient, during rehabilitation in the water, adopts a vertical position and holds on to the bars located on the sides of the pool. We have already mentioned that the load varies according to the direction of movement exerted on the kickboard. For different angles we suggest studying resistance according to the aforementioned formula.

A complete description of the WAT-JOB method requires a classification of the type of pathology dealt with. We shall thus describe only two exercises, which we believe to be the most revealing.

1. *Rehabilitation of hip flexion movement.* The kickboard should be placed parallel to the thigh, at a distance of 15 cm from the hip joint, before commencing the exercise (Fig. 4).

In light of everything that has been said above, with a kickboard measuring 20 × 20 cm subjected to a semi-rotating movement along a fixed axis (in this case the axis passes through the hip joint) at around 2 m/s, the patient must overcome a resistance of 3.32 kg at every rotation, thus after ten rotations the patient will have moved around 33 kg.

2. *Kinetic chain type movement entailing nearly full flexion of the hip and extension of the knee.* The femoral quadriceps is a hip flexor and knee extensor. Placing a kickboard as shown in the plate and another in the area above the ankle, a complete kinetic chain movement of the quadriceps will be achieved (Fig. 5).

Clearly the kickboards used can be of different sizes in order to administer different loads.

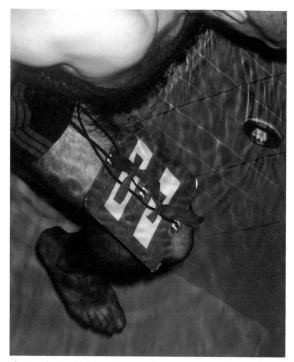

Fig. 3. Plastic kickboard immersed in water and monitored with a strain gauge in order to quantify force/velocity relationship

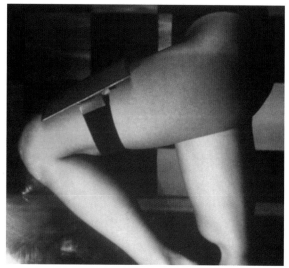

Fig. 4. Hip flexion with kickboard

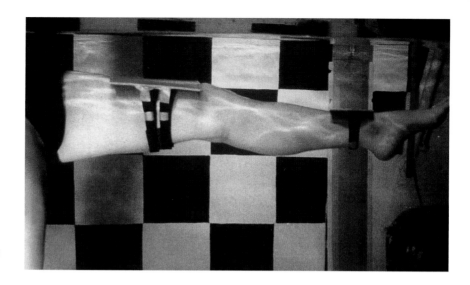

Fig. 5. Hip flexion and knee extension with kickboard

Briefly, the two conditions that can help raise the work load are thus: an increase in the speed of movement in water and an increase in the surface area size subjected to the kickboard resistance. For this purpose, some side appendices can be applied to the kickboard.

Rehabilitation of Knee After ACL Reconstruction Using the WAT-JOB Water Method

Day-to-day experiences concerning the rehabilitation of athletes that have been operated on, usually marked by the urgent need to resume competitive activity, have led us to prepare some exercises that can complement traditional rehabilitation methods and, if applied correctly, speed up treatment times and offer unquestionable advantages in medical and practical terms, without harming the patient.

To give a more complete picture, we shall describe a traditional rehabilitation method after ACL reconstruction which include in the various phases the new techniques we have proposed.

The functioning of the injured knee during the rehabilitation process is very different from the kinesiological behaviour of a healthy knee. The therapist must therefore fix the general biomechanical concepts of healthy joint movement and compare them with the knee undergoing rehabilitation, carefully observing that a pathological knee basically differs from a sound one in terms of joint defence mechanisms in respect of external agents, such as the force of gravity [5, 10]. A pathological knee is a knee at risk: if for example it does not possess the full ROM as we have said, it will also have shortcomings in the final 5° of the maximum combined rotation that the femur exerts on the tibia (if the foot is resting on the ground). This action of the femur with a healthy knee makes it possible to give tension to

all joint elements and to counteract, for example, the unevenness of the terrain, since in this phase of full extension the joint is closed. It should be added that exercises generating a load at 45° (perpendicular to the centre of rotation at the height of the tibial plate) may be harmful owing to their tendency to further damage the tibia, thus strain the new ligament, especially if they are applied in an early phase. A classical example is the leg-extension in both isokinetic and isometric form [9]. This is why gravity-based load will not be easily allowed in the first days of rehabilitation, barring recourse to special methods such as pool work using kickboards.

The therapist should not limit his action to passive kinesiological aspects, but should also study the exercises and the choice of training contrivances, especially in the first period of rehabilitation [11]. Of extreme importance, therefore, is the *rehabilitation method* adopted, namely the quantity of work to be administered and its quality, taken to mean the choice of rehabilitation devices.

Rehabilitation Phases

Rehabilitation of the knee with reconstructed ACL involves five or six working phases.

Pre-operation Phase

This period, which seldom involves the practical involvement of the physical therapist, is of fundamental importance for the success of rehabilitation, and it usually consists of a series of exercises performed by the patient according to instructions supplied by the physician or kinesiologist, designed to recover the full ROM of the knee, improve strength of the limb and the normal gait pattern.

The duration of this pre-phase varies from 2 to 3 weeks starting from the resolution of the inflammation of the joint, and it is of course dependent on the muscular state of the patient being operated on. Unfortunately, for a variety of reasons, the patient tends to neglect this phase, often for understandable psychological reasons, unless motivation is very high (professional athlete).

Phase 1 (From 1st to 15th Day)

In the first few days (2 or 3) after the operation, the patient is usually in hospital, immobilised in a post-op brace in full extension with a painful and swollen joint.

He can start immediately the use of CPM (continuous passive movement) systems to regain passive extension and flexion usually in 2 weeks.

The optimisation of knee therapy begins in the first days after leaving hospital with exercises for maintaining good muscular strength of the lower limb. By including exercises for the leg, hip and ankle, the patient is able to have full weight-bearing at the end of the third week. We recommend pool exercises right from an early stage of rehabilitation, making sure that the patient dips only the part of the leg below the wound, whose scar is still fresh at this time. Using a fin of moderate width, flexion, extension and ankle circumduction, exercises can be performed. In addition to work in the pool, we also recommend assisted active exercises of the ankle with and without the aid of rubber bands.

These techniques should be viewed as complementary to traditional techniques, such as isometric contraction of the quadriceps and active isotonic flexion of the knee flexors, as well as the two previous exercises combined. In this phase the patient usually walks with the aid of crutches, and the orthopaedist sets the knee-pad at a still-closed angle of extension.

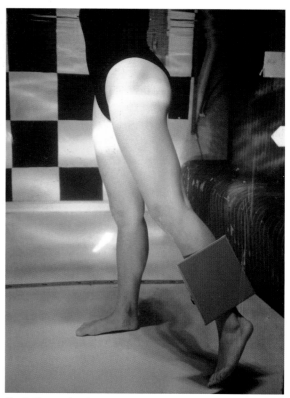

Fig. 6. Circumduction movement

In addition to the previous methods, it is now possible to begin isometric 'circuit' exercises, or isodynamic exercises, using rubber bands: the former can be performed by the patient himself, while the latter require the therapist's assistance. We are of the opinion that the latter method is preferable, allowing greater control over loads and execution techniques.

Phase 2 (From 15th Day to End of 1st Month)

We believe that this is the 'critical' phase, on which the success of rehabilitation depends.

In full agreement with recent studies on the strain measurements of ACL during rehabilitation exercises in vivo [4, 14], which do not allow open kinetic chain exercises in this period, we start pool exercises which, exploiting the buoyant nature of humans in water, make it possible to perform thigh-hip and leg-thigh flexion-extension exercises, overloading movements through the use of kickboards: in other words, what is not permitted out of water can safely be done in it. In the water it is also possible to perform adduction, abduction and circumduction exercises (Fig. 6).

From the 15th day (after stitches have been removed) until the 30th day, a WAT-JOB measuring 20 × 20 cm for the thigh and one measuring 10 × 10 cm for the leg will be used.

Phase 3 (Second Month)

In this phase it is possible to include exercises to stimulate the active knee extension, advancing the strengthening of the lower limb muscles. In the pool, work loads are intensified by increasing the size of the kickboard (30 × 20 cm) and the width of the fin.

Out of the water, passive extension exercises can be continued, supplemented by the use of more complex machines: the *treadmill*, both by flat and uphill exercises, at low speeds, interspersed by pauses for the re-coordination of pace (heel-toe exercises) and running, the *ergometric bicycle* for work on vastus medialis and lateralis muscles exercises with rubber bands to develop greater tensions, especially for the movement of thigh abductors and adductors.

In this period, moreover, Kotz electrical stimulation currents can be used. These manage to employ a greater number of muscular fibres [14].

Phase 4 (Third Month)

This phase is very similar to the previous one, the main difference being an increase in the number of times exercises are repeated.

In this phase pool exercises are no longer training-intense, since oversized kickboards or considerable speed of movement would be needed to increase the load. But having arrived at this phase of rehabilitation without undue problems, we believe that the patient can perform any movement and use all machines (including open kinetic chain for leg-extension). The physical therapist must use his own imagination and the means at his disposal to make relative rehabilitation effective and stimulating.

Phases 5 and 6 (Reconditioning)

In these phases we can begin to start with reconditioning exercises, including increasingly complex out-of-water exercises in terms of coordination and kinetics. If, for example, the athlete is a footballer, it may be possible to implement running circuits with changes of direction (like relay runs) or, using a lightweight ball, perform ball-control exercises using the limb operated on and the healthy limb as a support. For other sports, exercises will be based on a knowledge of the motor requirements of the specific sporting activity.

Our use of the technique on 20 high-level athletes (Table 1), compared with a control group (20 subjects, Table 2) undergoing the classic programme, confirmed its validity, i.e. the first group (using the new hydrotherapy technique) had a mean period of rehabilitation of 105 ± 9 days while the second (using the usual technique) had a mean period of 182 ± 7 days. The follow-up after 12 months, carried out with orthopaedic tests, such as the Jerk and Lachman test, and applying the KT 1000 knee arthrometer (Table 3), demonstrated an optimal response of the group after their return to athletic activity.

Table 2. Control group

20 subjects, 16 male and 4 female: Male: 7 soccer, 4 basketball, 1 taekwondo, 3 volleyball and 1 handball Female: 2 basketball, 1 volleyball, 1 soccer	
Presurgical period	No preventive physical training performed because all the subjects were operated on within 15 days of ACL injury
Postsurgical period	
1 – 14 days	CPM 60 – 90 – 110° Isometric contractions – flex/ext co-contractions Deambulation (7 days) with 20% load with DON-JOI
15 – 30 days	Stop CPM and stitches avulsion Isometric contraction Skate for flexion Deambulation with total load with DON-JOI Massage, patella round mobility, passive extension
30 – 60 days	Isometric exercises Cyclette, treadmill, side step up Isotonic exercises Passive extension Stop DON-JOI
60 – 120 days	Leg press Swimming (no breaststroke) Treadmill, open air bycycle Free extension
120 – 240 days	Running on soft court with DON JOI and start recondition and training Isokinetic exercises

Table 1. Remark group

20 subjects, 17 male and 3 female: Male: 9 soccer, 3 basketball, 4 volleyball and 1 judo Female: 1 basketball, 1 volleyball, 1 soccer	
Presurgical period	No preventive physical training performed because all the subjects were operated on within 15 days of ACL injury
Postsurgical period	
1 – 14 days	Like control group and more In 10 days foot flex/extension in water with a flipper (knee at 45°)
15 – 30 days	Like control group and more 3 water workout stages (Flex/ext-AB/AB-DUC) of the hip with a 20 × 20 tablet
30 – 60 days	Like control group and more 4 water workout stages (Flex/ext-AB/AB-DUC) of the hip with a 20 × 20 tablet Interval training run 2:1 on soft court or treadmill Reconditioning exercises (balloon foot, jumping on elastic mat)
60 – 120 days	Like control group and more Knee water workout continues with 20 × 20 tablet upper the knee and 10 × 10 on ankle Running on different courts No isokinetic work or leg press Start specific training (day 105)

Table 3. Remark group

	Jerk test	Lachman test	KT 1000 (manual maximum test)
Presurgery test: mean of all the group	++	+++	Knee difference: 5 – 7 mm
12-month follow-up	Negative	Negative	Knee difference: 2 mm

References

1. Abbot IH (1945) Theory of wings. Dover, New York
2. Berta C (1985) Aerodinamica computazionale. C.R.F., Torino
3. Edlich RF, Towler MA, Goitz RJ, Etal H (1987) Bioengineering principles of hydrotherapy. Int J Burn Care Rehabil 8:580–584
4. Faccini P, Zanolli S, Dalla Vedova D, Besi M, Candela V, Dal Monte A (1997) Simulation software and dummy test to quantify the water overload of a new rehabilitation tecnique. The 9th European Congress of Sport Medicine Porto, Portugal
5. Genuario SE, Vegso JJ (1990) The use of a swimming pool in the rehabilitation and reconditioning of athletic injuries. Contemp Orthop20: 381
6. Golland A (1981) Basic hydrotherapy. Physiotherapy 67 : 258–262
7. Karamcheti K (1966) Principles of ideal fluid aerodynamics. Wiley, New York
8. Keuthe AM (1976) Foundations of aerodynamics. Wiley, New York
9. Irrgang JJ, Harner CD (1997) Recent advances in ACL rehabilitation: clinical factors that influence the program. J Sports Rehabil 6: 111
10. Noyes FR (1977) Functional properties of knee ligaments and alteration induced by immobilisation. Clin. Orthop. 123: 210–214
11. Prins J, Cutner D (1999) Aquatic therapy in the rehabilitation of athletic injuries. Clin Sports Med 18: 447–461
12. Rieghels FW (1961) Aerofoil sections. Butterworths, London
13. Shanebrook JR, Jaszczak RD (1974) Aerodynamics of human body. In: Biomechanics. University Park Press, Baltimore MD pp 567–571 (Fourth International Series on Sport Science, vol 1)
14. Snyder-Mackler L, Delitto A, Daily SL et al (1995) Strength of the quadriceps femoris muscle and functional recovery after reconstruction of the anterior cruciate ligament: a prospective, randomize clinical trial of electrical stimulation. J Bone Joint Surg Am 77: 1166
15. Zanolli S, Faccini P, Dalla Vedova D (1996) Rehabilitation in water after reconstrution of knee ACL using quantifiable overload. In: Medicine and science in sport and exercise. World Congress of American College of Sport Medicine, Cincinnati USA
16. Besi M, Leonardi LM, Dalla Vedova D, Faccini P, Zanolli S R.O.S.S. Rehabilitation overload simulation software. Institute of Sport Science (CONI, Italy) Software

CHAPTER 19

Hyperthermia and Shock Waves: New Methods in the Treatment of Sports Injuries

Arrigo Giombini, Vittorio Franco, Alberto Selvanetti

Definition of Hyperthermia

Hyperthermia is the therapeutic technique which raises a pre-established part of the body to a temperature range between 41.5°C and 45°C, and maintains it at this range, for a given period of time.

Introduction and Historical Background of Diathermy

The primary rationale for the employment of therapeutic heat in physical medicine is the inducement of blood flow (BF) increase, which is anticipated to occur with the increase of temperature in the treated region.

This rationale is so because the mechanism for healing is thought to be highly dependent upon the transport of blood-nurturing substances and removal of toxic waste products [1]. The secondary rationale is the increase of the metabolic rate of a specific tissue volume, assuming that this behavior is comparable to the increase of the overall body metabolic rate on the basis of a 13% increase per degree above the normal temperature [2].

Shortwave (27.33 MHz) and microwave (2450 MHz) diathermy, together with ultrasound therapy, have been used over the decades as major heat methods for stimulating various beneficial physiological responses, and for the relief of a variety of pathological conditions.

Despite the widespread use of these methods in routine clinical practice, it appears that the major problem has been the lack of a correct scientific approach in the design and use of diathermy apparatus for optimal results.

Interest in the interaction of electromagnetic (EM) energy with biological tissues dates back to the first man-made EM sources. A. D'Arsonval, a French physiologist, found in 1892 that currents of frequency 10 KHz or greater would produce an increase of temperature without painful muscular contractions [3].

The word 'diathermy' was introduced by Nagelschmidt in 1907 to describe the relatively uniform heating produced in the tissue by the conversion of high frequency currents into heat [3]. Between 1900 and 1935 in fact, physicians were using high frequency currents of between 0.5 – 3 MHz and 10 MHz (long-wave diather-

my: 118 cm in muscle tissue at 10 MHz) for the above purposes.

In 1928, EM radiation as high as 100 MHz (short wave diathermy: 27 cm in muscle tissue at 100 MHz) was being produced by Esau, and used clinically by Schliephake [3]. Holmann in 1939 discussed the possible application of radio-waves of 25 cm wavelength for therapeutics, and predicted that these waves could be focused to produce heating of the deep tissues without excessive heating of the skin [3, 4].

The first therapeutic application of microwaves was at the Mayo Clinic (USA) in 1946 by Krusen and Leden, and involved the exposure of test animals to 65 W of 3000 MHz radiation (microwave diathermy: 1.45 cm at 3000 MHz). Despite the fact that the average temperature rise was greater in the skin and subcutaneous fat than in the deep muscle tissue, this work launched the use of microwave diathermy for application to physical medicine [5, 6]. It must be remembered, however, that these conclusions were based on the use of microwaves in dogs, which have thinner layers of subcutaneous fat and muscle than humans.

As a result of this study and the research done at MIT (Massachusetts Institute of Technology) in 1947, the FCC (Federal Communications Commission) assigned the frequency of 2450 MHz to physical medicine based on its alleged superiority in therapeutic value.

In 1950, Schwan demonstrated that 2450 MHz was not a good choice of frequency for the following reasons [7]:

1. Excessive heating in the subcutaneous fat
2. Poor penetration of energy into the muscle tissue due to small skin depth
3. Poor control of energy absorption due to large variation in the electrical thickness of subcutaneous tissues

Schwan recommended a frequency of 900 MHz or less. Lehmann and Guy, between 1960 and 1980, verified experimentally that 900 MHz or lower frequencies could produce better heating patterns than obtained with 2450 MHz or with other natural and technological heating modalities [8, 9].

In 1972, Johnson and Guy measured the properties of short-waves and microwaves in biological media in terms of depth of penetration of each frequency in tissue with a high water content (muscle and skin) and low water content (fat and bone [10]). As a result of this study it was noted that, in the range of frequency from 1 to 10,000 MHz, the depth of penetration was inversely correlated with frequency: the higher the frequency, the lower the penetration depth; the lower the frequency, the higher the penetration depth.

From 1980 to 1990, some studies showed that ultrasound could cause an increase of temperature in exposed human tissues and for this reason it became the most widely used deep heating method in physical medicine [11–15].

Knowledge of this historic evolution is important in the elucidation of the present-day problems encountered in the medical use and biological effects of short waves, microwaves, and ultrasound. Lack of physics and engineering knowledge in medicine has produced scientific research which did not consider the fact that electrical properties and geometry of tissue, as well as wave length, are far more important than the absorption and the focusing characteristics of waves in the generation of therapeutic heating patterns.

Benefits of Therapeutic Heating

The responses of therapeutic heating are:

1. Increase of blood flow due to vasodilatation accompanied by increase in capillary pressure [16–19]
2. Increase of cellular membrane permeability [20]
3. Increase of metabolic reaction rate [2]
4. Alteration in sensory nerve conduction [21]
5. Increase of viscous flow properties of collagenous tissues in tendon, joint capsule and scarred synovium [22–25]

Due to these effects, heating can promote tissue regeneration, oedema reduction, relaxation in muscle spasm and reduction of tendon and muscle pain.

The most important factors, mandatory for the number and intensity of biological reactions of heat, are:

1. The therapeutic temperature threshold: approximately from 41.5°C to 45°C
2. The duration of the therapeutic temperature threshold: from 3 to 30 min
3. The speed of the temperature rise: the faster it is, the better is the effect
4. The proper heating of the target volume [9, 16, 26, 27]

It must be stressed that one of the most important factors in determining the extent of the above physiological responses to heat is the blood flow rate(BFR).

Scientific studies published in the 1980s in the fields of oncology, biomechanical engineering and physical medicine, have proved that the increase of blood perfusion response is a function of temperature threshold: to produce a significant rise in blood perfusion, at least 41.5°C must be reached, and the maximum blood rate is achieved when the temperature reaches approximately 45°C [1, 28–30].

Although the mechanism regulating the blood perfusion process is complex and not easily summarized in few lines. Sekins and colleagues made possible the examination of the interplay between local temperature, muscle blood flow, specific absorption rate and temperature gradients (Figs. 1, 2). The following table may help to understand the average hyperemia values modified by the rise of temperature in a thigh muscle heated with hyperthermia prototype equipment:

Temperature	Blood perfusion
36°C	2.7 ml/min/100g
37°C approximately	2.7 ml/min/100g
38°C approximately	2.7 ml/min/100g
39°C approximately	2.7 ml/min/100g
40°C approximately	2.7 ml/min/100g
41°C approximately	2.7 ml/min/100g
42°C approximately	10 ml/min/100g
43°C approximately	20 ml/min/100g
44°C approximately	30 ml/min/100g
45°C approximately	40 ml/min/100g

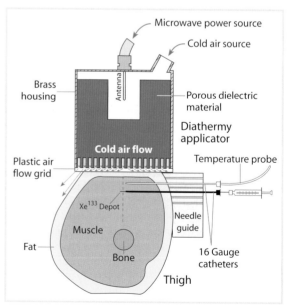

Fig. 1. Schematic of the experimental setup used to study human muscle temperatures and blood flow rates during 915-MHz direct contact diathermy. (From [1])

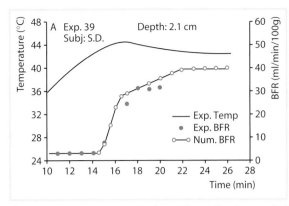

Fig. 2. Transient temperature and experimental and numerical blood flow rate (*BFR*) response at site of xenon injection depot. (From [28])

It is curious to note that there is no significant improvement in BFR in the range of temperature from 37°C (average normal temperature) to 41°C and only hyperthermic temperatures above 41°C are effective in producing significant hyperemia in the tissue targets.

Physics and Heating Technology Comparison

In 1972, Johnson and Guy published data regarding the main factors determining the energy absorption in human tissues [10]. Dielectric properties of the tissues, size, geometry, and depth, together with amplitude, frequency, duration, polarization, size, and shape of applicators, as well as space and coupling between the applicators and the tissue, are mandatory elements for transferring electromagnetic energy at depth to produce a proper heating effect.

It must be stressed that the heating effect is mainly due to the attenuation of transferred energy in tissue. Energy attenuation is a complex phenomenon due to the interaction of dielectric tissue properties (dielectric constant, conductivity, dissipation factor, permittivity), which vary as a function of the frequency [31], (Fig. 3).

As the frequency of the energy transferred in the tissue increases, the dielectric constant of the tissue decreases and the conductivity increases. So the higher the frequency is, the higher is the attenuation of the energy transferred in the tissue and consequently the lower is the penetration depth. The penetration depth is the depth at which the electromagnetic field is reduced to 37% and the power to 14%. Tables 1 and 2 clarify the ratio between Frequency (FQZ) and tissues with high and low water content.

The heating pattern in tissue is synonymous with the specific absorption rate (SAR) pattern. The SAR, mandatory for the evaluation of the heating efficiency of all hyperthermia applications, is physically defined as "the time derivative of the incremental energy absorbed by an incremental mass contained in a volume element of a given density" (NCRP 1981: National Council on Radiation Protection and Measurements).

The applicator efficiency can be quantified by measuring the SAR in the sagittal and coronal planes or on a given surface parallel to the applicator plate (effective fields size: EFS) and at depth perpendicularly to the applicator plate. The result of each of the three measurements gives a graphic design representing an isotherm showing the energy transferred from applicator into the tissue.

These studies are generally performed on phantoms having the same dielectric properties as human tissues [32].

It is strongly recommended to avoid FQZ and applicators since, due to difficult coupling and poor homo-

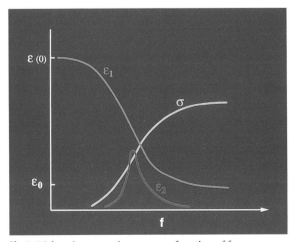

Fig. 3. Dielectric properties vary as a function of frequency. ε_1, dielectric constant; σ, conductivity; ε_2, dissipation factor. (From [31])

Table 1. Muscle, skin and tissues with high water content

Frequency	Dielectric constant	Conductivity [s/m]	Penetration depth [cm]
27.16 MHz	113	0.602	14.3
433 MHz	53	1.18	3.57
915 MHz	51	1.28	3.04
2450 MHz	47	2.17	1.70
10000 MHz	39.9	10	0.343

Table 2. Fat, bone and tissues with low water content

Frequency	Dielectric constant	Conductivity [ms/m]	Penetration depth [cm]
27.16 MHz	20	10.9 – 43.2	15.9
433 MHz	5.6	37.9 – 118	26.2
915 MHz	5.6	55.6 – 147	17.7
2450 MHz	5.5	96.4 – 213	11.1
10000 MHz	4.5	324 – 549	33.9

geneity of absorbed energy, hot spots are produced. Hot spots are in fact points at which the energy deposition is much higher than that absorbed in the irradiated volume, which raises temperature over 48/50°C.

One has to remember that temperature distribution is also a function of thermal diffusion, blood circulation and time. Since the heating/SAR pattern may vary considerably over a three-dimensional volume, due to the geometrical shape, and tissue composition of the body section to be irradiated, strong attention may be paid to the average size, depth, and tissue type of the targets usually treated in rehabilitation.

With the exception of the hip joints, average depth in physical medicine goes from 1 to 5 cm, average size goes from a few cubic centimeters to 200–300 cm³ and tissues to be heated are mainly muscles and tendons with respectively high and low blood perfusion.

Since 1966, a group of researchers, led by Lehmann and Guy, investigated the heating patterns of each technology or method used to increase the temperature in physical medicine during clinical practice [33].

In January 1974, a masterpiece of the contemporary *Therapeutic Application of Electromagnetic Power*, published in the Proceedings of the IEEE Transaction, made a comparison between different heating modalities like hot packs, infrared lamp, short-wave diathermy (27.13 MHz), microwave diathermy (2450 MHz), and microwave diathermy (915 MHz with surface cooling: hyperthermia prototype). Each heating pattern of the above modalities has been investigated, measuring the muscle temperatures every 1 cm (approximately) from the skin to 4–5 cm at depth in a thigh [26]. The results confirmed that:

1. Hot packs (conductive heating) increases the temperature only at the skin level and not at the therapeutic value.
2. Infrared increases the temperature to a therapeutic value only at the skin level.
3. Short wave diathermy (27.13 MHz) with an inductive applicator, increases the temperature to the therapeutic value only in the first 1.6 cm, without overheating the skin tissue.
4. Microwave diathermy (2450 MHz) reached the therapeutic value at 1.85 cm with the skin temperature above 45°C.
5. Microwave diathermy (915 MHz with surface cooling: hyperthermia prototype) reached the therapeutic temperature level (42–45°C) from 1 to 4 cm deep, keeping the skin temperature under 36°C.

On the other hand, ultrasound (US) technology for physical therapy does not permit ideal HT treatments, and consequently an ideal increase of blood flow rate, due to the physical behavior of sound waves on human tissue, the presence of hot spots, discomfort [34–36], and low power energy usable in commercial equipment.

The Ideal System for Proper Heating Patterns on Human Tissues

The choice of the ideal heating system depends on the medical requirements as regard to the therapeutic effects produced by hyperthermia. Physical medicine requirements dictated from physiology and physics applied to human tissues to produce effective hyperthermia treatments are subjected to the average three-dimensional target volumes, the average depth and average tissue damage of the lesions.

For this reason, a modern hyperthermia system for thermotherapy in orthopedics, sports medicine, and rheumatology needs the following characteristics:

1. The correct frequency to reach at least 3–4 cm in depth
2. 50% SAR depth around 2–2.5 cm
3. 50% SAR at the surface around 50 cm²
4. An efficient cooling system to keep the superficial tissue (skin, fatty tissue) under 42°C
5. A multipoint thermometry system to control the temperature
6. A computerized system to control and memorize the treatment

Actually, the medical equipment market offers devices with such requirements. Currently used in oncology for the treatment of superficial cancer [37–40], these hyperthermia systems have been developed to increase and maintain the temperature of a target volume of up to 300–400 cm³ from 41.5 to 45°C at a depth of 1–5 cm.

Figure 4 shows hyperthermia equipment built according to the 43/92 EEC (European Economic Community) rules, supplied with a microwave power generator at 434 MHz, an applicator at 434 MHz with a water bolus, a temperature-controlled system for invasive and non-invasive temperature measurement and specific software to control and memorized the temperature reached in the treated target.

The heating of three target volumes placed at three different depths, calls for a progressive increase of power (Watts) followed, within certain limits, by a lowering of the water temperature (WT), necessary to lower the temperatures of the surface tissues.

If the target is very superficial (<10 mm), the water bolus will be maintained at a temperature close to the target temperature, to facilitate the heating patterns produced at depth by the electromagnetic energy.

Temperature sensors placed at the surface or, if

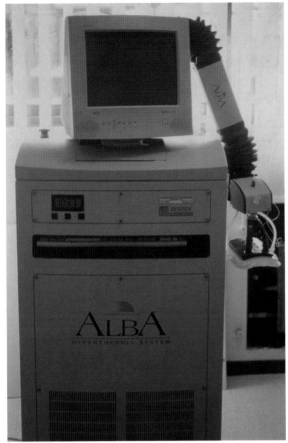

Fig. 4. Hyperthermia equipment supplied with a microwave power generator at 434 MHz (Alba System)

1. Increase of tendon extensibility
2. Reduction of pain and relief of muscle spasm
3. Increase of blood flow
4. Hematoma relief
5. Decrease of muscular and articular stiffness

A few experimental studies have shed some light on the clinical efficacy of microwave diathermy.

In an experimental study, Lehmann investigated the methods of elongating collagenous tissue to produce maximum length increase under therapeutic conditions [22]. He demonstrated that the exclusive use of heat or stretch does not produce elongation of the rat tail tendon, whereas combining the application of a sustained load and temperature of 45°C, produces significant residual length in the tendon.

In clinical practice, therefore, it seems reasonable to treat contractures using heat at therapeutic temperatures, (from 41°C to 45°C) while applying sustained stretch, and to maintain this stretch well after the heating period, in order to retain the achieved elongation. It is common practice to use heat to treat joints which have been damaged by trauma or disease.

In the last decade, a growing body of clinical evidence suggested that a local deep microwave hyperthermia (LDMWH) may be of therapeutic value in treating patients with different rheumatic conditions, because it has the advantage of heating the target organ (e.g., synovium), inhibiting several enzymatic systems (e.g., collagenase, cyclo-oxygenase, etc.), while sparing the surrounding tissues [41, 42].

In particular, the beneficial effects of LDMWH were demonstrated by Weinberger et al. [43] on seven rheumatoid arthritis patients with knee effusion who were treated with a 915 MHz device for 1 h twice a week for 2 weeks, reaching an intra-articular temperature of 41.3°C. Walking time for 50 feet, knee circumference, pain score index, together with synovial fluid samples were determined before and after each treatment.

The results demonstrated an improvement in the walking time ($P = 0.04$) and a significant decrease in pain ($P = 0.01$) at the end of treatment.

The exact mechanism of the hyperthermia effect in inflammatory joint diseases is not completely understood. It was suggested that an increase in tissue temperature up to 42°C might cause an intracellular metabolic arrest with an inhibition of DNA and protein synthesis, accompanied by an enhanced permeability of the cell membrane. A decrease in hyaluronate synthesis at 42°C has also been demonstrated in synovial fluid [43].

The efficacy and safety of LDMWH was further confirmed in a study on normal and Zymosan-induced arthritis in rabbits [44]. It was demonstrated that a repeated therapeutic dose of hyperthermia at 42.5°C for 1 h is well tolerated by the periarticular mesenchymal

needed, at depth, measure the temperature reached in the target and give feedback to the computerized system to optimize each hyperthermia treatment.

Regarding the safety and quality requirements dictated by government, it is important to note that some ISM (industrial scientific medical) frequencies are different in the EU (European Union) compared with the USA. The frequency of 434 MHz is allowed in the EU and is forbidden in the USA, while 915 MHz is allowed in the USA and is forbidden in the EU.

Therapeutic Applications of Hyperthermia

Hyperthermia equipment is used to treat both acute and chronic conditions, to facilitate healing and for the relief of pain. The rationale of hyperthermia as a therapeutic method in physical medicine has been supported by Lehmann (1970–1983) and Weinberger (1989–1992) with studies made on animals and humans. The use of hyperthermia in musculo-skeletal pathologies produces one or more of the following effects:

tissues and that after 1 month, no damage could be observed in normal rabbit knees, whereas in the arthritic joints it brought about a reduction in the degree of granulomatous reaction, decreasing the inflammatory process.

Muscle injuries quite often involve the development of intramuscular hematomas and these are a common occurrence in the athletic population [45]. So, during the resolution phase, the purpose of the physical therapy is to accelerate the healing process and the absorption rate of the hematoma. Even if heat application has been advocated by several authors to accelerate this resolution, no experimental data were available until 1983, when a study showed that selective heating of the muscle could increase the rate of intramuscular hematoma absorption [46].

Lehmann [46], first quantified the resolution rate of hematomas produced in the musculature of experimental animals comparable in size to humans; hematomas in the biceps femoris muscle were created in pigs by bilateral injections of blood, labeled with CR[51]. One side was treated with microwave diathermy at 915 MHz and the other side was used as a control.

The results demonstrated that tissue temperature achieved at the treated hematoma site was in the therapeutic range between 42°C and 45°C, the optimal temperature to elicit a maximal local vascular response [1, 46]. A decay curve for the radioisotope, showed that the time to the half-life value was significantly shorter for the treated side. This study supports the use of heat as an adjunct to other therapies aimed at resolution of muscular hematomas.

In a recent clinical study, the efficacy of hyperthermia at 434 MHz in the early treatment of muscle injuries in a group of 62 patients was evaluated and compared with conventional diathermy like ultrasound [47], (Fig. 5). All the patients underwent pain measurement with a VAS scale and ultrasonography before, at the end, and after 1 month.

The results demonstrated how the percentage of improvement was greater in the group treated with hyperthermia together with a faster resolution of the hematoma after 2 weeks of treatment, as compared with the ultrasound group. There were neither complications nor reoccurrences at the follow-up in the hyperthermia group while two reoccurrences and one calcification occurred in a case of pectoralis major injury in the ultrasound group.

This investigation confirms that hyperthermia at 434 MHz is a highly innovative, safe, and reliable method in the treatment of acute sport muscle injuries. The use of local hyperthermia (LH) has also been recently advocated in the treatment of neuropathies. Compression of the median nerve in a fibro-osseus canal on the palmar surface of the wrist is one of the most frequently described tunnel syndromes.

A recent study evaluated the efficacy of hyperthermia as a treatment in 32 patients affected by primary carpal tunnel syndrome (CTS), comparing the clinical results with instrumental examinations such as electroneurography (ENG), ultrasonography (US), and teletermography (TTG) [48].

The results demonstrated an improvement in the clinical score in 90% of the patients treated, and in ENG (P < 0.05), especially in the conduction velocity of the sensory median nerve in the third and the fourth fingers. The treatment was equally highly effective in the group that received only five applications instead of ten.

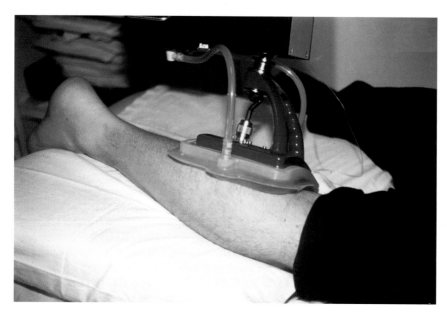

Fig. 5. Hyperthermia application in a case of medial gastrocnemius muscle injury

The indication for LH in the management of carpal tunnel syndrome could be questioned, since there is no controlled study comparing LH with the other widely accepted methods of treatment (e.g., local infiltration with corticosteroids or hand surgery). However, LH is not an invasive procedure and these primary results support its use in the early stages of CTS, in particular whenever standard treatments are contraindicated.

The use of heat methods in the treatment of tendon injuries has long been an accepted part of treatment protocols [49]. A wide variety of methods, including ultrasound and lasers are still employed to treat tendinopathies. Such methods are claimed to decrease inflammation and promote healing, but there is only limited evidence as yet to support many of these claims [50].

Treatment of any organic medical condition is ideally based on an understanding of the pathophysiology. Unfortunately, chronic overuse tendon conditions in athletes have been treated as inflammatory conditions when the histopathology clearly reveals, in most of the cases, degenerative tendinosis. Of course, many etiological factors may lead to degeneration, thereby reducing the tensile strength of the tendon.

There is evidence suggesting that decreased arterial blood flow, with resulting local hypoxia and impaired metabolic activity and nutrition, may be the key factors [51, 52], together with a failed cell matrix adaptation to excessive changes in load [53].

A study recently reported on the effectiveness of hyperthermia at 434 MHz in the treatment of 67 athletes affected by chronic painful tendinopathies, compared with an ultrasound-treated group [54]. Both groups were clinically (VAS scale) and instrumentally (ultrasonography) evaluated before, at the end and after 1 month.

The hyperthermia group showed a significant reduction of pain ($P < 0.001$) with a percentage of improvement of 68% as compared with the ultrasound group. The overall outcome, based on the resolution of pain and return to sports activity, demonstrated excellent and good results in 87% of the hyperthermia group compared with 43% of the ultrasound group. The early results of this study are encouraging, supporting the use of hyperthermia in the treatment of chronic tendinopathies.

Unfortunately, in this study the ultrasonography imaging was unable to demonstrate significant changes in tendon structure, due to its technical and diagnostic limitation and because of the short follow-up, despite the fact that many authors have suggested that in chronic tendinopathies the healing process is best indicated by relief of pain and abnormal imaging was absolutely compatible with excellent clinical results [55]. If microwaves at 434 MHz are to continue to be used as a therapeutic method, it is clearly essential that their efficacy must be evaluated with further well-designed controlled studies, in a variety of clinical conditions, as well as with long-term follow-ups.

Conclusions and Future Directions

It is particularly curious, that experimental and clinical work on the use of electromagnetic power to produce therapeutic temperatures (range 41–45°C), demonstrated by some authors more than 25 years ago, have not had, until today, a large following from the physical medicine world community.

In most countries, including the USA, heat therapy is still performed utilizing devices such as ultrasound, short wave or microwaves and lasers of different powers, although the physical characteristics of such systems have been proved to be inefficient to reach the necessary therapeutic heating levels in the range of depth of the damaged tissues.

Recently, in a few EU countries such as Italy, Spain, and the UK, hyperthermia equipment, operating at a frequency of 434 MHz and developed according to the requirements described by Lehmann and Guy in the 1980s, and by the EEC in the 1990s, have been employed for clinical use in sport traumatology, rheumatology, and sport medicine.

After 2 years of clinical work and analysis of almost 30 years of worldwide scientific literature on the use of heat in physical medicine, it is our opinion that this hyperthermia equipment will permit a better comprehension of the biological mechanisms which regulate the relationship between the thermal dose and the healing process of soft tissues with low or high water content or with low or high blood flow perfusion.

The knowledge of the in situ real time blood perfusion rate increase during a hyperthermia treatment, together with the in situ tissue sample biopsies performed at the end of a hyperthermia treatment session or cycle will be of paramount importance to better define the biological cell response to a heat 'dose'.

Up-to-date advanced scientific work on hyperthermia in cancer therapy is now suggesting a fascinating association between hyperthermia and anti-inflammatory drugs to potentiate each other's therapeutic effects, thanks to the increased (several fold) cell uptake of drugs which happens at high temperatures compared with normal temperature [56].

Extracorporeal Shock Waves in Orthopaedics

In 1980, the first patient with renal calculi was successfully treated with minimally invasive extracorporeal shock wave lithotripsy (ESWL). Since then the medical field of application of this form of energy has been extended. The most recent result of the medical and technical development of application is extracorporeal shock wave therapy (ESWT) for the treatment of orthopaedic pathologies.

At the beginning of the 1990s the first reports were published on the use of ESWT beyond nephrolithiasis and colelithiasis. The sonic sources and systems employed in ESWL and ESWT are very similar, which is no wonder, as the first ESWT trials were undertaken with conventional kidney and gallbladder lithotriptors.

Valchanov and Michailov [57] and Sukul et al. [58] inaugurated ESWT for the treatment of delayed and non-union of fractures, describing local decortication and fragmentation with stimulation of osteogenesis. These positive aspects were corroborated by Haist et al. [59], who noticed bony consolidation in 32 out of 40 cases with a pseudoarthrosis. In case reports, Dahmen et al. [60] and Loew and Jurgowski [61] achieved good results in calcifying tendinitis of the shoulder.

The indications for ESWT are progressively moving to cover a large part of the rest of the tendinous pathologies, especially at the insertional areas, and their limits of application, on the bone side of the orthopaedic diseases, have already reached the field of osteochondritis and osteonecrosis of the hip and the knee as a new promising technique of treatment.

Definition

A shock wave is scientifically defined as an acoustic or sonic wave, at the wave front of which the pressure above atmospheric rises from ambient pressure to maximum pressure (amplitude) within a few nanoseconds (10^{-9}). Current therapeutically used pressure amplitudes, range between 10 MPa and more than 100 MPa [62] (1 MPa = 10 bar, approximately tenfold atmospheric pressure). As a shock wave propagates at a specific speed – as do all sonic waves – determined by the medium in which it propagates and the intensity of the shock wave itself, one can calculate the shock front thickness. This is the spatial dimension between the locations where the pressure amplitude has been reached. In tissue, for example, the shock front thickness is in the range of 1.5 – 6 μm [63]. During transition of, for example, a cell wall, which has a thickness of a few molecular layers, significant forces can already come to bear on the wall, as there are immediate differences in pressure in front of and behind it. The pressure gradient, i.e., the change in pressure between two locations, reaches its maximum at a given wave amplitude in the shock front as compared with other forms of sonic signals, e.g., sinusoidal ultrasound.

Sources

In practice, all extracorporeal shock wave (ESW) generators consist of an electrical energy source, an electroacoustic conversion mechanism and a device for focusing the sound waves.

There are three methods of generating shock waves, namely by piezoelectic, electrohydraulic, or electromagnetic means.

Without entering into a detailed discussion on the technical data about the ESW generators, it is important to know that the electrohydraulic system produces high energy ESW, but with marked oscillations in the values of the energy flux density through the tissues, which do not remain constant during the therapeutic application. They need a spark electrode to work, but a fast deterioration in use reduces its life to about 1000 sparks [64, 65] before the electrode needs to be changed, while a single application, lasts some thousands of impulses, on average.

The piezoelectric device is very precise and has a long life but, in spite of a very sophisticated technology, produces only low-energy ESW, often requiring, repeated treatments to reach the desired result [64].

The more actual electromagnetic generators are mainly differentiated into two types because of their shapes: flat and cylinder coils. The average value of pressure, expressed in terms of energy flux density, is almost constant and the coil is a very long-lasting device.

To achieve a specific effect, the sound waves must be focused. When employing point sources (e.g., sparks) or cylinder sources, a focusing mirror is used. When employing areal sources, lenses or a self focusing appliance of partially spherical shape are used.

ESW in Medical Practice

Shock waves employed in medical practice are characterized by high positive pressures up to 80 – 100 MPa and negative pressures of 5 – 10 MPa Furthermore, they have a short rise time of 30 – 120 ns and a shorter pulse duration (5 μs),. In contrast to ultrasound, shock waves have low frequencies. Just in this respect, there is less absorption by the tissue. Moreover, the shock waves are applied with a lower repetition frequency of 1 – 2, maximum 4 Hz, which means that they have a low time-averaged intensity. The only thing that can be said for sure is that the shock wave does not cause tissue warming [66]. None of the known shock wave effects are due to thermal effects.

During the ESWT, it is important to know the energy dose administered for each treatment. All the authors, under a general agreement, distinguish the ESW into high-energy waves and low-energy waves; the level of energy turns out to be a complex parameter which is defined by the ratio between the applied power and the tissue density [64, 67].

Treatments with intermediate and high energy levels produce energy flux densities which range from those used for treatment of nephrolithiasis to many times this energy level, i.e., densities from 0.37 to 1.2 mJ/mm^2. This form of treatment nearly always requires analgesia or anesthesia. The indications are represented by pseudoarthrosis and some species of tendinosis calcharea.

Low-energy treatment employs 10% – 20% of the dose used for renal calculi, i.e., densities between 0.08 and 0.23 mJ/mm^2. In most cases anesthesia or analgesia is not required. The low energy range is mainly reserved for the treatment of localized soft tissue disorders.

Modes of Action

Regarding the action of shock waves on tissue, four phases have been postulated:

1. *Physical phase:* extracellular cavitations, ionized molecules and an increase of membrane permeability are direct effects of the shock waves.
2. *Physical-chemical phase:* diffusible radicals and interactions with biomolecules (in both phases mitochondrial lesions were observed).
3. *Chemical phase:* may be accompanied by intracellular reactions and molecular changes.
4. *Biological phase:* noted if these changes persist.

Many of the shock wave tissue interactions are not yet completely understood.

Several theories have been formulated to explain the mechanism of action of ESW on bone-related soft tissue pain:

1. The shock wave locally alters the chemical environment in such a way, that pain-inhibiting substances are produced.
2. The shock wave damages the cell membrane; no more generator potential is produced in the pain receptor for the formation of the pain signals.
3. The shock wave stimulates the pain receptor to emit a high frequency of nerve impulses. The retransmission of pain impulses is inhibited as it is subject to external stimuli (gate-control theory).
4. The shock wave induces a release of endorphin resulting in the reduction of (local) sensitivity to pain.

Therefore, there seem to be two possible modes of action in tissue; direct effects, or those caused by cavitation.

Direct Effects. Direct effects are mechanical effects caused by temporary positive pressure amplitudes during the propagation of a pressure pulse. The stability under load of the material (tissue) may be exceeded at the interface between the materials with different acoustic impedances. At such interfaces, the shock waves lead to changes in the excursion, which result in tensile and shearing loads. In soft tissue, where there are no great differences in acoustic impedance, the direct effects of shock waves do not appear to play a significant role.

Cavitation. The definition of cavitation is: expansion and oscillation of gas-filled cavities (pre-existing as cavitation nuclei) due to the tensile portion of a pressure wave with subsequent collapse. The cavitation results in mechanical and chemical effects:

1. Mechanical: shearing loads develop due to the oscillation of the developed cavitation bubbles. Due to the collapse of the bubbles, there is an inflow of water (jet streams). These inflowing water masses can reach velocities of between 400 and 700 ms^{-1} [66], which correspond to the velocity of bullets. One can surely imagine an effect of this jet stream on a mechanical basis.
2. Chemical: during the collapse of the cavitation bubbles, high temperatures develop locally inside the bubbles, which lead to the development of radicals. The induced radicals can subsequently lead to damage in the tissue.

The discussion as to which of the above types of effect is responsible for the biological effects is currently still under way.

In experiments on cells in suspension, Brümmer [68] and Smits [69] found a cell damage pattern which is dependent on the number of shock waves and the shock wave energy applied:

1. Transient membrane rupture (permeability) with secondary damage (cell edema)
2. Transient damage to endoplasmatic reticulum and cell nucleus
3. Dose-dependent vacuolization of the cytoplasma
4. Lesion in cytoskeleton (actin and vimentin fibers)
5. Complete cell rupture (e.g., hemolysis)

To understand the mode of action of the ESW on the bone tissue we need to consider their mechanical effects on the bone trabeculae. When the shock wave hits the anterior surface of a trabecula, because the impedance inside it (II medium) is lower compared with the one outside it (I medium), at the level of the I interface (I medium/II medium), part of the energy is reflected back (stretching force), while the remaining energy (compressing force) advances through the trabecula (II medium) to reach the posterior surface of it up to the II interface (II medium/I medium), where the acoustic impedance gradient is inverted and the reflected wave is negative.

At the level of both interfaces, the cavitation bubbles are formed and are then submitted to a deforming compression by the gradient of pressure, with a consequent reduction of the volume and increase in energy; they collapse progressively, the anterior wall hit by the shock wave introflects, while the posterior wall is extroflected by the stretching components, until the bubble releases part of the stored energy generating the jet streams directed toward the gradual shattering of the trabeculae.

According to Sukul and Johannes [58] these effects on the bone structures are comparable to the effects of lithotripsy on kidney and gallbladder stones. In the literature, several hypotheses have been considered:

1. Microfissures at the fracture ends
2. Development of a hematoma
3. Development of small cortical/spongiosa chips
4. Transformation of local connective-tissue cells

Steinbach [66] observed that in the focus center, the endotelial cells were no longer monolinearly next to each other, but were scattered around, partly ripped down to the basilemma and unica muscularis. A further effect was an increase in the fibrillic actin content in the endotelial cell; the closer the cells had been to the focus, the greater the fibrillic actin content in the cytoplasm (so-called stress fibers develop due to a variety of stimuli). Owing to the increased content of fibrillic actin in the endothelial cells, the latter retract and the intercellular distances increase, which might explain a higher vessel permeability.

Also, the phenomenon of neoangiogenesis might be related to the presence of chemiotactic factors, very close to the ESAF (endothelial stimulating angiogenetic factor), released by the stress fibers.

ESW has important effects on nerves and nerve cells. It could be hypothetically assumed that the mode of action is based on a direct mechanical effect of the shock wave on the axon membrane in the sense of an increase in permeability with consecutive depolarization and triggering of an action potential. However, it appears more probable that a cavitation-based effect plays a role in the triggering of the cumulative action potentials. A hyperpolarization of the neurons is achieved by means of shock wave treatment, whereby an energy dependency was discovered, i.e., the higher the energy of the emitted shock wave, the greater the polarization. These effects lasted for approximately 1 h after the shock wave. During hyperpolarization, a stimulus is necessary which is larger than that required before shock wave treatment, to excite an action potential. Whether this effect could play a role in palliative therapy will require further study.

Indications and Protocols of Therapy

From the first reports of Valchanou and Michailov [57] who inaugurated high energy ESWT for the treatment of delayed and non-union fractures, the clinical indications have been largely expanded toward other orthopaedic disorders, both in hard tissue pathology, i.e., osteonecrosis and osteochondritis or the problems of osteointegration at the metal-bone interface of the loose cementless prosthesis, and the soft tissue pathologies, i.e., almost all the insertional tendinitis and enthesopathies or muscles strains.

There is a general agreement among the authors that high energy treatments should be reserved for bone affections whereas low energy ESWT is the most indicated treatment for soft tissues lesions.

During soft tissue therapies, usually without any form of analgesia or anesthesia, the application of shock waves is also based on a sort of 'pain feedback', by asking the patient when he recognizes his symptomatology, and the quality and the site of pain; but it must always be remembered that there are algogenic structures, i.e., the periosteum of the superficial bones or the sensitive nerve bundles, easily stimulated by the ESW: their activation always induces strong pain and it might confuse the operator. For this reason it is important that an in-line ecographic aiming device is available to precisely individuate the site of pathology.

The high energy ESWT almost always requires pain control by means of analgesic/anesthetic treatment. An image intensifier is absolutely necessary to position the focus of the ESW right on the site of pathology, otherwise it is impossible to individuate it exactly.

Pseudarthrosis

Delayed union is defined when a fracture is not healed completely within 4 months. Healing that does not happen within 6 months is called pseudarthrosis. Congenital forms of pseudarthrosis are known. According to radiological criteria, pseudoarthrosis can be hypertrophic or atrophic. The present studies show that ESWT is not indicated in cases of congenital non-unions, and that results are better in hypertrophic forms than in atrophic ones.

The protocol schemes according to Russo et al. [70] distinguish between small bones and other bones.

In the first case, two applications, the latter 24–48 h after, 4000 impulses, 0.7–1.0 mJ/mm², are recommended.

Non-unions of the long bones are treated with ESW in four sessions, each second day, 4000/5000 impulses, 1.0 mJ/mm². The decision to cease the treatment or to continue it with the second phase is based on the evidence of osteogenic response in the X-rays and magnetic resonance imaging (MRI) controls. A second and a third phase are only needed when partial fusion or no fusion at all are observed. Modalities and energy rates are the same as for the first phase.

Prosthesis Loosening

During the last few years, the application of ESW for hip prosthesis failure was advocated from two different, almost opposite, points of view. Haupt [71] and other authors [72, 73] have considered the possibility of using it to facilitate the removal of cement at the interface with bone in the revision of cemented prostheses.

On the other hand, Schaden [74] believes that the application of ESW for loosening of the femoral component in cementless hip prostheses might effectively help to re-fix the stem bone, as he observed at least in three case reports. What he advises is to utilize a high energy device (28 kV) for a number of applications of between 4000 and 8000 impulses.

Osteochondritis, Osteochondrosis, and Osteonecrosis

Osteochondritis dissecans of the knee or talus was treated with ESW by Schleberger [75], resulting in integration of the dissecating bone piece, but success rates have not been reported yet. Few treatments with promising results have been performed in patients with Köhler's, Perthes's, or Osgood-schlatter's disease [75, 76]. To date, these therapies must be considered experimental.

Some authors have started, in the last 2 or 3 years, to employ ESW in the therapy of earlier forms of osteonecrosis of the femoral head and femoral condyles of the knee. Unfortunately, we have not yet had results or technical information about these procedures.

Tendinosis Calcarea of the Shoulder

Probably, calcifying tendinitis of the shoulder represents the first field of application of ESW in orthopaedic soft tissue pathologies.

According to Rompe [77], high energy ESW are expected to exert a direct, mechanically disintegrating effect on hard surfaces such as calcareous deposits in the supraspinous tendon. Low energy ESWT, however, is regarded as a form of hyperstimulation analgesia. In the low energy treatment the patient receives 1500 impulses of 0.06 mJ mm⁻² of energy density. The high energy treatment consists of 1500 impulses of 0.28 mJ mm⁻² administered under regional anesthesia.

Gigliotti, Russo et al. propose a different protocol of treatment for calcifying tendinitis: 2000–2500 impulses set at a level of density energy of 0.07–0.11 mJ mm⁻² in a series of 5-weekly sessions.

Insertional Tendinitis

Insertional tendinitis is a very common pathological picture in athletes. Among these, patellar tendinitis and epicondylitis humeri (radialis more often than ulnaris) have the higher rates of incidence. Haist [78] proposes a treatment protocol based on three to four sessions of about 25 min (1500 impulses at a frequency of 1 Hz) with the energy density between 0.06 and 0.12 mJ mm⁻². We had promising results in patellar tendinitis after submitting the patients to a four-session cycle of treatment: 1500 impulses at an energy level of 0.11 mJ mm⁻² each seventh day. No patient needed analgesia for it.

Contraindications and Side Effects

ESWT is absolutely contraindicated in pediatric or adolescent patients under the age of 18 years, during pregnancy, if there are pathological neurological, or vascular findings, if there are local infections, tumors, or blood coagulation diseases.

Rotator cuff tears, arthritic degenerative changes of the gleno-humeral joint, and ligamentous articular instability should also be considered relative contraindications for treatment.

When properly performed, ESWT is free from general side effects in healthy subjects.

Regional reactions have been observed since the first urological employment. They are usually temporary and limited to small local swelling, hematomas and petechial hemorrhages.

Conclusions

According to the opinion of the several authors involved up to now in ESWT, shock wave application in orthopaedics has to be considered as minimally invasive, and a safe method of treatment as regards traditionally difficult and problematic bone and tendinous pathologies, like non-unions and enthesopathies.

Almost no side effects whatsoever have been observed in hundreds of thousands of therapy sessions all over the world since the very early beginnings of this treatment.

However, due to the high cost of the equipment, and consequently of the treatments, this therapy should be restricted to patients who do not experience considerable pain relief after a defined period of established conventional treatment.

When non-union of a fracture occurs, either in operated and non-operated patients, ESWT should be considered, and eventually administered, before resorting to a surgical treatment, as a revision or completely new procedure.

References

1. Sekins KM, Emery AF, Lehmann JF, McDougall JA (1982) Determination of perfusion field during local hyperthermia with the aid of finite element thermal models. J Biom Engineering, 104: 272–279.

2. Brown AC, Brengelman G (1965) Energy metabolism. In: Ruch and Patton (eds) Physiology and biophysics. Philadelphia PA: Saunders, 1030–1049.

3. Licht S (1965) History of therapeutic heat. In: Licht S (ed) Therapeutic heat and cold. Waverly Press, Baltimore 6:196–231

4. Hollmann HE (1939) Zum Problem der Ultrakurzwellen. Behandlung durch Anstrahlung. Strahlen Therapie, 64: 691–702

5. Krusen FH, Herrick JF, Leden U, Wakim KG (1947) Microkymatotherapy: preliminary report of experimental studies of the heating effect of microwaves (radar) in living tissues. Proc Staff Meet Mayo Clin, 22:209–224

6. Leden UM, Herrick JF, Wakim KG, Krusen FH (1947) Preliminary studies on the heating and circulating effects of microwaves (radar). Br J Phys Med 10:177–184

7. Schwan HP, Piersa GM (1954) Absorption of electromagnetic energy in body tissues. Am J Phys Med 33:371–404

8. Lehmann JF, Guy AW, Johnson VC, Brunner GD, Bell JW (1962) Comparison of relative heating patterns produced in tissues by exposure to microwave energy at frequencies of 2450 and 900 megacycles. Arch Phys Med 43:69–76

9. Guy AW, Lehmann JF (1966) On the determination of an optimum microwave diathermy frequency for a direct contact applicator. IEEE Trans Biomed Eng 13:76–87

10. Johnson C, Guy AW (1972) Nonionizing electromagnetic wave effects in biological materials and systems. Proc IEEE 60:692–718

11. Ter Haar G, Dyson M, Oakley EM (1987) The use of ultrasound by physiotherapists in Britain. Ultrasound Med Biol 13:659–663

12. Draper DO, Castel JC, Castel D (1995) Rate of temperature increase in human muscle during 1 MHz and 3 MHz continuous ultrasound. J Orthop Sports Phys Ther 22:142–150

13. Dyson M, Pond JB, Joseph J, Warwick R (1968) The stimulation of tissue regeneration by means of ultrasound. Clin Sci 35:273–285

14. Kramer JF (1984) Ultrasound: evaluation of its mechanical and thermal effects. Arch Phys Med Rehabil 65:223–227

15. Chan AK, Myrer JW, Measom GJ, Draper DO (1998) Temperature changes in human patellar tendon in response to therapeutic ultrasounds. J Athletic Training 33:130–135

16. Lehmann JF, Delateur BJ (1990) Therapeutic heat. In: Lehmann JF (ed) Therapeutic heat and cold, 4th edn. Williams and Wilkins, Baltimore, 417–581

17. Abramson DI, Burnett C, Bell J, Tuck S (1960) Changes in blood flow, oxygen uptake and tissue temperatures produced by therapeutic physical agents. Am J Phys Med 47:51–62

18. Akyurekli D, Gerig LH, Raaphorst GP (1997) Changes in muscle blood flow distribution during hyperthermia. Int J Hyperthermia 13:481–496

19. Baker RJ, Bell GW (1991) The effect of therapeutic modalities on blood flow in the human calf. J Orthop Sports Phys Therapy 13:23–27

20. Fox HH, Hilton SM (1958) Bradykinin formation in skin as a factor in heat vasodilatation. J Physiol 142:219–222

21. Kanui TI (1985) Thermal inhibition of nociceptors-driven spinal cord nerves in rats. Pain 21:231–234

22. Lehmann JF, Masock AJ, Warren CG, Koblaski JN (1970) Effect of therapeutic temperatures on tendon extensibility. Arch Phys Med Rehabil 51:481–487

23. Weinberger A, Fadilah R, Lev A, Levi A, Pinkhas S (1988) Deep heat in the treatment of inflammatory joint disease. Med Hypoth 25:231–233

24. Lentell G (1992) The use of thermal agents to influence the effectiveness of a low-load prolonged stretch. J Orthop Sports Phys Ther 16:200–205

25. Le Ban MM (1962) Collagen tissue: implications of its response to stress in vitro. Arch Phys Med Rehabil 43461

26. Guy AW, Lehmann JF, Stonebridge JB (1974) Therapeutic applications of electromagnetic power. Proc IEEE 62:65–75

27. Guy AW, Chou CK (1983) Physical aspects of localized heating by radio waves and microwaves. In: Storm KF (ed) Hyperthermia in cancer therapy. GK Hall Medical Publishers, Boston

28. Sekins KM, Dundore D, Emery AF, Lehmann JF, McGrath PW, Nelp WB (1980) Muscle blood flow changes in response to 915 MHz diathermy with surface cooling as measured by Xe 133 clearance. Arch Phys Med Rehabil 61:105–113

29. Song CW, Kang MS, Rhee JG, Levitt SH (1980) The effect of hyperthermia on vascular function, pH, and cell survival. Radiology 37:795–803

30. Song CW (1984) Effect of local hyperthermia on blood flow and microenvironment: a review. Cancer Res (suppl.) 44: 4721–4730

31. Chou CK (1987) Phantoms for electromagnetic heating studies. In: Chou CK (ed) Physics and technology of hyperthermia, Martinus Njhoff Publ Boston, pp 294–318

32. Guy AW (1971) Analysis of electromagnetic fields induced in biological tissues by thermographic studies on equivalent phantom models. IEEE TransMicrowave TheorTech 19:205–214

33. Lehmann JF, Silverman DR, Baum BA (1966) Temperature distributions in the human thigh produced by infrared, hot pack and microwave applications. Arch Phys Med Rehabil 47:291–299

34. Ziskin MC (1993) Fundamental physics of ultrasound and its propagation in tissue. Radiographics 13:705–709

35. Falconer J (1990) Therapeutic ultrasound in the treatment of musculo-skeletal conditions. Arthritis Care Res 3:85–91

36. Gam AN, Johannsen F (1995) Ultrasound therapy in musculo-skeletal disorders: a meta-analysis. Pain 63: 85–91

37. Kim JH, Hahn EW, Ahmed SA (1982) Combination hyperthermia and radiation therapy for malignant melanoma. Cancer 50:478–452

38. Overgaard J, Gonzalez G, Hulshof MCMM, Arcangeli G, Dahl O, Mella O (1995) Randomized trial of hyperthermia as adjuvant to radiotherapy for recurrent or metastatic malignant melanoma. Lancet 345:540–543

39. Perez CA, Nussbaum G, Emani B, Vongerichten D (1983) Clinical results of irradiation combined with local hyperthermia. Cancer 52:1597–1603

40. Gabriele P, Amichetti M, Orecchia R, Valdagni R (1995) Radiation therapy and hyperthermia in advanced or recurrent parotid tumors. Cancer 75:908–913

41. Fadilah R, Lev A, Pinkhas S, Weinberger A (1987) Heating rabbit joint by microwave applicator. Arch Phys Med Rehabil 68:710–712

42. Spiegel TM, Hirschberg J, Taylor J, Paulus HE, Furst DE (1987) Heating rheumatoid knees to an intra-articular temperature of 42.1°C. Ann Rheum Diseases 46:716–719

43. Weinberger A, Fadilah R, Lev A, Shohami E, Pinkhas J

(1989) Treatment of articular effusions with local deep microwave hyperthermia. Clin Rheum 4:461–466

44. Weinberger A, Abramonvici A, Fadilah R, Levy A, Giler S, Lev A (1990) The effect of local deep microwave hyperthermia on experimental zymosan-induced arthritis in rabbits. Am J Phys Med Rehabil 69:239–244

45. Garrett WE (1990) Muscle strain injuries. Clinical and basic aspects. Med Sci Sports Exercise 22:436–443

46. Lehmann JF, Dundore DE, Esselman PC (1983) Microwave diathermy: effects on experimental muscle hematoma resolution. Arch Phys Med Rehabil 64:127–129

47. Sorrenti D, Casciello G, Dragoni S, Giombini A (2000) Applicazione della termoterapia endogena nel trattamento delle lesioni muscolari da sport: studio comparativo con ultrasuoni. Med Sport 53:59–67

48. Sabatini L, Giannini F. Karradsheh S, Ravenni R, Cioni R (1996) Local hyperthermia: a new treatment for carpal tunnel syndrome. Proc 7th Int Congr on hyperthermic oncology, vol. II. Rome C3C:370–373,

49. Rivenburgh DW (1992) Physical modalities in the treatment of tendon injuries. ClinSports Med 11:645–659

50. Stanish WD, Curwin S, Rubinovich M (1985) Tendinitis: the analysis and treatment for running. Clin Sports Med 4:593–609

51. Kannus P, Jòzsa (1991) Histopathological changes preceding spontaneous rupture of a tendon. A controlled study of 891 patients. J Bone Joint Surg (Am) 73:1507–1525

52. Archambault JM, Preston Wiley J, Bray RC (1995) Exercise loading of tendons and the development of overuse injuries; a review of current literature. Sports Med 2:77–89

53. Laedbetter WBC (1992) Cell-matrix response in tendon injury. Clin Sports Med 11:533–578

54. Casciello G (1999) Application of microwave diathermy in the treatment of tendinopathies in sport. Thesis of Post-Graduate School in Sport Medicine, University of Rome 'La Sapienza'

55. Astrom M, Gentz CF, Nilsson P, Rausing A, Sjoberg S, Westlin N (1996) Imaging in chronic achilles tendinopathy: a comparison of ultrasonography,magnetic resonance imaging and surgical findings in 27 histologically verified cases. Skeletal Radiol 25: 615–620

56. Kong G, Dewhrist MW (1999) Hyperthermia and liposomes. Int J Hyperthermia 5:345–70

57. Vachalnov V, Michailov P (1991) High energy shock waves in treatment of delayed and non-union of fractures. Int Orthop (SICOT) 15:181–184

58. Sukul K, Johannes E (1993) The effect of high energy shock waves focussed on cortical bone: an in vitro study. J Surg Res 54:46

59. Haist J, Steeger D (1992) The extracorporeal shockwave therapy in the treatment of disturbed bone union. 7th Int. Conference on Biomedical engineering, Singapore, 222–224

60. Dahmen GP, Meiss L (1991) Extracorporale Stosswellentherapie (ESWT) im knochennahen Weichteilbereich an der Schulter. Extracta Orthop 15:25–28

61. Loew M, Jurgowski W (1993) Extracorporale stosswellen-lithotripsie bei tendinosis calcarea. Z Orthop 131:470–473

62. Ueberle F (1998) Shock wave technology. In: Siebert W, Buch A (eds) Extracorporeal shock waves in orthopaedics. Springer, pp 59–87

63. Stranne SK, Cocks FH (1990) Mechanical property studies of human gallstones. J Biomed Mater Res 24:1049–1057

64. Basaglia N, Bertocchi A, Carli S (1999) 'Shock waves' in medicina riabilitativa. MR vol 13, 2:11–24

65. Wess O, Feige A (1997) Introduction to the physics and technology of extracorporeal shock wave therapy (ESWT). Storz Medical Ag, Kreuzlingen

66. Buch M (1998) Review. In: Siebert W, Buch A (eds) Extracorporeal shock waves in orthopaedics. Springer, pp 3–58

67. Russo S, Canero R (1998) Meccanismo di azione dell'onde d'urto sul tessuto osseo. Atti del Corso Interdisciplinare, Parma 27 febbraio, pp 12–16

68. Brümmer F, Suhr D (1990) Standardisierte in vitro-Modelle zur Charakterisierung von Stosswellen. Biomed Tech, 35:237

69. Smits G, Jap P (1994) Biological effects of high energy shock waves in mouse skeletal muscle. Correlation between 3P magnetic resonance spectroscopic and microscopic alteration. Ultrasound Me Biol 19(5):339

70. Russo S, Gigliotti S (1998) Results with extracorporeal shock wave therapy in bone and soft tissue pathologies. In: Siebert W, Buch A (eds) Extracorporeal shock waves in orthopaedics. Springer, pp 149–155

71. Haupt G (1997) Use of extracorporeal shock waves in the treatment of pseudoarthrosis, tendinopathy and other orthopaedic diseases. J Urol 158:4–11

72. Karpman RR, Magee FP (1987) Work in progress. The lithotripter and its potential use in the revision of total hip arthroplasty. Orthop Rev 16:38

73. May TC, Krause WR (1990) Use of high energy shock waves for bone cement removal. J Arthroplasty 5:19

74. Schaden W (1998) Clinical experience with shock wave therapy of pseudoarthrosis, delayed fracture healing, and cement-free endoprosthesis loosening. In: Extracorporeal shock waves in orthopaedics. Springer, pp 137–148

75. Schleberger R (1995) Anwendung der extrakorporalen Stosswelle am Stütz- und Bewegungsapparat im mittelenergetischen Bereich. In: Chaussy C, Eisenberger F (eds) Die Stosswelle, Forschung und Klinik. Attempt Verlag, Tübingen, p 166

76. Haist J, von Keitz-Steeger D (1995) Stosswellentherapie knochennaher Weichteilschmerzen. Ein neues Behandlungskonzept. In: Chaussy C, Eisenberger F (eds) Die Stosswelle, Forschung und Klinik. Attempt Verlag, Tübingen, p 162

77. Rompe JD, Rumler F, Hopf C, Nafe B, Heine J (1995) Extracorporeal shock waves therapy for calcifying tendinitis of the shoulder. Clin Orthop Rel Res 321:196

78. Haist J, Steeger D (1994) Die ESWT der epikondylopathia radialis et ulnaris. Ein neues Behandlungskonzept knochennaher Weichteilschmerzen. Orthop Mitteilungen 3:173

Subject Index